Taking Action

Taking Action

Cognitive Neuroscience Perspectives on Intentional Acts

edited by Scott H. Johnson-Frey

A Bradford Book
The MIT Press
Cambridge, Massachusetts
London, England

This book was set in Bembo by Achorn Graphic Services, Inc.
Printed and bound in the United States of America.

Library of Congress Cataloging-in-Publication Data

Taking action : cognitive neuroscience perspectives on intentional acts / edited by Scott H. Johnson-Frey.
  p. cm.
  "A Bradford book."
  Includes bibliographical references and index.
  ISBN 0-262-10097-5 (hc. : alk. paper)
  1. Cognitive neuroscience. 2. Intention. I. Johnson-Frey, Scott H.
QP360.5 .T35 2003
153—dc21
                                   2002029583

10 9 8 7 6 5 4 3 2 1

Contents

Preface

In the quest to understand mechanisms of behavior, neurologists, neuro-scientists, and psychologists have adopted a divide-and-conquer strategy, partitioning the complex terrain of brain functions into three principal domains: perceptual, cognitive, and motor. Although such a scheme is a logical outgrowth of viewing the brain as three largely separable component systems, each responsible for a particular domain, overly rigid adherence to this scheme has created artificial boundaries between research domains, impeding progress in understanding phenomena that involve complex interactions among perceptual, cognitive, and motor processes—especially intentional actions. As illustrated by the chapters to follow, there are at least three reasons why scientists interested in these phenomena need to think across traditionally defined domains.

First, the very premise that the brain can be neatly partitioned into perceptual, cognitive, and motor systems is obsolete. Indeed, the more we learn about functional organization, the less clear the demarcations between these systems become. Jeannerod (chapter 5) shows that many brain regions believed to be exclusively involved in perception or motor control—including primary motor cortex—can be engaged by internal action simulations: purely cognitive processes that involve no overt movements. Likewise, Iacoboni (chapter 4) presents evidence that similar brain regions are involved in both the perception and production of particular motor acts. These and other findings expose the futility of exclusively assigning areas to perceptual, cognitive, or motor systems.

Second, the behavior of processes taking place in one system is often affected by those occurring within other systems. Milner and Dyde (chapter 1) demonstrate that, even though perceptual judgments are subject to illusions, visuomotor actions seem impervious to such effects. Danckert and Goodale (chapter 2) show that pointing movements are considerably more accurate when based on perceptual representations arising from input to the lower visual field, whereas representations computed from input to the upper visual field are better suited to shifts of visual attention. That a process within one system can behave very differently in the context of processes within another raises serious concerns about the validity of studying perceptual, cognitive, or motor processes in isolation.

Finally, any reasonably complex action involves processes that span multiple systems. As detailed by Kruse, Port, Lee, and Georgopoulos (chapter 12), how we catch moving targets can only be understood in terms of complex interactions between perceptual, cognitive, and motor processes. I argue (chapter 7) that the same goes for our unique ability to use tools. In short, whether viewed through the lens of single-unit electrophysiology, transcranial magnetic stimulation, psychophysics, or functional neuroimaging, understanding the processes and mechanisms that underlie actions requires thinking across traditionally defined borders.

This volume represents a diverse sampling of the ways in which cognitive neuroscientists are successfully meeting this challenge—*taking action*. Thus, in addition to the contributions mentioned above, Helmuth and Ivry (chapter 8) provide readers with recent insights into how the brain flexibly sequences individual movements; Franz (chapter 9), into how it coordinates multiple limbs; Desmurget and Grafton (chapter 10), into how it utilizes feedforward and feedback mechanisms; Padoa-Schioppa and Bizzi (chapter 11), into how it enables the acquisition of new actions; and Rotte (chapter 13), into how it copes with the challenges of controlling actions when compromised by disease. Readers are also treated to groundbreaking attempts to chart the relatively unexplored, yet fundamental, issues of how the brain formulates intentions to act, by Rosetti and Pisella (chapter 3), and how it expresses ideas through manual gestures, by Sirigu, Daprati, Buxbaum, Giraux, and Pradat-Diehl (chapter 6).

My thanks go, first of all, to the contributors themselves, who graciously rose to the challenge of preparing original chapters, honored their deadlines, and patiently acceded to my requests for revisions, and second, to editor Tom Stone and his very able staff at MIT Press, for their invaluable support and encouragement. I dedicate this volume to my wife, Margaret Anne, who is the inspiration for all that I do, and my son, George Whit, who in his two years has taught me a lifetime's worth about action, and my daughter, Louisa Scott, who reminds me how much I still have to learn.

I

Perception and Action

Beginning with the pioneering work of Ungerleider and Mishkin in the early 1980s, there has been considerable interest in identifying the functional significance of a gross division between two processing pathways in the primate visual system: the ventral (occipitotemporal) stream and the dorsal (occipitoparietal) stream. A particularly influential model by Milner and Goodale states that the ventral stream participates in perceptual judgments, whereas the dorsal (visual) stream is involved in visuomotor transformations necessary for sensory-guided movements. Over the past several years, researchers have reported a striking behavioral dissociation consistent with this position: Subjects' conscious perceptual judgments may be influenced by visual size illusions even though their reaching and grasping actions remain unaffected. One interpretation of these results is that the ventral stream is subject to illusory perceptions, whereas the dorsal stream constructs veridical representations of the world, on which actions are then based. Milner and Dyde (chapter 1) reconsider this issue and report findings on orientation illusions and action that suggest limited interactions between ventral and dorsal streams through their numerous interconnections.

Although much attention has been devoted to distinguishing between dorsal and ventral stream processes, comparatively little work has been done on effects related to the location of stimuli in the visual field. Danckert and Goodale (chapter 2) argue that, when it comes to action, where stimuli fall in the visual field may be of considerable importance. Specifically, they report evidence for a lower visual field advantage for controlling prehensile movements in peripersonal space, which appears to reflect higher resolution of spatial attention. By contrast, they argue that shifts of visual attention are more efficient to targets occurring in the upper visual field, possibly to allow for vigilance to events in extrapersonal space.

1

Orientation and Disorientation: Illusory Perception and the Real World

A. David Milner and Richard T. Dyde

1.1 Introduction

The areas within the primate neocortical mantle devoted to visual processing are highly interconnected, but not uniformly so. In tune with the earlier conclusions of Ungerleider and Mishkin (1982), connectional analyses have shown that these areas segregate into two broadly separate concatenated clusters or "streams" (Felleman and Van Essen, 1991; Morel and Bullier, 1990; Baizer et al., 1991; Young, 1992). In Milner and Goodale's conceptualization (1995), based on a wide range of evidence, much of which accumulated during the 1980s and 1990s, these two anatomical pathways are dedicated to distinctively different functional end points: The "dorsal stream" plays a rather direct and automatized role in the visual control of action, whereas the "ventral stream" underlies the construction of our conscious visual percepts and provides inputs into cognitive processing systems. The ventral stream enables the initial storage and later recognition of objects, scenes, and events, and the evocation of visual imagery about them. Consequently, it can inform actions carried out at a temporal or spatial distance from the visual input. The dorsal stream is concerned, not with the past or future, but with the successful implementation of goal-directed motor acts in the "here and now." Milner and Goodale's conceptualization contrasts with the traditional "two visual systems" model, which distinguishes not so much between different functional end points as between separate domains of visual input—objects and locations (Ungerleider and Mishkin, 1982).

The evidence for a duality of the kind proposed by Milner and Goodale is derived chiefly from neuroscience:

- the properties of single neurons recorded in the two visual streams;
- the deficits (and—crucially—the preserved abilities) that follow lesions to the two streams;

• the anatomical outputs of the two streams; and most recently,
• the differential activation of human visual areas within the two streams as measured by functional neuroimaging.

This evidence from neuroscience is both strong and convergent, but it is lent additional independent support by evidence of a different kind. Since the early 1980s, studies with normal human subjects have revealed dissociations between perception and action, first in the domain of visual location processing (see Bridgeman et al., 1997), and later in the domain of visual size processing (see Haffenden and Goodale, 2000; Hu and Goodale, 2000). These discoveries have been made through the use of perceptual illusions of different kinds, most of which turn out to have little if any influence on the visual processing that guides action. The illusions that show such a dissociation can be plausibly interpreted as operating at a level of the perceptual system beyond the separation of the two visual streams in the cortex. That is, their illusory influence on the observer's perceptual experience probably depends mainly on mechanisms located deep in the ventral stream per se, leaving the visuomotor mechanisms of the dorsal stream largely untouched.

The illusions that reveal the clearest dissociations result from the influence of distal elements in the visual scene on the perception of a target object. For example, Bridgeman and colleagues (1981) used the "induced motion" effect, in which a fixed visual target surrounded by a frame that shifts laterally consistently appears to move in a direction opposite to that of the frame. Despite the power of this illusion, their subjects persisted in pointing to the real location of the target. Bridgeman and his colleagues have argued that the perceptual system is designed to deal with the relative location of a stimulus within the visual array rather than with its absolute egocentric location. For action systems, however, where the relevant effector must be directed unerringly to the stimulus, the absolute position of the stimulus is critical. Thus, although a perceived shift in the position of a target can occur as a function of a misleading visual context, the motor output needs to remain unaffected. In more recent research, Bridgeman and his colleagues have used an illusion where location is misperceived without the need for relative motion. In the "Roelofs illusion," it is sufficient merely for the surrounding frame to be asymmetrically located within the visual field. When the frame is offset leftward, a central target will appear to be rightwardly located, and vice versa. Again the general result (providing the response was made rapidly) was that pointing was aimed accurately, in defiance of the illusion. When observers were required to delay a few seconds, however, then the Roelofs illusion did affect their pointing behavior, to much the same extent as it affected their perceptual report. Evidently, when the response was not made immediately, the perceptual system (Bridgeman et al.'s "cognitive system") took control of it, with predictably erroneous consequences.

The conclusions of Bridgeman and colleagues can be extended well beyond the domain of target location. The visual surroundings play a major role in perceptual processing in general, whether in our perception of shape, size, orientation, motion, or location. That the metrics of perception are relative, not absolute, explains why we have no difficulty perceiving objects on television, a medium in which there are no absolute metrics at all. When we perceive the size, location, orientation, and geometry of an object, we implicitly do so in relation to other objects in the scene we are looking at. In contrast, this relative visual coding is of only limited use in the control of our actions. The brain systems for programming and controlling our reaching and grasping movements must have access to reliable metrical information about the real size and shape of an object, and about its three-dimensional disposition with respect to the observer.

A powerful recent demonstration of the difference between the frames of reference used by the perception and action systems has been provided by Hu and Goodale (2000), who used virtual reality displays, where artificial "objects" of different sizes could be displayed without the possibility of familiarity with particular real objects obscuring the interpretation of the experiment. The investigators presented subjects with a series of three-dimensional virtual images of target blocks, each of which was paired with an image of another block that was always 10% wider or narrower than the target block. The blocks were never visible for more than half a second. The subjects were asked either to reach out and grasp the target block (marked with a red spot) or to indicate the size of the block manually, using their forefinger and thumb. To ensure natural grasping movements, the display was designed so that there was a real but unseen block in the same location as the virtual target (see figure 1.1).

The distracter block induced a strong "size-contrast effect": The observers consistently judged a target block as smaller when accompanied by a large block than when accompanied by a small block. In contrast, when they reached out to grasp that target object without delay, they opened their hand to an identical degree during the reach, no matter which distracter it

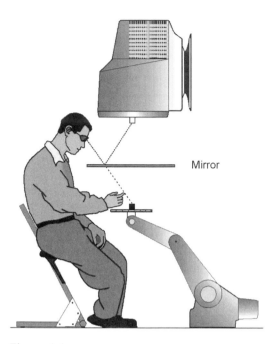

Mirror

Figure 1.1
Virtual reality setup used by Hu and Goodale (2000). Subjects were asked to reach out and grasp a block (ranging from 30 mm to 50 mm in width), which was visually paired with either an adjacent larger or smaller block. (Reprinted with permission from Hu and Goodale, 2000.)

was paired with (figure 1.2a). In other words, the anticipatory scaling of grip size to the size of the target object was not at all subject to the size-contrast effect that dominated perceptual judgments. This result confirms that the scene-based coding of size that is such a ubiquitous feature of our perceptual experience does not apply at all to the visual coding of size used to guide the action of grasping. Of course, it makes good sense to have a visuomotor system that works with real size rather than relative size, and therefore it should perhaps not be so surprising that the system is immune to the size-contrast illusion. Strikingly, however, when Hu and Goodale asked their subjects not to grasp the target object immediately, but only to do so after a 5 s delay, when there was no longer a visual image present, the illusion clearly affected the anticipatory scaling of their hand grip (figure 1.2b).

Like the findings of Bridgeman and colleagues, those of Hu and Goodale point to an essential relativity in the processing of size for perceptual

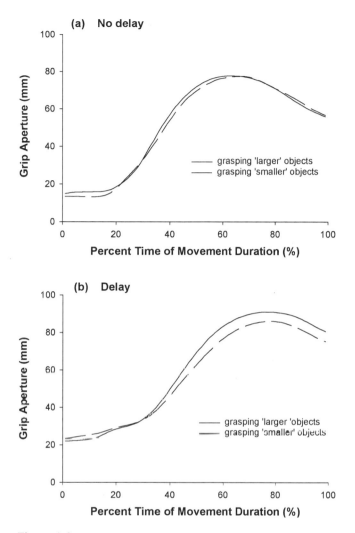

Figure 1.2
Specimen grasp profiles while subjects reached out to grasp either for a block paired with a larger one ("grasping smaller") or a similar block paired with a smaller one ("grasping larger"). The maximum opening of the hand gives an index of the visual calibration of the grip during the course of reaching. (Reprinted with permission from Hu and Goodale, 2000.)

purposes, but a stubborn objectivity in the processing of size for direct action. They interpret their results firmly within the framework of Milner and Goodale's model (1995), whereby the dorsal stream is identified as the mediator of direct visuomotor transformations for immediate action, whereas the ventral stream governs our perceptual experience and visual memory.

There are other visual illusions that, like induced motion, the Roelofs effect, and the size-contrast effect, may turn out to be more correctly referred to as "perceptual" than as "visual" illusions. Recent years have seen a large number of studies comparing "perceptual" measures of geometric visual illusions with "visuomotor" measures. The illusions studied have included the Muller-Lyer (e.g., Mack et al., 1985; Gentilucci et al., 1996), the Ponzo (e.g., Brenner and Smeets, 1996; Jackson and Shaw 2000), and the horizontal-vertical (e.g., Vishton et al., 1999) illusions. In the study that provided the impetus for much of this work, however, Aglioti and colleagues (1995) made the striking claim that visually guided grasping of solid disks was immune to the Ebbinghaus (or "Titchener circles") illusion. The authors used pairs of poker chips, one of which was surrounded by an annulus of smaller circles printed on the background surface, and the other by an annulus of larger circles. Although these surrounds induced a powerful contrast illusion whereby the disk surrounded by large circles appeared smaller, and vice versa, they had no significant effect on the grip aperture during reaching to grasp one or the other disk. Perhaps not surprisingly given its theoretical interest, this study has spawned a small cottage industry of further studies of the Ebbinghaus/Titchener illusion, with varying results according to the precise methodology used. It has become clear that the phenomenon described in Aglioti et al., 1995, is not as straightforward as it first seemed, and is subject to a range of complicating factors that influence the likelihood and extent of observing an effect of the surround stimuli.

It is clear from recent reviews of the literature (Carey, 2001; Dyde, 2001), that the general result of these various studies of visual size illusions is not a clear-cut dissociation between "perception" and "action." Instead, the usual pattern is an intermediate one, whereby—to varying degrees—the visuomotor as well as the perceptual measures used are affected by the illusion-inducing surround. Often this visuomotor effect is not significant and usually it is very small. In other cases, however, it may be of a magnitude approaching that of the perceptual illusion. How do we explain this variability of outcome? There are of course specific factors that pertain to particular illusions, for example, the space between the target stimulus and the surrounding circles in the Ebbinghaus/Titchener illusion (Haffenden and Goodale, 2000). This factor plays an additive role in influencing hand grip aperture quite independent of the illusion per se, probably because the visuomotor system is designed to take into account stimuli that could constitute obstacles during prehension (McIntosh et al., 2000). But there still seems to be evidence for some residual influence of the various size illusions on hand grip during prehension. How can this be explained if, as argued above, the metrics of reaching and grasping are guided by a dedicated brain system (the dorsal stream) separate from the system that furnishes our conscious perception of the stimuli? The answer may well be that separateness does not imply that the two systems are entirely independent of each other. After all, Canada and the United States are separate sovereign nations with clear mutual borders, but that does not prevent them from interacting. Analogously, we know that there are multiple anatomical interconnections between the dorsal and ventral visual systems (Felleman and Van Essen, 1991). These interconnections might allow an illusion arising in the ventral stream to be passed to visual processing areas within the dorsal stream, causing consistent visuomotor errors to occur. We also know that the two visual streams are each furnished with information from the same optic nerve, the same optic tract, and the same primary visual cortex. Indeed, they are both fed from the same secondary cortical areas that receive visual information directly from primary visual cortex, such as areas V2, V3, and the middle temporal (MT) area. If an illusion arises, not—or not only—at a high level in the ventral stream, but in part at least in one of these earlier cortical areas, then the inevitable result will be a distorted input passing to both visual streams.

In examining this idea within the domain of visual orientation perception, our starting point was a well-known illusion first studied systematically during the 1940s (Witkin and Asch, 1947) and called the "rod and frame" illusion (figure 1.3). Like the other illusions discussed above, it is dependent on the surrounding features of the scene, which induce a relative percept of the target object that dominates our conscious judgments. Just as we can judge the size of an object on a TV screen by comparison with other familiar objects present in the scene (e.g., buildings), so we will judge a lamppost

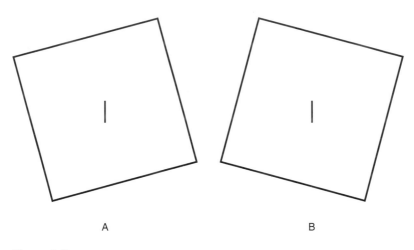

A   B

Figure 1.3
Rod and frame illusion (RFI). The two central target rods in each array (*A* and
B) are parallel, but appear convergent as a result of the effect of the surrounding
frame. On any given trial, observers were presented either with display *A* or display *B*.

to be vertical on a TV screen if it is parallel to the walls of a building. In
neither case do we have *absolute* information about the size or orientation
of the object: The size and orientation on the screen will depend on factors
such as the distance and orientation of the TV camera during the filming.
In general, our perceptual system implicitly assumes that large items present
in the array have a stability that allows other stimuli to be measured against
them. Indeed, research has shown that when the target is surrounded by
more than one frame, it is the *outermost* frame that determines the rod and
frame illusion (Di Lorenzo and Rock, 1982).

    Just like the Roelofs and the size-contrast illusions, therefore, the rod
and frame illusion seems likely to depend primarily on the relationship between the surrounding scene or visual framework on the one hand, and
the target stimulus on the other. Each of these illusions, of location, size,
and orientation, would seem to be paradigmatically related to the intrinsically *relative* nature of perceptual processing. Currently, we know of no
direct evidence on environmental versus egocentric coding of orientation
in different cortical visual areas. In the standard monkey visual electrophysiology experiment, the orientation selectivity of cortical neurons is assessed
quite straightforwardly by presenting oriented lines, edges, or gratings to
the animal within the confines of a stable screen with fully visible edges,

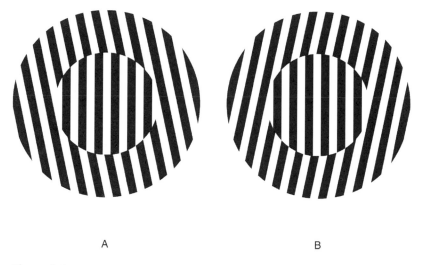

A   B

Figure 1.4
Simultaneous tilt illusion (STI). The two central target gratings in each array (*A* and *B*) are parallel, but appear convergent as a result of the effect of the surrounding gratings. On any given trial, observers were presented either with display *A* or display *B*.

set in the gravitationally vertical plane. Accordingly, we do not know whether a neuron in primary visual cortex (V1; Hubel and Wiesel, 1968) or inferior temporal cortex (ITC; Gross, 1973) or posterior parietal cortex (PPC; Sakata et al., 1992) would respond the same if the screen were to be tilted while the stimulus remained constant, or indeed, if its edges were to be made invisible. The theoretical position set out by Milner and Goodale (1995) would clearly predict that such context effects would play a major role on orientation selectivity within the ventral stream, and only a minor one elsewhere.

But contextual effects cannot explain all visual illusions of orientation. In particular, they seem unlikely to play a major role when the inducing surround is immediately contiguous to the target, as in the simultaneous tilt illusion (Gibson and Radner, 1937; see figure 1.4). In this case, it makes much more sense to appeal to local contour interactions to explain the illusion. Neurons selective for orientation are grouped together in V1 in columns, such that neighboring columns favor stimulus orientations slightly different from each other, and the closer two neurons lie along the surface of the cortex (within a range of around 0.5 mm), the more similar their orientation preferences will be. Recent research has shown that there are extensive lateral connections between these orientation columns, most of them inhibitory in nature (Sengpiel et al., 1997). One major function of these inhibitory connections is probably to sharpen the orientation selectivity of individual neurons, by making them less responsive to contours at dissimilar orientations (Sengpiel et al., 1997). At the same time, however, an accidental by-product of this mechanism would be to cause a shift in the distribution of neurons responding to a target grating pattern when it is surrounded by a grating set at an orientation a few degrees away from it. Thus the percept, if assumed to be conveyed by the mode of the distribution of orientationselective neurons, would shift away from the inducing tilt. This would parallel the kind of account often given for the tilt aftereffect.

Given the plausibility of this kind of mechanism operating in V1, it may be assumed that its biased results would be passed on via secondary visual areas such as V2 and V3 to orientation-selective neurons throughout the cortex. Neurons responding to oriented contours are found not only in ventral stream areas such as V4, TEO and inferior temporal cortex (ITC), but also in the dorsal stream areas including V3A, V6, PIP, and AIP. In short, a simultaneous tilt illusion (STI) generated in V1 would infect the entire cortical visual system. Some neurons in AIP, for example, are selective for the orientation of a lever that the monkey has to grasp and pull— these should be affected by the STI every bit as much as neurons in ITC that are responsive to passively viewed patterns like colored rectangles. Unless, of course, the striped surround that elicits the STI also operates to some extent as a "context" for the target—which it might do if it were large enough to occupy a wide expanse of the visual array. If so, then there should still be a large STI present in the visuomotor system, but an even larger one in the perceptual system. Conversely, of course, one could imagine a situation where the rod and frame illusion (RFI) might recruit lateral contour interactions, especially if the frame were reduced in size relative to the rod (Das and Gilbert, 1995). If so, then one would predict an increased tendency for the illusion to extend to visuomotor as well as perceptual measures. In the following experiments (Dyde and Milner, 2002), we took care to minimize the annulus size in our STI presentations to reduce the likelihood of the surround acting as a frame for the target, and vice versa: We made the frame in the RFI as large as possible to reduce the likelihood of direct contour interactions.

1.2   Experiment 1: The Simultaneous Tilt Illusion

Each of the two simultaneous tilt illusion patterns A and B (see figure 1.4) were presented in turn on a computer monitor. Subjects were asked to respond to the orientation of the central grating either by "mailing" a square plastic card up against the screen as if passing it through the bars of the target grating or by rotating the card in a separate location below the monitor in such a way as to match the perceived orientation of the target grating. The "mailing" response was designed to be a visually guided act that should be controlled by dorsal stream processing. This processing is assumed to transform the egocentrically coded target orientation rather directly into effector coordinates (mediated through wrist rotation). Because of its separate location, the matching response should preclude the direct transformation of visual information into action coordinates and is assumed to be guided by a perceptual representation mediated by ventral stream processing.

The inner (target) grating was 75 mm in diameter, whereas the outer inducing grating had a diameter of 115 mm. The outer grating was oriented 12° clockwise or counterclockwise to form stimuli A and B (figure 1.4). A torus-shaped mask was fixed to the monitor in order to mask the inner screen edge and the outer monitor casing. The stimuli were presented within the masking torus aperture (215 mm in diameter). An identical torus was affixed below and vertically aligned with the upper torus, its central aperture providing the location where the card was held by the subject when making "matching" responses.

Stimuli consisted of a composite of two square-wave, monochrome gratings of half a cycle per centimeter. The patterns were presented for 1,000 ms in a pseudo-random sequence, interspersed with "filler" trials where the central grating was veridically inclined from the vertical (4° clockwise or counterclockwise) in order to maintain the naïveté of the subjects as to the nature of the illusion and to discourage response perseveration. The subject's cue to respond (from a constant start position) was given at stimulus offset, to preclude any on-line corrective feedback regarding the target's true orientation. Simultaneously with this cue, three visual noise patterns were briefly presented (each for 50 ms) to remove retinal afterimages of the stimulus pattern.

The orientation of the handheld card was continuously recorded by using an Optotrak movement-tracking system (Northern Digital, Inc.) to

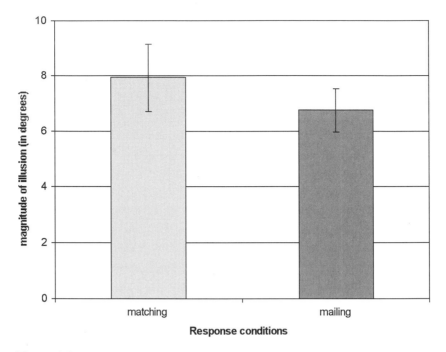

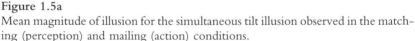

Figure 1.5a
Mean magnitude of illusion for the simultaneous tilt illusion observed in the matching (perception) and mailing (action) conditions.

monitor the positions of two infrared emitting markers embedded in the card. The final orientation of the card was computed as the mean orientation of the markers for the 500 ms following movement end time. The end of the Optotrak sampling period was indicated by an auditory tone. This tone acted as the cue for the subject to return the card to the start position. The presence of the visual illusion was determined by comparing the mean responses to stimuli A and B. The magnitude of illusion (measured in degrees) for each subject for both test conditions was derived from the difference between the mean response to stimulus A and mean response to stimulus B. The 12 subjects (6 male, 6 female; age range 19–53) were undergraduate psychology students who received course credit for participation. All were right-hand dominant, with normal or corrected-to-normal vision, and were naive to the illusion.

The results of this experiment are summarized in figure 1.5a–b. From figure 1.5a, we can see that there was a substantial illusory effect both in the perceptual condition (with a group mean of 7.92° of illusion) and in

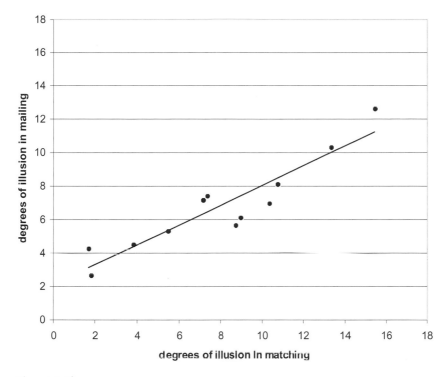

Figure 1.5b
Correlation between the magnitudes of illusion of the simultaneous tilt illusion seen in the matching and mailing conditions. Error bars indicate one standard error of the mean.

the visuomotor condition (with a group mean of 6.75° of illusion), the effect being significantly different from baseline ($p < .001$) in both conditions. Although there was a suggestion of a smaller illusory effect for the mailing task, the mean difference between conditions failed to reach statistical significance.

The apparent pattern of association between the perceptual and visuomotor measures for the simultaneous tilt illusion is further strengthened by the large and highly significant correlation between the two illusion magnitudes across subjects (Pearson's $r = .967$; $p < .01$), as illustrated in figure 1.5b. This correlation suggests a large degree of shared causality in the illusion magnitude across measures, as would be predicted if both measures were dependent on information from a shared "misprocessing" of the target orientation. Despite the slightly stronger illusory effect on the perceptual measure (figure 1.5a) and the resulting regression slope of less than unity (figure 1.5b), the overall pattern of results gives clear support for an early siting of the STI and therefore a comparable influence on both dorsal and ventral visual streams.

1.3   Experiment 2: The Rod and Frame Illusion

In a second experiment we used a specially constructed apparatus to present in turn each of the two rod and frame patterns illustrated in figure 1.3. Subjects responded either by grasping the central rod between forefinger and thumb or by adjusting a separately located rod to match the stimulus rod to indicate their perception of the rod orientation. As in experiment 1, the orientation of the hand during the grasping task was assumed to be a goal-directed response governed by the dorsal visual stream, whereas the matching response was assumed to express a subject's perceptual experience, mediated by the ventral stream.

The stimuli were presented within a large adjustable frame (70 cm × 70 cm) made from translucent white plastic sheeting. All but the outer 2 cm of the sheet was painted opaque matte black, leaving a white frame at the outer edges. The frame was mounted on a pivot that allowed its orientation in the frontal plane to be adjusted. Fixed to this common pivot and in front of the frame was a rod 100 mm long, 15 mm wide, and 5 mm deep, which could also be independently adjusted in orientation. The separation between rod and frame was approximately 37° of retinal arc. A measure on the reverse of the apparatus allowed the rod and frame to be set to given orientations within ±0.5°. The study was conducted in a darkened room with the apparatus backlit, making the frame dimly luminescent, and with enough residual light to make the rod clearly visible. An identical rod and frame (the matching apparatus) was placed to the right of the stimulus frame. The matching frame was fixed at gravitational vertical with a rod that could be adjusted by the subjects to express their perceived orientation of the target rod.

The test stimuli (a vertical rod with the frame at either 15° clockwise or counterclockwise from vertical) were presented for 2,000 ms in a pseudo-random sequence, interspersed with filler trials in which the rod was veridically inclined 2° clockwise or counterclockwise from vertical. In the grasping condition, an auditory tone sounded immediately after the presentation period signaling the subject to reach for the rod. This tripped a switch that extinguished the only light source, so that reaching was per-

formed in darkness (open loop). No visual persistence of the frame or rod
was reported. The orientation of the hand was recorded using the Optotrak
system to monitor the position of markers attached to subjects' forefinger
and thumb. Final hand orientation was calculated at a fixed point (50 ms)
before movement end time, to ensure that haptic feedback did not act as
a cue. On contacting the target, subjects returned their hand to the switch,
which acted as the fixed starting position. In the matching condition the
auditory tone again acted as the cue to respond, whereupon the subject
adjusted the rod in the separate frame to match that of the stimulus rod.
A 5 s time limit was set to complete this task. The orientation of the matching rod was recorded manually from the scale on the rear of the apparatus.

The 12 subjects (8 female, 4 male; age range 19–34) were undergraduate psychology students who received course credit for participation. All
were right-hand dominant, with normal or corrected-to-normal vision, and
were naive to the illusion. The presence of an illusion for each subject was
determined by comparing the mean responses to stimuli A and B (figure 1.3). The magnitude of illusion (measured in degrees) for each subject
in each condition was derived from the difference between the mean response to stimulus A and mean response to stimulus B.

Figure 1.6 illustrates the summary of results and shows the presence
of a clear and statistically significant illusion in the matching condition
($t[11] = 2.91$; $p < .01$), whereas the small residual effect in the grasping
condition fails to reach statistical significance. The mean difference in magnitude between these two measures of illusion strength is also highly significant ($t[11] = 2.98$; $p < .01$). This indicates a strong illusory effect of
the frame on the perceptual measure, whereas the visuomotor measure was
largely refractory to the illusion. A correlational analysis of the magnitude of illusion across subjects between the two conditions was undertaken, and this showed no evidence for a significant shared effect between
measures ($r^2 = .14$; n.s.).

The presence of a strong illusory effect on the perceptual measures,
in the absence of any apparent effect on the visuomotor measure, again
confirmed our predictions. The context dependence of perceptual processing causes our experiences to be highly sensitive to the frame of reference within which a stimulus is presented, in this case resulting in a false
processing of the target orientation. However, the visuomotor system does
not seem to integrate the frame into the processing involved in computing
the necessary orientation of the hand for a successful grasp.

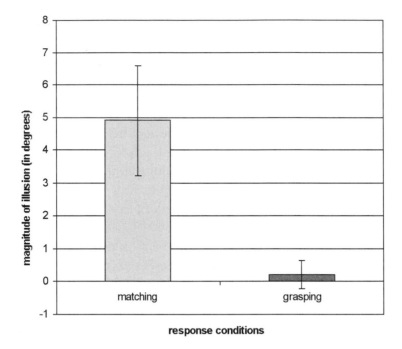

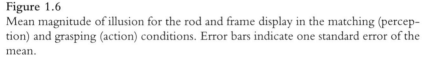

Figure 1.6
Mean magnitude of illusion for the rod and frame display in the matching (perception) and grasping (action) conditions. Error bars indicate one standard error of the mean.

1.4   Interim Summary of Experiments 1 and 2

These two experiments present evidence for predictable patterns of association and dissociation for the simultaneous tilt illusion and rod and frame illusion, respectively; predictions that are based on the suggested causal mechanisms involved in the illusions and their likely neutral site of effect. Experiment 1 specifically rebuts the potential criticism that visuomotor measures will *always* return smaller illusory effects than perceptual ones, due to differences in the attentional characteristics of the two response conditions, rather than from any underlying differences in visual processing. Yet experiment 2 demonstrates that even within that same stimulus feature domain (orientation), a perceptual illusion that results from the integration of scene-based cues can leave visuomotor responses relatively unaffected. Evidently the grasping response is tuned exclusively to the veridical characteristics of the target stimulus, whereas the perceptual system finds the wider contextual information compelling and irresistible.

Thus we found a clear and predicted *dissociation* between perceptual and visuomotor tasks within one visual illusion, and a clear and predicted *association* within another. Would it be possible to find a dissociation in the *opposite* direction? To attempt to do this, and at the same time to strengthen our interpretation of the findings thus far, a third experiment was undertaken. This involved a combination of the two illusions, with a methodology and design that was a hybrid of the two previous experiments.

1.5   Experiment 3: The Simultaneous Tilt Illusion within a Frame

In experiment 1 (STI) an illusory effect was evident in both visuomotor and perceptual measures, whereas in experiment 2 (RFI) the illusory effect was evident only in perception. We reasoned that if the simultaneous tilt pattern was embedded within a tilted frame in such a way as to induce opposing illusions, then in measures of perception the two effects should largely nullify one another, with a resultant small magnitude of illusion, whereas in visuomotor testing the nullifying influence of the rod and frame illusion should be much less, leaving the net simultaneous tilt illusion relatively large. In other words, the composite illusion should yield a greater magnitude of illusion for the visuomotor measure than for the perceptual measure: precisely the opposite pattern to that seen in experiment 2. Figure 1.7 illustrates the form of the stimuli that we used.

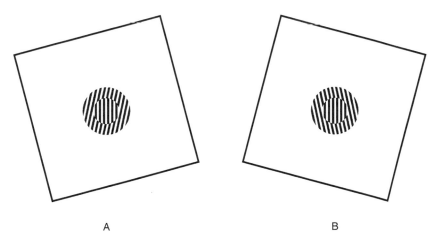

A   B

Figure 1.7
"STI within a frame": The simultaneous tilt illusion embedded within an opposing frame, such that the two perceptual illusions tend to cancel each other out (experiment 3).

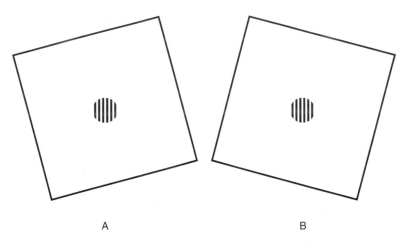

A   B

Figure 1.8
"Rods and frame" illusion: The RFI display used in experiment 3 incorporating a central grating stimulus instead of a single rod.

As an additional control, a variant of the rod and frame illusion was formed by taking the central target grating of the simultaneous tilt illusion and embedding it alone within a frame (forming a "rods and frame" illusion; see figure 1.8). According to our interpretation of experiment 2, this array should still return a higher magnitude of illusion in measures of perception than in visuomotor control. The four patterns shown in figures 1.7 and 1.8 were presented in turn to subjects, who responded either by mailing a card against the central target grating (the visuomotor measure) or by adjusting a separate grating to match the perceived orientation of the central stimulus.

The combined illusion stimulus consisted of a printed version of the simultaneous tilt pattern (with a central target grating 93 mm in diameter and an inducing outer grating 166 mm in diameter), which was mounted at the center of the frame as in experiment 2, in place of the rod. The outer inducing grating was set at 15° clockwise or counterclockwise from gravitational vertical. A matching frame (similar to that described in experiment 2) was located to the right of the stimulus frame. This was fixed at gravitational vertical, with a response grating identical to the stimulus grating, which could be rotated to match the orientation of stimulus grating. Lighting and room conditions were identical to those for experiment 2. To form the control "rods and frame" stimuli, the inducing outer grating was masked leaving only the central grating visible within the frame. The frame was tilted 15° clockwise or counterclockwise from vertical.

Within each test condition, the patterns were presented for 2,000 ms in pseudo-random order, interspersed with filler trials where the central stimulus grating was veridically inclined away from gravitational vertical (2° clockwise or counterclockwise). In the two visuomotor conditions, a tone sounded at the end of the stimulus presentation and the lights were extinguished, whereupon the subject mailed the card against the central target grating. The orientation of the card was recorded using the Optotrak system to monitor the two markers attached to the card. The response was taken as the orientation of the card computed 10 ms before the end of movement. In the two perceptual conditions, the tone indicated the start of a 2 s response window within which the subject adjusted the response grating in the second frame so as to indicate the perceived orientation of the stimulus grating. The response was recorded manually by means of a scale on the reverse of the apparatus. The 17 subjects (11 female, 6 male; age range 19–42) tested were undergraduate psychology students, who received course credit for their participation. All subjects were right-hand dominant, with normal or corrected-to-normal vision, and were naive to the illusion, not having taken part in any related studies.

It had been our prediction that the combined array would return a higher illusion magnitude in the visuomotor condition than in the perceptual condition. As can be seen from the summary of results in figure 1.9, there was indeed a larger mean net effect on the visuomotor measure than on the measure of perception. This difference is statistically reliable ($t[16] = 2.63$; $p < .01$, uncorrected). We also predicted that in the "rods and frame" variant of the experiment 2 paradigm, a higher illusion magnitude would still be found for the perceptual than the visuomotor measure. As figure 1.9 also illustrates, we did find a similar pattern of results to those found in experiment 2, namely a larger mean illusion in perception than in the visuomotor measure, and this difference is statistically reliable ($t[16] = 3.25$; $p < .01$, uncorrected).[1]

It should be noted that there was now a statistically significant, though comparatively small, illusion in the visuomotor measure in the "rods and frame" task, that was not apparent in the "rod and frame" data of experiment 2. Although this result suggests that the mailing measure may have been more susceptible to the illusion than the grasping measure had been, the overall pattern of results in experiment 3 still shows a reversing pattern of effects between the two illusion types used (combined STI-RFI versus "rods and frame"). The two-way interaction is highly significant

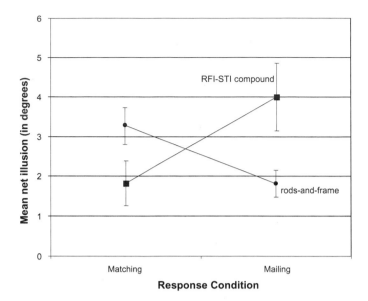

Figure 1.9
Mean magnitude of illusion for the rods and frame–simultaneous tilt compound illusion (STI plus frame) observed in the matching (perception) and mailing (action) conditions, depicted as filled squares. The contrasting results for the control rods and frame illusion (RFI) in matching and mailing conditions is depicted as filled circles. Error bars indicate one standard error of the mean. Note that the compound illusion is in the direction indicating a stronger STI than RFI, in broad agreement with the results of experiments 1 and 2.

($F[1,16] = 16.09$; $p < .001$). This "double dissociation" is difficult to account for except on the basis of the hypothesized separation of the neural mechanisms responsible for the constituent illusions.

1.6   General Discussion

As anticipated in section 1.1, clearly different patterns of results were evident in the two orientation illusions we studied. The simultaneous tilt illusion (STI) of our experiment 1, which, we argued, is probably generated wholly or mainly at early stages of visual cortical processing, was found to influence not only perceptual judgments, but also visually guided "mailing" behavior directed toward the central target grating. The magnitude of the illusion was comparable between the perceptual and visuomotor measures, and highly correlated in the two tasks across subjects. This pattern argues strongly for a common mechanism underlying both the perceptual and the visuomotor STI effects. In contrast, the rod and frame illusion (RFI) of our experiment 2 influenced perception much more than visually guided grasping directed at the target rod. Furthermore, the small and non-significant visuomotor illusion was not at all correlated with the much larger illusion reported in the perceptual version of the task. Thus it seems most unlikely that the illusions seen in the two tasks in experiment 2 were determined by a common underlying mechanism. Instead, the results of experiment 2 support our prediction: Whereas perception should be strongly influenced by distal visual elements creating a "frame of reference" for orientation (Witkin and Asch, 1947; Howard, 1982), visuomotor control should be relatively unaffected by such contextual influences.

Our conclusions regarding the STI agree closely with independent work carried out by two groups of researchers. Van der Willigen and colleagues (2000) report equal effects of the illusion on both perceptual and mailing behavior (although they do not report magnitudes). Glover and Dixon (2001), who monitored the orientation of their subjects' hand during reaches to grasp a "handle" target embedded within a grating annulus of varying relative orientations, report a clear illusory effect of the background on the reaching response. The effect appeared early in the response and diminished over time (presumably being corrected on-line using visual feedback, which was unavailable in our experiment 1).

Neither of these two reports (contrary to the claim of Glover and Dixon, 2001) provides evidence against the Milner and Goodale (1995) hypothesis that has been offered as a way of understanding the various published dissociations between perceptual and visuomotor measures of location and size illusions. To the contrary, they are readily explained within the Milner and Goodale conception of separate visual processing streams for perception and action because these flow largely from a single source. As first proposed by Ungerleider and Mishkin (1982), the dorsal and ventral streams both emanate from primary visual cortex, V1. Accordingly, if the simultaneous tilt illusion is mediated within V1 (or its immediate cortical projection areas), then a lack of dissociation between perceptual and behavioral measures of the illusion is precisely what would be predicted from the theory. Furthermore, this interpretation is bolstered by the results of our experiment 2, in which we found a clear dissociation between the perceptual and behavioral effects of the rod and frame illusion, which was hypothesized to be generated, not in V1, but later in the perceptual system.

In our experiment 3, we pitted the two illusions of our experiments 1 and 2 against each other, using the same manual task (mailing) as in our experiment 1. We argued that if our interpretation were correct, then the two opposite perceptual illusions should tend to nullify each other, whereas the two opposing visuomotor illusions should not. In the visuomotor condition, the much larger illusion generated by the simultaneous tilt annulus should drown out any small converse visuomotor illusion caused by the frame. Consequently, the mailing response, already shown in our experiment 1 to be highly sensitive to the simultaneous tilt illusion, should still reveal a strong illusion, despite the absence of a net perceptual illusion in the display. This pattern of results was precisely what emerged in our data.

In experiment 3 we used a mailing rather than a grasping task to examine a grating variant of the rod and frame illusion. Our replication of the same dissociative pattern as found in experiment 2, combined with the reverse dissociation of the combined RFI-STI for the same subject group, represents what can be regarded as a "double dissociation" of illusory effects between the two conditions. This double dissociation argues strongly for the differential processing of visual orientation for use in perception and visuomotor control, and directly echoes the findings of neuropsychological studies in the domain of orientation (Perenin and Vighetto, 1988; Goodale et al., 1991) and, as far as we are aware, is the first instance where a direct analogue of the double dissociation between neuropsychological syndromes has been demonstrated in the healthy visual cortex.

It is true, however, that the "rods and frame" task used in experiment 3 showed a statistically significant, though small, visuomotor illusion effect. Why should the very same frame elicit a visuomotor illusion effect in experiment 3 but not in experiment 2? One explanation would be that there was a small "simultaneous tilt illusion" present in experiment 3 even with the large frame used in our rod and frame illusion tasks, perhaps due to distant lateral influences in VI (Das and Gilbert, 1995). But then, why was the task in experiment 3 more susceptible to such an effect than that used in experiment 2? The answer may lie in the nature of the responses made in the two experiments. Hand orientation during rod grasping may not be guided wholly by the visual orientation of the rod, but also guided in part by the spatial locations of the ends of the rod.[2] The mailing task, for its part, must depend entirely on orientation information, which may explain why the small orientation illusion seen in the mailing task (experiment 3), where there is no unique pair of points for the visuomotor system to code, virtually disappears in the grasping task (experiment 2).

The important point is that the use of location information in experiment 2 cannot account for the small magnitude of visuomotor illusion found even in the "rods and frame" task of experiment 3, where there were no local points for the visual system to identify in guiding the response. The grating target in the mailing task did not afford such location information, nor could the mailing response readily use it.[3]

In this chapter we have argued that the site of origin of visual illusions may be at any point within the progression from the retina to the highest realms of the perceptual system. The novelty of what we are saying lies only in the refinement of this statement to take account of the splitting off of a separate visual processing pathway (the dorsal stream) after the initial analysis of the visual scene that takes place in primary visual cortex (V1) and its adjacent early cortical areas. In the dorsal stream, we have implied, because, by its nature, the system has to deliver a set of veridical metrics for guiding action, no distortion of the input should take place. But of course, this may be an oversimplification. However well designed these structures may be for their purpose within the normal world where they evolved, sufficiently *abnormal* inputs may create distorted outputs. Interestingly, Van der Willigen and colleagues (2000) report having carried out a three-dimensional version of the simultaneous tilt illusion, which involved an annulus tilted in the depth plane relative to the target disk (using stereoscopic viewing). In this task, there was a paradoxically *larger* magnitude of illusion in the "mailing" measure than in the perceptual matching condition, though a substantial illusion was present in both conditions. These results suggest that although, like the two-dimensional version of the STI, this illusion may be initially generated in early cortical areas, there is then some further processing in the visuomotor system that may exacerbate this early effect. One possibility is that the neurons with three-dimensional orientation selectivity that are located in posterior parts of the intraparietal sulcus in the monkey (roughly, the posterior intraparietal or PIP area; Sakata et al., 1997) are subject to inhibitory interactions comparable to those seen between two-dimensional orientation coding neurons in primary visual cortex. At present, it is unknown whether this might be so.

Notes

1. A Bonferroni correction for these two planned comparisons of magnitude differences in experiment 3 returns statistically significant differences for both comparisons at the .05 level.

2. Brenner and Smeets (1996; Smeets and Brenner, 1999) have even argued that whenever we reach out to grasp an object, the brain may code *only* the individual locations of the potential grasp points, and direct the fingers to those points to achieve the grasp.

3. Thus the "positional coding" argument of Brenner and Smeets would have no reason to predict other than the full "perceptual" illusion in the visuomotor "rods and frame" task of experiment 3. Indeed, if this were otherwise, then we should not have found a large visuomotor STI illusion using a similar mailing task in experiment 1.

References

Aglioti, S., Goodale, M. A., and DeSouza, J.F.X. (1995). Size-contrast illusions deceive the eye but not the hand. *Curr. Biol.* 5: 679–685.

Baizer, J. S., Ungerleider, L. G., and Desimone, R. (1991). Organization of visual inputs to the inferior temporal and posterior parietal cortex in macaques. *J. Neurosci.* 11: 168–190.

Brenner, E., and Smeets, J. B. J. (1996). Size illusion influences how we lift but not how we grasp an object. *Exp. Brain Res.* 111: 473–476.

Bridgeman, B., Kirch, M., and Sperling, A. (1981). Segregation of cognitive and motor-oriented systems of visual perception. *Percept. Psychophys.* 29: 336–342.

Bridgeman, B., Peery, S., and Anand, S. (1997). Interaction of cognitive and sensorimotor maps of visual space. *Percept. Psychophys.* 59: 456–469.

Carey, D. P. (2001). Do action systems resist visual illusions? *Trends Cogn. Sci.* 5: 109–113.

Das, A., and Gilbert, C. D. (1995). Long-range horizontal connections and their role in cortical reorganization revealed by optical recording of cat primary visual cortex. *Nature* 375: 780–784.

Di Lorenzo, J. R., and Rock, I. (1982). The rod and frame effect as a function of righting of the frame. *J. Exp. Psychol. Hum. Percept. Perform.* 8: 536–546.

Dyde, R. T. (2001). Perceptual and visuomotor studies of illusions of orientation. Ph.D. diss., University of Durham, England.

Dyde, R. T., and Milner, A. D. (2002). Two illusions of perceived orientation: One fools all of the people some of the time, but the other fools all of the people all of the time. *Exp. Brain Res.* 144: 518–527.

Felleman, D. J., and Van Essen, D. C. (1991). Distributed hierarchical processing in the primate cerebral cortex. *Cereb. Cortex* 1: 1–47.

Gentilucci, M., Chieffi, S., Daprati, E., Saetti, M. C., and Toni, I. (1996). Visual illusion and action. *Neuropsychologia* 34: 369–376.

Gibson, J. J., and Radner, M. (1937). Adaptation and contrast in perception of tilted lines. *J. Exp. Psychol.* 20: 453–469.

Glover, S., and Dixon, P. (2001). Motor adaptation to an optical illusion. *Exp. Brain Res.* 137: 254–258.

Goodale, M. A., Milner, A. D., Jakobson, L. S., and Carey, D. P. (1991). A neurological dissociation between perceiving objects and grasping them. *Nature* 349: 154–156.

Gross, C. G. (1973). Visual functions of inferotemporal cortex. In *Handbook of Sensory Physiology*. Vol. 7/3, *Central Processing of Visual Information*. Part B, *Visual Centers in the Brain*, R. Jung (ed.). Berlin: Springer-Verlag, pp. 451–482.

Haffenden, A. M., and Goodale, M. A. (2000). Independent effects of pictorial displays on perception and action. *Vision Res.* 40: 1597–1607.

Howard, I. P. (1982). *Human Visual Orientation*. New York: Wiley.

Hu, Y., and Goodale, M. A. (2000). Grasping after a delay shifts size-scaling from absolute to relative metrics. *J. Cogn. Neurosci.* 12: 856–868.

Hubel, D. H., and Wiesel, T. N. (1968). Receptive fields and functional architecture of the monkey striate cortex. *J. Physiol.* 195: 215–243.

Jackson, S. R., and Shaw, A. (2000). The Ponzo illusion affects grip-force but not grip-aperture scaling during prehension movements. *J. Exp. Psychol. Hum. Percept. Perform.* 26: 418–423.

Mack, A., Heuer, F., Villardi, K., and Chambers, D. (1985). The dissociation of position and extent in Müller-Lyer figures. *Percept. Psychophys.* 37: 335–344.

McIntosh, R. D., Dijkerman, H. C., Mon-Williams, M., and Milner, A. D. (2000). Visuomotor processing of spatial layout in visual form agnosia. Presented at meeting of Experimental Psychology Society, Cambridge. July.

Milner, A. D., and Goodale, M. A. (1995). *The Visual Brain in Action*. Oxford: Oxford University Press.

Milner, A. D., Perrett, D. I., Johnston, R. S., Benson, P. J., Jordan, T. R., Heeley, D. W., Bettucci, D., Mortara, F., Mutani, R., Terazzi, E., and Davidson, D. L. W. (1991). Perception and action in visual form agnosia. *Brain* 114: 405–428.

Morel, A., and Bullier, J. (1990). Anatomical segregation of two cortical visual pathways in the macaque monkey. *Vis. Neurosci.* 4: 555–578.

Perenin, M. T., and Vighetto, A. (1988). Optic ataxia: A specific disruption in visuo-motor mechanisms: 1. Different aspects of deficits in reaching for objects. *Brain* 111: 643–674.

Sakata, H., Taira, M., Mine, S., and Murata, A. (1992). Hand-movement-related neurons of the posterior parietal cortex of the monkey: Their role in the visual guidance of hand movements. In *Control of Arm Movement in Space*, R. Caminiti, P. B. Johnson, and Y. Burnod (eds.). Berlin: Springer-Verlag, pp. 185–198.

Sakata, H., Taira, M., Kusunoki, M., Murata, A., and Tanaka, Y. (1997). The parietal association cortex in depth perception and visual control of hand action. *Trends Neurosci.* 20: 350–357.

Sengpiel, F., Sen, A., and Blakemore, C. (1997). Characteristics of surround inhibition in cat area 17. *Exp. Brain Res.* 116: 216–228.

Smeets, J. B., and Brenner, E. (1999). A new view on grasping. *Mot. Control* 3: 237–271.

Ungerleider, L. G., and Mishkin, M. (1982). Two cortical visual systems. In *Analysis of Visual Behavior*, D. J., Ingle, M. A., Goodale, and R. J. W. Mansfield (eds.). Cambridge, Mass.: MIT Press, pp. 549–586.

Van der Willigen, R. F., Bradshaw, M. F., and Hibbard, P. B. (2000). 2-D tilt and 3-D slant illusions in perception and action tasks. *Perception* 29: 52.

Vishton, P. M., Rea, J. G., Cutting, J. E., and Nunez, L. N. (1999). Comparing effects of the horizontal-vertical illusion on grip scaling and judgment: Relative versus absolute, not perception versus action. *J. Exp. Psychol. Hum. Percept. Perform.* 25: 1659–1672.

Witkin, H.A., and Asch, S. E. (1947). Studies in space orientation: 4. Further experiments on perception of the upright with displaced visual fields. *J. Exp. Psychol.* 38: 762–782.

Young, M. P. (1992). Objective analysis of the topological organization of the primate cortical visual system. *Nature* 358: 152–155.

2

Ups and Downs in the Visual Control of Action

James A. Danckert and Melvyn A. Goodale

2.1   Introduction

Why do we see things in detail in only the central part of our visual field? The main reason is almost certainly the cost of processing. It is estimated that if as much cortex were devoted to processing information from our peripheral as from our foveal vision, our brains would weigh more than 15 tons (Eric Schwartz, cited in Aloimonos, 1994)! Fortunately, by moving our gaze from one part of the world to another, we can bring to bear the considerable processing power of the part of the visual system that deals with the few degrees of central vision.

Despite the dramatic overrepresentation of the central visual field in perceptual processing, visual information in the periphery plays an important role in the control of human behavior (for review, see Goodale and Murphy, 1997). For one thing, the visual periphery is exquisitely sensitive to visual movement and other stimuli of potential importance. Once these stimuli are detected, we then redirect our gaze toward the stimuli to examine them in greater detail (e.g., Posner and Dehaene, 1994). But this is not the only contribution that peripheral vision makes. Optic flow in the visual periphery plays an important role in the control of posture and locomotion (e.g., Bardy et al., 1999; Crundall et al., 1999). Moreover, vision of the moving limb in the peripheral visual field is used for the on-line control of reaching and grasping movements: In "visual open-loop" conditions, where a view of the moving limb is denied, reaching and grasping movements are typically slower and less accurate than they are in "visual closed-loop" conditions, where full vision of the moving limb is always available (e.g., Connolly and Goodale, 1999; Prablanc et al., 1979).

The role of the visual periphery in the control of actions such as locomotion and manual prehension is reflected in its differential representation

in the two main pathways of visual processing identified in the primate
cerebral cortex (Ungerleider and Mishkin, 1982). The ventral "perception"
pathway, which runs from primary occipital cortex (area V1) to inferotemporal cortex, has primarily a foveal representation of the visual field—
a fact consistent with its crucial role in the perception and recognition of
objects and scenes (Milner and Goodale, 1995). In contrast, the dorsal "action" pathway, which runs from area V1 to posterior parietal cortex and
plays a critical role in the control of actions such as goal-directed limb
and eye movements, has a full representation of the visual field (Goodale
and Milner, 1992; Milner and Goodale, 1995; Ungerleider and Mishkin,
1982; figure 2.1), presumably necessary for efficient visual control of behavior patterns where the effector, the controlling stimuli, or both are often
present in the peripheral visual field. Although the functional separation of
the two visual pathways is by no means complete, with regions such as the
middle temporal (MT) area, for example, sending afferents to both pathways (Maunsell and Newsome, 1987), the perception-action distinction
provides a compelling explanation for why ventral stream processing concentrates on central vision (particularly the fovea), whereas dorsal stream
processing appears to involve the entire visual field, including the far
periphery.

In his theoretical account of how three-dimensional visual space is
processed in the primate brain, Previc (1990, 1998) divides the visual field
into peripersonal (close to the body) and extrapersonal (beyond reaching
distance) space, suggesting that there may be even greater complexities in
the representation of the central and peripheral visual fields.[1] In general,
actions such as grasping or manipulating tools are carried out in peripersonal
space, particularly in the region of space below eye level. For this reason,
Previc argues, there is a lower visual field advantage in the processing of
visual information for the control of many goal-directed actions, whereas
processes such as visual search or scene perception are generally carried out
in extrapersonal space and may be more efficient in the upper visual field
(see also Skrandies, 1987 for a discussion of upper, lower visual field differences in humans).

Previc's functional distinction parallels to some extent the division of
labor between action and perception proposed by Goodale and Milner
(1992; Milner and Goodale, 1995) for the dorsal and ventral visual pathways
in the cerebral cortex. One might expect therefore that the dorsal stream,
crucial for the visual control of prehensile movements, would demonstrate

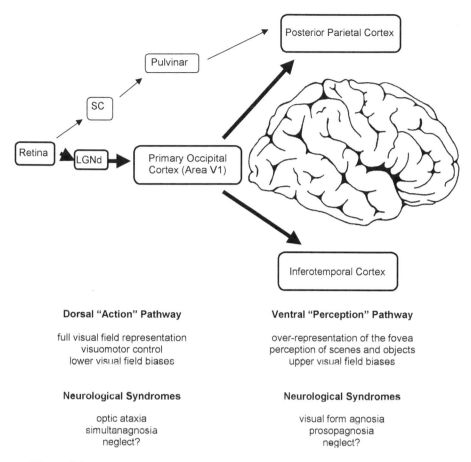

Dorsal "Action" Pathway

full visual field representation
visuomotor control
lower visual field biases

Ventral "Perception" Pathway

over-representation of the fovea
perception of scenes and objects
upper visual field biases

Neurological Syndromes

optic ataxia
simultanagnosia
neglect?

Neurological Syndromes

visual form agnosia
prosopagnosia
neglect?

Figure 2.1
Schematic representation of the dorsal "action" and ventral "perception" pathways. Neuropsychological impairments resulting from lesions at various points of these pathways are indicated at the bottom of the figure. SC, superior colliculus; LGNd, dorsal lateral geniculate nucleus.

a bias toward processing information in the lower visual field, whereas the ventral pathway, important for scene and object perception, would demonstrate a bias toward processing information in the upper visual field. It is perhaps both premature and simplistic, however, to suggest a one-to-one mapping of the lower and upper visual fields onto the dorsal "action" and the ventral "perception" pathways. As we discuss later, because processing in the ventral stream seems heavily biased toward central vision, any upper visual field bias would not extend far into the periphery. Nevertheless, it seems likely that the visual control of action, which is mediated by the dorsal stream, would be mapped onto neural circuits that are biased toward processing visual information in those parts of space where actions typically occur. In other words, it seems likely that the neural substrates of actions that usually unfold in the lower visual field, such as manual prehension, also have a stronger representation of that part of the visual field.

After a brief account of what is known about anatomical and physiological anisotropies in the representation of the upper and lower visual fields in the monkey and human cerebral cortex, this chapter reviews the behavioral evidence for an asymmetry in the processing of visual information in the lower and upper visual fields, focusing largely on evidence for a lower visual field bias in the visual control of manual prehension.

2.2   Anatomical Considerations

Differential Representation of the Upper and Lower Visual Fields in the Retina

Differences in how the central and peripheral visual fields are represented in the central nervous system are evident even at the level of the retina. Although the fovea occupies only an extremely small region at the back of the eye, it has a much higher ganglion cell density than the rest of the retina. Indeed, there is a rapid decline in ganglion cell density as one moves away from the fovea (Curcio and Allen, 1990; Curcio et al., 1987). But the decline in density of ganglion cells beyond the fovea and parafovea is not uniform. Two main anatomical anisotropies have been observed in both the human and the monkey retina: There is a greater density of ganglion cells, first, in the nasal hemiretina (which receives visual information from the temporal visual field) than in the temporal hemiretina (which receives visual information from the nasal visual field); and second, in the superior hemiretina (which receives information from the lower visual field) than in the inferior hemiretina (which receives information from the upper visual field). The nasal-temporal asymmetry is the larger of the two with the density of ganglion cells in the nasal hemiretina exceeding that of the temporal hemiretina by approximately 300%, whereas the superior-inferior asymmetry is on the order of 60% (Curcio et al., 1987). In the monkey, these asymmetries, including the upper and lower visual field asymmetry, are also evident at the level of the lateral geniculate nucleus (Schein and de Monasterio, 1987).

Beyond the Retina: Differential Representation of the Upper and Lower Visual Fields in Cerebral Cortex of the Monkey

It is well known that the fovea has a much larger representation in striate cortex than one might expect given the tiny part of visual space this part of the retina subtends. This "cortical magnification" of the fovea is even more exaggerated as one moves further along the ventral stream of visual processing. At the level of the inferotemporal cortex, for example, the receptive fields of visually responsive neurons almost always include the fovea and very little of the far periphery (Gross et al. 1971), reflecting the role of this region in object recognition (which almost always occurs in central vision). But cortical magnification is not present in all visual areas beyond striate cortex. Some regions of the dorsal stream of visual processing, such as the parieto-occipital area, have essentially no cortical magnification at all (Colby et al., 1988). The amount of cortex devoted to the fovea in this region is no larger than would be expected on the basis of the extent of the visual field it subtends, which is exactly what one might expect to see in a pathway dedicated to the visual control of action (for a review of this literature, see Goodale and Murphy, 1997).

Anisotropies of representation in visual areas of the cerebral cortex are less marked for the upper and lower visual fields than for the central and peripheral visual fields. Areas V1 and V2 maintain a full representation of the visual field, although the lower and upper visual fields are represented in distinct anatomical regions above and below the calcarine fissure, respectively. If there are differences in how information from the upper and lower visual fields is coded in these regions, they are not evident in gross anatomy. Beyond areas V1 and V2, there are some regions that maintain an exclusive representation of either the upper or the lower visual field, but not both. For example, area V3 maintains an exclusive lower visual field representation, whereas area VP maintains an exclusively upper visual field representation (Burkhalter et al., 1986). Area V3 is reciprocally connected with the dorsal portion of area V1 (which represents the lower visual field). It used to be thought that there was no corresponding set of projections from the ventral portion of area V1 to area V3v; recently, however, Lyon and Kaas (2001) have demonstrated such a connection.

Area MT, a region that plays a primary role in the processing of visual motion, has a greater representation of the lower visual field (Maunsell and Van Essen, 1987). A similar difference in visual field representation has been observed in area V6A, a region of the dorsal parieto-occipital cortex. Only 14% of neurons within area V6A appear to have receptive fields that include the upper visual field; the remaining 86% include some representation of the lower visual field (Galletti et al., 1999). Neurons in this region have been shown to be related to eye, head, and arm position (Galletti et al., 1997), although some neurons code spatial coordinates in a gaze-independent manner (Galletti et al., 1993). Given that it is reciprocally connected with area MT and maintains a large representation of the central visual field, area V6A may be important for the visual monitoring of ballistic movements and the central control of the final stages of limb movements (Galletti et al., 1999; see also Battalia-Mayer et al., 2000).

Functional Neuroimaging of Visual Field Representation in Humans
Although asymmetries in the representation of the visual field have been observed in many visual areas of monkey cortex, we know much less about how they are manifested in the human visual system. Humans, like monkeys, show cortical magnification of the central 4–6° of the visual field in area V1. There is also evidence from neuroimaging that some early visual areas in the human brain have an exclusive representation of either the upper or the lower visual field. For example, there is a strong upper visual field representation in the ventral region of area V4 (V4v) and a corresponding lower visual field representation in the dorsal region of the same area (area V4d) (Tootell et al., 1996, 1998a).[2] But for areas that have a representation of the entire visual field, there is little reliable neuroimaging information about upper and lower visual field asymmetries—in part because retinotopic mapping studies have not explored the peripheral field beyond 15° from the fovea. Moreover, no neuroimaging studies have explicitly compared upper and lower visual field activation. Thus, for example, although area V8 has representations of both the upper and lower visual fields, it is not known whether the *extent* of those representations is equivalent

(Hadjikhani et al., 1998). Furthermore, these studies cast no light on the question of differential *functions* within these regions: Although it is clear that different anatomical regions of area V8 process visual information from the upper and lower visual fields, respectively, it is not clear whether these regions are also specialized for different visual processes. Functional magnetic resonance imaging (fMRI) studies of other visual areas, such as area MT and the lateral occipital (LO) region, have also revealed a coarse representation of both the upper and lower visual fields (Tootell et al., 1998b). But again, it is not clear whether the lower visual field bias observed in the monkey area MT exists in humans and, if it does, whether it also reflects a functional asymmetry.

Electrophysiological Studies of Visual Field Representation in Humans

Evoked potentials offer another way of studying how the human visual system responds differentially to upper and lower visual field stimulation. Fioretto and colleagues (1995) found increased amplitudes and decreased latencies for the so-called P100 component of the visual evoked potential (VEP) to lower visual field stimuli as compared to upper visual field stimuli. In addition, they also observed the same anisotropy in amplitude and latency for the later P300 component of the VEP. Whereas the P100 component of the VEP is thought to reflect early "sensory" processing in area V1, the later P300 component is thought to represent a more cognitive component associated with attentional processing (Brecelj et al., 1998; Jones and Blume, 2000). Similar asymmetries between responses to upper and lower visual field stimulation have been observed in early visual areas using magnetoencephalographic (MEG) recordings (Portin et al., 1999). Rather than suggesting that these results indicate a greater *area* of cortex subserving the lower visual field, it has been argued that there may be greater neuronal *synchrony* for stimuli appearing in the lower visual field. Interestingly, a recent MEG study also demonstrated stronger links between areas V1 and MT for lower than for upper visual field stimulation (Tzelepi et al., 2001), providing tentative but tantalizing support for the claim that moving stimuli are processed more efficiently in the lower visual field. More research is needed to support this claim, but there is no doubt that electrophysiological studies have revealed clear differences in the way early areas of the visual system respond to stimuli presented in the lower and upper visual fields. It is important to remember, however, that, even though they provide excellent temporal resolution for the study of human neural mechanisms, the spatial resolution of event-related potentials (ERPs) is not as fine-grained as that of fMRI. The study of the functional differences in cortical representation of the upper and lower visual fields would benefit from a combination of these two techniques.

2.3   Action and Perception in the Upper and Lower Visual Fields

Most of the considerable research into visual information processing in the peripheral visual field (for review, see Goodale and Murphy, 1997) has focused on differences in processing along the *horizontal meridian*. Only a few studies have compared differences in performance as a function of the position of stimuli along the vertical extent of the visual field. Moreover, little attention has been paid to possible differences in visuomotor performance in the upper and lower visual fields. The following subsection reviews the evidence for differences in perceptual processing in the upper and lower visual fields and describes work in our own laboratory on differences in visuomotor processing in these fields.

Perception in the Upper and Lower Visual Fields

When they compared right-left visual field differences in reading English and Yiddish, Mishkin and Forgays (1952) found an unexpected advantage for word recognition in both languages in the lower over the upper visual field. More recent studies, however, have not demonstrated a consistent lower visual field advantage in reading words: Some have shown the opposite advantage, and others have shown no difference at all between the upper and lower visual field (Heron, 1957; Kajii and Osaka, 2000), although discrepancies in the results may be due in part to differences in methodology. Moreover, in the case of reading (and perhaps many other skilled visual routines), the fact that there are differences in performance in the upper and lower visual fields may be due as much to prior experience and behavioral context as to any fundamental differences in visual processing in the two fields (for a discussion of these issues, see Efron, 1990).

Beyond the highly learned task of reading, there are substantial asymmetries in perceptual processing across the upper and lower visual fields that cannot simply be explained by retinal factors. It has been suggested that processing of "local" visual information may be carried out more efficiently in the upper visual field, whereas processing of more "global" information may be carried out more efficiently in the lower visual field (Christman, 1993; for review, see Previc, 1998). There is certainly evidence that discrimination of global patterns, such as spatial frequency gratings, is superior in the lower visual field (Berardi and Fiorentini, 1991). It remains to be seen whether the global-local distinction in processing in the lower and upper visual fields, respectively, can be usefully mapped onto the more familiar global-local asymmetry proposed for visual processing in the right and left hemispheres, respectively (for a discussion of some of the implications of the traditional global-local distinctions made in attentional literature, see Allport, 1994).

Edgar and Smith (1990) have suggested that people more often overestimate the spatial frequency (whether high or low) of gratings presented in their lower than in their upper visual field. Again, this finding would appear to suggest that the asymmetry arises centrally rather than at the level of the retina.

With more complex stimuli, asymmetries in perceptual abilities across the vertical extent of the visual field are somewhat more difficult to interpret. Rubin and colleagues (1996) explored the perception of illusory contours in both the upper and lower visual fields using Kaniza figures and a display designed to induce an illusory occlusion effect. Based on the finding that illusory conjunctions were perceived more frequently in the lower than in the upper visual field for both types of stimuli, they postulated a lower visual field bias for segmentation processes, arguing that the ability to segregate figures from their background might be more efficiently carried out in the lower visual field (Rubin et al., 1996). It is possible that such a bias may also be explained in attentional terms (He et al., 1996). That is, if attentional resolution is greater in the lower visual field, one may also expect that processes requiring fine-grained attentional resolution, such as figure-ground segmentation, may also be superior in the lower visual field. Finding that attentional tracking and conjunction detection were more accurate when carried out in the lower than in the upper visual field, He and colleagues (1996) suggested that visual attention operated more efficiently in the lower than in the upper visual field, which may explain many of the advantages in processing lower visual field information discussed thus far. It may be the case that advantages in processing lower visual field information may actually reflect biases in how visual spatial attention is directed (He et al., 1996), although this point has also been recently disputed (Carrasco et al., 1998; Talgar and Carrasco, 2001). We shall return to the thesis that the deployment of attention may be more fundamentally linked to processing in the lower than in the upper visual field.

Grasping Objects in the Upper and Lower Visual Fields

Over the last two decades, considerable information has accumulated about the functional organization and the neural substrates of grasping movements (for review, see Jeannerod, 1997). As has been the case with the oculomotor system for some time, it is now possible to record kinematics of actual movements made in real time and three-dimensional space (for review, see Goodale and Servos, 1996). Furthermore, the constraints of the physical plant and many of the neural circuits subserving skilled movements are reasonably well understood (Andersen, 1987; Andersen et al., 1990, 1997; Decety et al., 1994; Grafton et al., 1996; Snyder et al., 1997; Tweed and Vilis, 1987).

The first to explore the control of prehension in the visual periphery and to compare the accuracy of that control with the accuracy of perceptual judgments of object size, Goodale and Murphy (1997) found that maximum grip aperture (typically achieved about 65% of the way into a reach-to-grasp movement) remained well scaled to the size of goal objects presented in the far periphery, even at eccentricities as far as 70° from the fovea. Moreover, variability in the scaling did not change as a function of eccentricity. Perceptual judgments of the object's size, on the other hand, became much more variable as the object was presented at greater eccentricities. When they compared grip scaling and perceptual judgments of object size in the upper and lower visual fields (Murphy and Goodale, 1997), they found that subjects took longer to initiate a grasping movement to goal objects in the upper visual field than in the lower visual field, although they found no differences in the perceptual estimations of size in the two fields. In addition, grip scaling was more tightly coupled to object width for targets presented in the lower visual field than for objects presented in the upper visual field. It should be pointed out that the target object was always presented in the same position with respect to the subject's arm and body. Only the fixation point was changed (i.e., subjects were required to fixate a light-emitting diode (LED) that was 15° above or below the target). In this way, the biomechanical constraints on movements of the upper limb were the same across all trials, even though the target was sometimes in the upper visual field and sometimes in the lower visual field.

Taken together, these results suggest that grasping movements made to targets in the far periphery are almost as efficient as those made to targets close to the fovea—and that this efficient control is more evident in the lower than in the upper visual field.

Speed-Accuracy Trade-Off Is Evident Only in the Lower Visual Field Murphy and Goodale's observations (1997) were extended in a more recent study in our laboratory that examined differences in visuomotor control in the upper and lower visual fields, but at much smaller eccentricities from the fovea. Because differences in factors such as ganglion cell density between the two fields are most dramatic beyond 30° from the fovea (Curcio and Allen, 1990), at smaller eccentricities, any differences in performance between the two fields are more likely to reflect differences in central rather than retinal processing of the visual information. In our study, subjects made repetitive pointing movements to targets that were presented in the near periphery approximately 10° from the fovea (Danckert and Goodale, 2000a, 2001). They were required to point to the center of the targets, which varied in size from trial to trial, while maintaining fixation on a point above or below the target display (figure 2.2). Thus, just as in Murphy and Goodale, 1997, the biomechanical constraints were the same for movements directed at targets in the lower and upper visual fields, which meant that any differences in performance would have to be due to differences in processing visual information from the two fields about the target, the moving hand, or both. The task we used has been shown to have a robust speed-accuracy trade-off, as defined by Fitts's law (1954), which states that movement duration increases linearly with an index of item difficulty (ID) calculated as a function of movement amplitude (A) and target width (W) using the following formula:

$$ID = \log_2(2A/W).$$

In other words, movement duration should increase as a function of the index of difficulty. As it turned out, this was exactly what we found—but only for movements made to targets in the lower visual field. In other words, when subjects made repetitive pointing movements to targets of different sizes that were presented in the lower visual field, movement time increased in a linear way with increases in item difficulty. When they made the same movements toward targets in the upper visual field, however, we

James A. Danckert and Melvyn A. Goodale

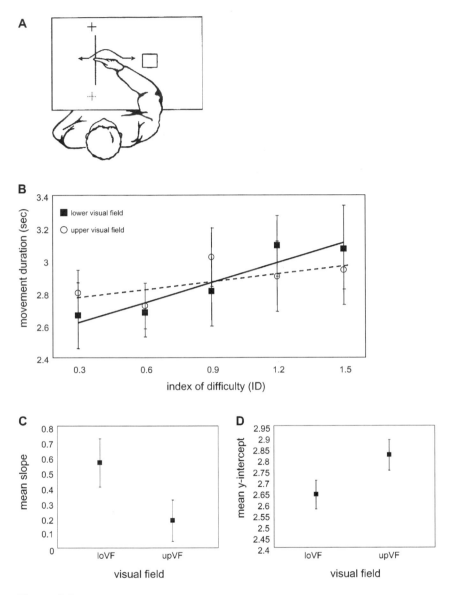

Figure 2.2
(A) Schematic representation of the stimulus display used in Danckert and Goodale,
2001. Subjects were required to make five pointing movements to the center of
the target within a given trial. The double-headed arrow indicates the directions
in which subjects pointed. Note that when fixating a cross in the upper portion
of the display (solid cross) movements and targets were perceived in the lower
visual field, whereas fixating a cross in the lower portion of the display (dashed
cross) ensured that movements and targets were perceived in the upper visual field.

found that there was no relationship between movement duration and item difficulty (figure 2.2). Indeed, as figure 2.2 shows, when an analysis of variance was carried out on the slopes of regression lines that had been separately fitted to each subject's data, the slope of the lines describing the relationship between movement duration and item difficulty was found to be significantly greater for movements to targets in the lower than in the upper visual field. As the y-intercept of the regression lines indicates, the overall movement duration was shorter for movements made to targets in the lower than in the upper (figure 2.2). Moreover, the peak velocity of movements showed a strong relationship with target width in the lower but not in the upper visual field (figure 2.3A).

Pointing movements made to targets in the lower visual field were also more accurate than those made to targets in the upper visual field (figure 2.3B). In other words, subjects were both faster and more accurate when pointing to targets in the lower visual field (Danckert and Goodale, 2001). Taken together, these results suggest that the visual control of skilled motor acts of the upper limb are more efficient in the lower than in the upper visual field.

Because the targets in this task were never more than about $10°$ from the fovea, where differences in ganglion cell density are not that apparent (Curcio and Allen, 1990), these results are unlikely to be purely "retinal." Instead, the difference in performance in the lower and upper visual fields is likely to reflect a functional specialization in central visual structures, probably in the dorsal "action" pathway, for the control of upper-limb movements made to goal objects in the lower visual field (and peripersonal space).

◄ Only one cross was present during any given trial. Subjects were instructed to emphasize speed and accuracy equally in their movements. The biomechanics of movements did not differ across conditions and the experimental setup and stimuli were designed such that targets would subtend the same degree of visual angle in each visual field. Movements were measured using a three-camera system that monitored infrared light emitting diodes placed on the subjects' finger and wrist. (B) Group mean movement duration for real movements plotted against an index of difficulty as calculated by Fitts's law (1954). Linear lines of best fit are plotted on this figure (open circles and dashed lines represent upper visual field targets, whereas filled squares and solid lines represent lower visual field targets). (C) Group mean slope as a function of visual field. (D) Group mean y-intercept as a function of visual field. loVF, lower visual field; upVF, upper visual field. Error bars in panels B–D indicate one standard error of the mean.

A

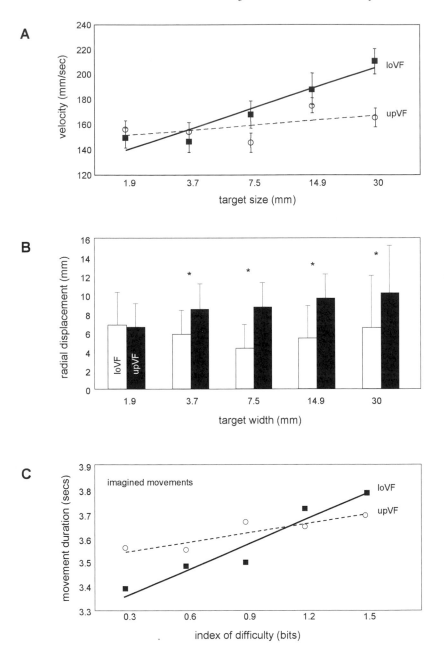

Imagery across the Upper and Lower Visual Fields   Additional support for the hypothesis that structures within the dorsal action pathway are specialized for the control of limb movements made to goal objects in the lower visual field comes from studies on imagined movements. It is generally accepted that mental imagery makes use of many of the same neural structures involved in the generation of real percepts or real movements (Farah, 1984; Jeannerod, 1994). For example, when subjects were asked to imagine a familiar face or a familiar place while their brains were being scanned, the corresponding areas in the ventral visual pathway that code actual percepts of faces and places were selectively activated (O'Craven and Kanwisher, 2000). Similarly, when subjects were asked to move their hand or, on other occasions, to imagine moving their hand, the same areas in the supplementary motor area, premotor cortex, the motor strip, and the cerebellum were activated (Decety et al., 1994; Lotze et al., 1999).

The evidence described above suggests that the brain mechanisms involved in transforming visual information into the required coordinates for guiding skilled, goal-directed movements might also be recruited when subjects are asked to imagine making such movements. As a consequence, if the required movement engages transformational mechanisms that are specialized for action in a particular part of space, subjects might find it easier to imagine performing a movement that engages those mechanisms than a similar movement that does not. Specifically, subjects might somehow be more "efficient" in carrying out a series of repetitive pointing movements they imagined to targets in their lower visual field than the same movements imagined to targets in their upper visual field. But how does one measure the efficiency of imagined movements?

◀ Figure 2.3
(*A*) Group mean peak velocity plotted against target width. Linear trend lines are fitted for both upper (dashed line) and lower visual fields (solid line). (*B*) Group mean radial accuracy data plotted at each target width for both the upper (filled rectangles) and lower (open rectangles) visual fields. ★ represents a significant difference in radial displacement across the visual fields at $p < .05$. Radial accuracy was measured by taking the square root of the sum of the squared x and y distances of the endpoints of each movement. (*C*) Group mean movement duration for imagined movements. The linear regression equations were significant for imagined movements made in both the upper and lower visual fields, although analysis of the slope and y-intercepts indicated that imagined movements were generally faster in the lower visual field and showed a steeper relationship with the index of difficulty. Error bars in panels A–B indicate one standard error of the mean.

The difficulty in measuring mental imagery is that only indirect measures can be used to make inferences about the nature of mental imagery. Subjects, for example, might be required to report when a series of movements they have been asked to imagine have been "completed." Using such a measure, a number of investigators have shown that the same kind of speed-accuracy trade-off observed for actual movements was also obtained when subjects were asked to imagine making such movements (Decety et al., 1989; MacKenzie et al., 1987; Maruff et al., 1999a, 1999b; Sirigu et al., 1996), the duration of imagined movements increasing in a linear fashion with the index of difficulty as defined by Fitts's law.

Using this kind of measure, we showed that imagined repetitive pointing movements "aimed" at lower visual field targets are more efficient than the same movements aimed at upper visual field targets (Danckert and Goodale, 2000a). Subjects were presented with targets of different sizes in the upper or lower visual field and required to fixate above or below the display, in same fashion as before (figure 2.2). But in this experiment, they were simply asked to imagine making repetitive pointing movements to the targets. The relationship between target size and the indicated duration of imagined movements was stronger for targets in the lower visual field (as indicated by a steeper slope and lower y-intercept calculated from individual regression lines fitted to each subject's data) than for targets in the upper visual field. Nevertheless, the relationship between target size and duration was not entirely absent for targets in the upper visual field (figure 2.3C). In other words, subjects demonstrated a significant speed-accuracy trade-off for imagined movements in this part of the field as well—in stark contrast to their actual movements to targets in the upper visual field, where there was no relationship at all between target size and movement duration (figure 2.2). As with all tasks investigating mental imagery, of course, we could not be sure that subjects were always complying with task instructions (i.e., to imagine pointing to targets in the upper visual field). But even with this lack of control over the strategies employed by individual subjects, there remained a large and significant advantage for imagined movements made to targets in the lower visual field. These results with imagined movements provide additional support for the suggestion that the lower visual field advantage for real movements reflects a bias in how the visuomotor mechanisms in the dorsal stream process information derived from the lower visual field—and is not due entirely to differences in ganglion cell density at the level of the retina.

Intercepting Moving Targets in the Upper and Lower Visual Fields

As mentioned earlier, monkey neurophysiology has demonstrated an over-representation of the lower visual field in area MT, an early visual area dedicated to motion processing (Maunsell and Newsome, 1987; Maunsell and Van Essen, 1987). Although we had demonstrated that subjects were better at pointing to or grasping static targets in the lower than in the upper visual field, we wondered whether they would show a similar lower visual field advantage when they were asked to intercept moving targets. To test this idea, we asked subjects to point to moving targets as rapidly and accurately as possible while fixating points either above or below the moving targets (again ensuring that the biomechanics of the interceptive movements were identical in each condition; figure 2.4A–B; Danckert et al., 2001).

Subjects showed shorter periods of deceleration (both in absolute terms and normalized for total movement duration) when they attempted to intercept targets moving in the lower than in the upper visual field (figure 2.4C). In other words, they spent less time closing in on the target when it was moving in the lower visual field. This advantage for movements directed toward targets in the lower visual field did not arise at the expense of accuracy; there was no difference between the fields in endpoint accuracy or variability. In short, subjects needed less time to intercept moving targets when those targets appeared in the lower visual field (Danckert et al., 2001).

In summary, for several different types of skilled actions of the upper limb (grasping, repetitive pointing, imagined pointing, and interceptive movements), we have demonstrated an advantage when those movements are directed at targets in the lower visual field. These behavioral observations converge nicely with data from neurophysiological studies in the monkey and electrophysiological and imaging studies in the human that show a stronger representation of the lower visual field in a number of cortical visual areas, including those involved in the visual control of reaching and grasping. Taken together, these findings suggest that the dorsal stream, known to be involved in the mediation of visually guided actions, has a bias toward processing visual information about the target (or the moving hand) that is derived from the lower visual field.

What Exactly Is Being Processed More Efficiently in the Lower Visual Field? The evidence reviewed above shows that there is a substantial advantage for visually guided movements executed in the lower over the

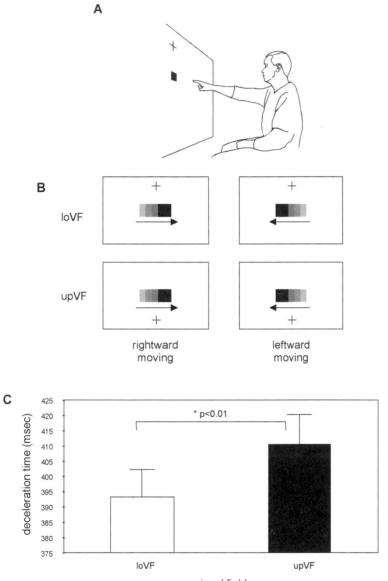

A

B

loVF

upVF

rightward
moving

leftward
moving

C

deceleration time (msec)

* p<0.01

loVF   upVF

visual field

upper visual field. The question remains as to whether this advantage represents a bias in processing visual information about the goal object, about the position or velocity of the moving hand as it approaches the target, or about both. The advantage for grasping objects in the lower visual field demonstrated by Murphy and Goodale (1997) was observed under visual open-loop conditions, in which the subjects' view of their hand was occluded after movement onset. Although this would appear to suggest that visual feedback of the moving hand is not necessary for demonstrating a lower visual field advantage in prehension, it does not mean that visual feedback from the moving hand is not processed more efficiently in the lower visual field. Indeed, the lower visual field advantage observed by Murphy and Goodale might have been even larger had they run the study under visual closed-loop conditions, where subjects *could* see their moving hand. Moreover, it is likely that some tasks will put greater demands on visual feedback from the moving hand than others. For example, in the visually guided pointing task used by Danckert and Goodale (2001), given the simultaneous requirements of speed and accuracy, feedback from the moving hand is likely to play a crucial role in controlling movements made to the different target sizes. Such feedback might be even more important in tasks where subjects are tracking a moving target. Further research is needed to explore just how movements in the lower visual field gain their advantage—and how the nature of that advantage might vary across different kinds of visuomotor tasks.

◀ **Figure 2.4**
(*A*) Schematic display of the experimental setup for intercepting moving targets. The display pictured has an upper fixation point so that the target and movement are perceived in the lower visual field. A lower fixation point equidistant from the target's *x*-axis path was used to explore movements in the upper visual field. Kinematics of movements were measured using infrared optoelectronic measuring systems as in Danckert and Goodale, 2001 (see figure 2.2). (*B*) Schematic representation of the four possible target types. An upper fixation point means that targets and movements are perceived in the lower visual field (loVF), whereas a lower fixation point means that movements and targets are perceived in the upper visual field (upVF); this ensures that the biomechanics of movements are identical across all trials. (*C*) Group mean deceleration time for interceptive movements made in the upper visual field (filled rectangle) and the lower visual field (open rectangle) averaged across direction of target movement. The difference was also significant when expressed as a percentage of total movement duration. Error bars indicate one standard error of the mean.

2.4   Neurological Disorders and Visual Field Representation

The visual deficits and spared visual abilities of neurological patients have also provided some insights into how visual information from the lower and upper visual fields might be differentially processed. Two types of patients are of particular interest with respect to possible differences in the representation of the upper and lower visual fields: Patients with hemianopia arising from lesions of primary occipital cortex (area V1), who nevertheless show some residual visual functions in their blind field ("blindsight"), and patients with damage to the temporal-parietal junction, who fail to acknowledge or attend to stimuli in contralesional space (unilateral neglect). A brief discussion of these two patient groups is presented here, with particular emphasis on how these disorders may shed some light on how the healthy brain might deal with visual information differently depending on whether it originates from the lower or the upper visual field. (For more general discussions of blindsight and neglect, see Stoerig and Cowey, 1997, and Rafal, 1998, respectively.)

Blindsight and the Lower Visual Field: The Case of G.Y.

Lesions of primary visual cortex lead to visual deficits in the contralesional hemifield that correspond topographically to the damaged region of cortex (for review see Stoerig, 1996; Stoerig and Cowey, 1997). Typically, patients are blind in the contralesional hemifield: They report seeing nothing at all in that part of their visual field. When tested carefully, however, some of these patients demonstrate residual visual capacities within their blind field. They might, for example, be able to point or saccade toward targets in their blind field, despite having no direct awareness that the targets are there (Weiskrantz et al., 1974; Weiskrantz, 1986; Zihl and Werth, 1984a, 1984b). In fact, they are often surprised they can localize targets they cannot "see." The term *blindsight* refers to the variety of residual visual capacities of the otherwise blind field (Weiskrantz, 1986). Since the phenomenon was first reported, a broad range of "unconscious" visual abilities have been described including relatively accurate pointing, saccades, or both; grip scaling and wrist orientation during grasping; motion discrimination; rudimentary form discrimination; and wavelength processing (Barbur et al.,1993; Danckert et al.,1998; Perenin and Rossetti, 1996; Weiskrantz, 1987). The phenomenon of blindsight suggests that visual pathways independent of the primary retinogeniculate pathway to area V1 retain the ability to perform some rudimentary analysis of visual information, despite the lack of input from area V1 (Stoerig and Cowey, 1997). One such pathway runs from the eye directly to the superior colliculus, which is typically spared following damage to area V1. This pathway and its indirect projections to extrastriate visual cortex via the pulvinar may mediate much of what has been designated "blindsight" (Danckert and Goodale, 2000b; Stoerig and Cowey, 1997).

Another pathway, from the superior colliculus to the pulvinar and from there to extrastriate cortex, projects predominantly to the dorsal visual stream (see Milner and Goodale, 1995, for a review). If the better visuomotor performance in the lower visual field described earlier is reflective of a bias in the dorsal stream for processing visual information in the lower visual field, then this bias should also be evident in the residual visual capacities in the blind field of hemianopic patients. In other words, if blindsight indeed depends in part on processing in the dorsal stream, then patients should do better with lower than with upper visual field stimuli. Recently, de Gelder and colleagues (2001) were able to demonstrate reliable spatial summation, namely, reaction times (RTs) to dual targets presented simultaneously to both the sighted and blind fields were shorter than those to single, sighted field targets (see Marzi et al., 1986) in blindsight patient G.Y., but only when targets appeared in the lower portion of his "blind" field. Furthermore, using ERPs, they were able to demonstrate a reliable electrophysiological response only to lower visual field targets. That is, when two targets were presented in G.Y.'s lower visual field, one in his sighted field and the other in his blind lower quadrant, his P1 response was observed to be earlier than when only one target was presented in the lower quadrant of his sighted field. This was not the case if targets were presented to his sighted and blind upper visual quadrants (de Gelder et al., 2001). An ERP study in normal observers also showed that the spatial summation effect was more robust in the lower visual field (Miniussi et al., 1998). That G.Y. showed a similar bias suggests that the effect is not entirely dependent on projections from area V1. In other words, the lower visual field bias may reflect the residual processing within intact dorsal stream structures that continue to receive input from the superior colliculus via the pulvinar.

A recent fMRI study attempted to construct retinotopic maps of G.Y.'s spared extrastriate cortex in the lesioned hemisphere (Baseler et al., 1999). With foveal stimulation, many extrastriate regions demonstrated conventional retinotopic organization. When stimuli were restricted to

G.Y.'s blind field, however, responses were found predominantly in dorsal extrastriate regions of his damaged hemisphere. Furthermore, regions of cortex in the damaged hemisphere that had previously demonstrated "normal" retinotopy to foveal stimulation now responded predominantly to stimuli presented in the lower portion of his visual field defect (Baseler et al., 1999).

Although these data are intriguing, one has to be certain, for example, that G.Y.'s lesion of area V1 has not selectively spared tissue representing the lower visual field. A recent fMRI investigation of the visual responsiveness of G.Y.'s damaged hemisphere shows that this is not the case (Kleiser et al., 2001). There was no evidence of activation in the perilesional region of area V1, even with a stimulus known to drive area V1 neurons optimally (a high-contrast reversing ckeckerboard). Nor was there any evidence of islands of activation within the lesion itself. This suggests that G.Y.'s lesion is quite complete (with the possible exception of the occipital pole, which could account for the spared macular vision in G.Y.). It is possible, of course, that more ventral extrastriate regions have been damaged in G.Y., a pattern of damage that could explain why some of his residual visual responses were better in the lower rather than the upper visual field. Moreover, it is not clear that some sort of reorganization of connections might not have taken place within the remaining extrastriate regions and these connections somehow favor the processing of lower visual field stimuli. (For a discussion of these possibilities and others, including the idea that collicular projections to dorsal extrastriate cortex from the pulvinar are responsible for the activation, see Baseler et al., 1999.)

Before speculating further about what might account for the lower visual field bias in some of G.Y.'s visual responses, however, it would be useful to know whether residual visual abilities in other blindsight patients, particularly spared visuomotor abilities, are more likely to be invoked by stimuli in the lower than in the upper visual field. Unfortunately, with the exception of G.Y., there have been no systematic explorations of how visual responsiveness varies as a function of position within the blind hemifield across a range of different visual responses.[3]

Finally, it should be mentioned that there is some evidence that the upper bank of the calcarine fissure, which represents the lower visual field, is more refractory to vascular lesions than the lower bank, which represents the upper visual field (Kitajima et al., 1998). It is well known that patients with lesions of primary visual cortex are more likely to exhibit a superior than an inferior quadrantanopia, probably because the upper bank of the calcarine fissure is more vascularized than the lower bank (Mohr and Pessin, 1992; Smith and Richardson, 1966), perhaps reflecting again the over-representation of the lower visual field.

Neglect of Peripersonal or Extrapersonal Space: Altitudinal Neglect
Patients with damage to the temporoparietal junction, usually in the right hemisphere, often fail to attend to or respond to stimuli appearing in their contralesional field. This so-called unilateral neglect is independent of any sensory disturbances and is therefore thought to reflect an impairment of spatial attention (Driver and Mattingley, 1998; Karnath et al., 2001; Rafal, 1998). Typical tests used to demonstrate neglect include cancellation tasks (e.g., the patient is asked to cross off lines, letters, or stars presented on a sheet of paper placed at their body's midline), copying or drawing tasks (e.g., the patient is asked to copy symmetrical drawings of flowers or to make free drawings of symmetrical objects such as a butterfly), and line bisection (see Rafal, 1998, for a review). Line bisection requires that the patient judge the midpoint of lines that vary in length, with neglect patients typically bisecting lines to the right of the true midpoint. Although the direction of the impairment in neglect patients is typically observed for left versus right space (e.g., canceling out only objects on the right side of a page, drawing only the right half of a flower), neglect can also occur within other frames of reference. For example, patients can demonstrate neglect for the right side of objects independent of their location in space (Driver et. al., 1994). Even the neglect of contralesional space can be played out in different frames of reference with respect to the observer, such that neglect can occur in personal space (e.g., failing to shave one side of the face), peripersonal space (e.g., neglecting the food on one side of a plate), or even in extrapersonal space (e.g., neglect for objects or scenes beyond reaching space; see Rafal, 1998, for a review).

But more important for the thesis being developed in this chapter, there is also intriguing evidence that some patients will neglect stimuli within a frame of reference that maps onto the distinction between the upper and lower visual fields we have been drawing. Rapcsak and colleagues (1988), for example, describe a patient with bilateral lesions that include the posterior parietal cortex who shows a deficit that the authors call "altitudinal neglect." In a vertically oriented line bisection task, the patient marked the perceived midpoint of the line well above the true midpoint for both visual and tactile presentations. Furthermore, she showed "extinction" to a lower visual field stimulus when that stimulus was accompanied by an upper visual field stimulus. In a later study (Mennemeier et al., 1992), the same patient, when presented with a line extending away from the body, tended to mark the perceived midpoint of the line *beyond* the true midpoint. In short, this patient appeared to neglect stimuli in the lower visual field and near (peripersonal) space. Similar cases have been reported by other groups of investigators (Butter et al., 1989; Pitzalis et al., 2001).

In contrast to the patients described above, Shelton and colleagues (1990) describe a patient with bilateral inferior temporal lobe lesions who bisected vertical lines *below* the true midpoint and bisected lines extending away from the body *nearer* to the body. In other words, this patient appeared to neglect the upper visual field and extrapersonal or far space. One major complication involved with interpreting deficits in such patients, however, is the coexistence of superior visual field quadrantanopias following temporo-occipital lesions. It may be the case that patients with superior visual field cuts demonstrate the biases they do, not because of neglect, but because of a sensory impairment in the upper visual field (Barton and Black, 1998; Kerkhoff, 1993). But superior field cuts cannot account for all instances of neglect of the upper visual field and extrapersonal space following temporo-occipital lesions (see Adair et al., 1995). Interestingly, a recent positron-emission tomography (PET) study explored changes in regional cerebral blood flow when subjects bisected lines in near versus far space (Weiss et al., 2000). Results demonstrated increased blood flow in dorsal parietal regions when subjects bisected lines in near space, and in more ventral occipito-temporal regions when lines were bisected in far space. This finding suggests that, even in healthy individuals, near and far space (and perhaps the lower and upper visual fields) are processed by the dorsal and ventral streams, respectively.

The data on neglect in the vertical dimension, though scanty, suggest that patients who neglect the lower visual field (and near space) tend to have lesions that involve the posterior parietal cortex, whereas patients who neglect the upper visual field (and far space) tend to have lesions in the temporo-occipital cortex. This double dissociation maps neatly onto the distinction between upper and lower visual field representation in the ventral and dorsal streams that has been suggested in this chapter (and more boldly by Previc, 1990, 1998), although a functional dissociation between the two kinds of neglect has not been established.

In fact, one must be extremely cautious in trying to map what are poorly understood syndromes onto different brain structures. There are just too few patients of this kind described in the literature. Moreover, almost all studies of neglect in the vertical dimension have used only the line bisection task, which may not be the most sensitive measure of neglect (Ferber and Karnath, 2001). It would be interesting to see whether patients with neglect would demonstrate similar upper or lower visual field biases on cancellation and copying tasks, and whether neglect in the visuomotor domain is more common in the lower than in the upper visual field, perhaps using a variation on the task used by Hussain and colleagues (2000), who showed that patients with typical left-sided neglect had a specific difficulty in initiating leftward movements toward visual targets on the left side of space. Finally, it would be interesting to explore in greater detail the defining attentional deficits in patients with neglect in the vertical dimension. As the next section indicates, the lower and upper visual fields may have biases in different aspects of attention. For this reason, the attentional problems shown by patients who neglect the lower visual field might be expected to be quite different from those shown by patients who neglect the upper visual field. All of this will remain speculation until more empirical studies are carried out.

2.5   Attention in the Upper and Lower Visual Fields

One variable invoked in discussions of lower and upper visual field differences is attention. It has been argued, for example, that attention has a higher resolution in the lower than in the upper visual field (Carrasco et al., 1998; He et al., 1996; Talgar and Carrasco, 2001). Thus tasks that require focused attention show a marked lower visual field advantage. An example of such a task is attentional tracking, in which two or more target disks are tracked by the observer as they move on the screen among several other randomly moving disks (Pylyshyn and Storm, 1998). The trick is that the target disks are physically identical to the nontarget disks, and are identified as targets only by a brief color change that occurs at the beginning of a trial. When there are two or more target disks, the only way they can be tracked is by deploying attention to multiple locations. In other words, because the target disks often move in quite different directions they cannot be followed with eye movements. He and colleagues (1996) showed that observers are able to track such targets much better when they are placed in the lower than the upper visual field. They argued that the superior performance in the lower visual field is due to the better attentional resolution in this part of the field. In other words, observers could keep their attention on the target disks even when the targets came very close to non-target disks.

He and colleagues (1996) also found a similar lower visual field advantage for detecting static targets presented in the visual periphery when those targets were defined by a conjunction of different features (shape and orientation) and were flanked by similar distracter items. Even though the position of the target is known ahead of time, observers typically find it difficult to attend only to the target and not to the distracters because the targets are "crowded" by the presence of the flanking items. The finer the grain or resolution of attention, of course, the easier it is to identify the target in one of these "crowding" tasks. Thus the finding that observers did better when the display was in the lower visual field in He et al., 1996, again suggests that attentional resolution is better in this part of the visual field.

More recently, Ellison and Walsh (2000) have claimed that the attentional differences between the upper and lower visual fields may not be as great as originally claimed by He and colleagues (1996). They found no difference in a conjunction search (where the targets were red forward slashes and the distracters were red back slashes and green forward slashes) when the array of items was presented to the entire visual field. Nevertheless, they did find a lower visual field advantage when the array was restricted to either the lower or the upper visual field. In some ways, the presence of the weak but significant lower visual field advantage in Ellison and Walsh, 2000, could be construed as a confirmation of He and colleagues' findings. In other words, because the demands on attentional resolution were not nearly as great in Ellison and Walsh, 2000, as they were in He et al., 1996, it is not surprising that the observed difference between the fields was also not as great. But the fact that Ellison and Walsh found a lower visual field advantage even with *reduced* demands on attentional resolution suggests that attention may indeed be somehow more efficient in this part of the visual field.

The thesis that there is an attentional bias for processing stimuli in the lower visual field receives further support from Rezec and Dobkins (2001), who measured thresholds for both direction-of-motion and orientation discrimination in the upper and lower visual fields. They found that when the target displays were presented alone in a single quadrant, a small lower visual field advantage was found for the motion task but not the orientation task. But when noise distracters (either randomly moving dots or vertically oriented lines, depending on the task) were presented in the other three quadrants, a dramatic lower visual field advantage emerged for both the motion task and the orientation task. This result again suggests attentional resolution is better in the lower visual field.

This lower-field bias in attentional resolution can be contrasted with a host of findings showing that shifts of attention in visual search tasks and other related paradigms are biased toward stimuli in the upper visual field (for review, see Previc, 1998). Indeed, in a recent study that explored the effects of manipulating a number of variables in visual search, Fecteau and colleagues (2000) found a robust upper visual field advantage in all tasks. A similar upper visual field advantage in visual search for three-dimensional targets has been reported by Previc and Naegele (2001; see also Previc and Blume, 1993). Indeed, there is evidence that saccadic eye movements, which are a physical instantiation of a shift of attention, show a shorter latency when directed to stimuli in the upper than in the lower visual field (Shelliga et al., 1997; see also Previc and Murphy, 1997; for similar data in monkeys see Li and Andersen, 1994; Schlykowa et al., 1996; and Zhou and King, 2002).

These findings suggest we might be more disposed to *shifting* attention to stimuli in the upper than in the lower visual field. But once we are engaged in a task that demands more detailed analysis—and perhaps more precise visuomotor control—we are better served by the greater attentional resolution in the lower visual field. According to this scenario, attention has better resolution in the lower visual field because the control of most of our skilled actions takes place there. In other words, most of our actions take place within arm's reach, in peripersonal space. We need good attentional resolution in this part of space so that we can select targets for action from other distracting items in the visual array and perhaps, more important, maintain precise on-line control of those actions in the presence of the distracters. At the same time, we need to remain vigilant so that our attention can be shifted rapidly to salient stimuli in extrapersonal space, which is largely represented in the upper visual field. Thus both visual fields show attentional biases—but those biases are quite different.

The distinction we are making between attentional resolution and shifts of attention cannot be mapped onto the division of labor between the dorsal and ventral streams. Indeed, numerous human neuroimaging studies have implicated regions in the posterior parietal cortex in a broad range of attention-demanding tasks (Culham and Kanwisher, 2001). The higher attentional resolution in the lower visual field may reflect the bias that already exists in the dorsal stream pathway for the control of visually guided movements in this part of the field. Shifts of attention can be driven in a bottom-up fashion by salient stimuli, such as transient changes in a stimulus or high-contrast edges, or in a top-down fashion by stored information about goal objects. How all of this unfolds is poorly understood at present, but it is likely that any top-down driven shifts of attention would use information derived from ventral stream processing. The relationship between these different aspects of attention and differential processing of information from the upper and lower visual fields is an area ripe for further experimentation.

2.6   Conclusion

Although studies across a broad range of experimental tasks support Previc's original proposal (1990) for a division of labor between visual processing in the upper and lower visual fields, we would argue that the asymmetry has largely been driven by the specialization of the lower visual field for the control of skilled actions in peripersonal space. There is a clear lower visual field advantage for the visual control of skilled movements, such as pointing and grasping; that the same bias is evident for imagined movements suggests the underlying asymmetry is central and not purely retinal. The perceptual asymmetries are not nearly so clear-cut and may reflect instead a difference in the deployment of attention across the vertical extent of the visual field. Thus attentional resolution appears to be higher for stimuli in the lower visual field, even though the focus of attention can be shifted more quickly to stimuli in the upper visual field. These reciprocal asymmetries in different aspects of attention may have evolved alongside a need to control actions directed toward objects in peripersonal space, while at the same time maintaining vigilance for stimuli in extrapersonal space. In short, it is the need to act, and not simply to perceive, that has driven the functional organization of the human visual system.

Acknowledgment

We wish to thank the Natural Sciences and Engineering Research Council of Canada for supporting much of the research reported in this chapter.

Notes

1. Extrapersonal space is further divided into *focal, action,* and *ambient* space. For detailed, full account of this theory, see Previc, 1998.

2. Recent fMRI studies have also been able to create topographical maps of smaller structures such as the dorsal lateral geniculate nucleus (LGNd), but have provided no insight into possible *functional* asymmetries in the representations of the upper and lower visual fields (e.g., Chen et al., 1999).

3. For a discussion of G.Y.'s abilities throughout his hemianopic field defect, see Kentridge et al., 1997.

References

Adair, J. C., Williamson, D. J., Jacobs, D. H., Na, D. L., and Heilman, K. M. (1995). Neglect of radial and vertical space: Importance of the retinotopic reference frame. *J. Neurol. Neurosurg. Psychiatry* 58: 124–728.

Allport, A. (1994). Attention and control: Have we been asking the wrong questions? A critical review of twenty five years. In *Attention and Performance XIV*, D. E. Meyer and S. Kornblum (eds.). Cambridge, Mass.: MIT Press, pp. 183–218.

Aloimonos, Y. (1994). What I have learned. *Comput. Vis. Image Understanding* 60: 74–85.

Andersen, R. A. (1987). Inferior parietal lobule function in spatial perception and visuo-motor integration. In *Handbook of Physiology*. Sec. 1, *The Nervous System*. Vol. 5, *Higher Functions of the Brain*. Part 2, F. Plum, V. B. Mountcastle, and S. R. Geiger (eds.). Bethesda, Md.: American Physiological Society, pp. 483–518.

Andersen, R. A., Asanuma, C., Essick, G., and Siegel, R. M. (1990). Corticocortical connections of anatomically and physiologically defined subdivisions within the inferior parietal lobule. *J. Comp. Neurol.* 296: 65–113.

Andersen, R. A., Snyder, L. H., Bradley, D. C., and Xing, J. (1997). Multimodal representation of space in the posterior parietal cortex and its use in planning movements. *Annu. Rev. Neurosci.* 20: 303–330.

Barbur, J. L., Watson, J. D. G., Frackowiak, R. S. J., and Zeki, S. (1993). Conscious visual perception without V1. *Brain* 116: 1293–1302.

Bardy, B. G., Warren, Jr., W. H., and Kay, B. A. (1999). The role of central and peripheral vision in postural control during walking. *Percept. Psychophys.* 61: 1356–1368.

Barton, J. J. S., and Black, S. E. (1998). Line bisection in hemianopia. *J. Neurol. Neurosurg. Psychiatry* 64: 660–662.

Baseler, H. A., Morland, A. B., and Wandell, B. A. (1999). Topographic organisation of human visual areas in the absence of input from primary cortex. *J. Neurosci.* 19: 2619–2627.

Battalia-Mayer, A., Ferraina, S., Mitsuda, T., Marconi, B., Genovesio, A., Onorati, P., Lacquaniti, F., and Caminiti, R. (2000). Early coding of reaching in the parieto-occipital cortex. *J. Neurophysiol.* 83: 2374–2391.

Berardi, N., and Fiorentini, A. (1991). Visual field asymmetries in pattern discrimination: A sign of asymmetry in cortical visual field representation. *Vision Res.* 31: 1831–1836.

Brecelj, J., Kakigi, R., Koyama, S., and Hoshiyama, M. (1998). Visual evoked magnetic responses to central and peripheral stimulation: Simultaneous VEP recordings. *Brain Topog.* 10: 227–237.

Burkhalter, A., Felleman, D. J., Newsome, W. T., and Van Essen, D. C. (1986). Anatomical and physiological asymmetries related to visual areas V3 and VP in macaque extrastriate cortex. *Vision Res.* 26: 63–80.

Butter, C. M., Evans, J., Kirsch, N., and Kewman, D. (1989). Altitudinal neglect following traumatic brain injury: A case report. *Cortex* 25: 135–146.

Carrasco, M., Wei, C., Yeshurun, Y., and Orduña, I. (1998). Do attentional effects differ across visual fields? *Eur. Conf. Vision Percept. Abstr.* 29.

Chen, W., Zhu, X.-H., Thulborn, K. R., and Ugurbil, K. (1999). Retinotopic mapping of lateral geniculate nucleus in humans using functional magnetic resonance imaging. *Proc. Natl. Acad. Sci. U. S. A.* 96: 2430–2434.

Christman, S. D. (1993). Local-global processing in the upper versus lower visual fields. *Bull. Psychonom. Soc.* 31: 275–278.

Colby, C. L., Gattass, R., Olson, C. R., and Gross, C. G. (1988). Topographical organisation of cortical afferents to extrastriate visual area PO in the macaque: A dual tracer study. *J. Comp. Neurol.* 269: 392–413.

Connolly, J. D., and Goodale, M. A. (1999). The role of visual feedback of hand position in the control of manual prehension. *Exp. Brain Res.* 125: 281–286.

Crundall, D., Underwood, G., and Chapman, P. (1999). Driving experience and the functional field of view. *Perception* 28: 1075–1087.

Culham, J. C., and Kanwisher, N. G. (2001). Neuroimaging of cognitive functions in human parietal cortex. *Curr. Opin. Neurobiol.* 11: 157–163.

Curcio, C. A., and Allen, K. A. (1990). Topography of ganglion cells in human retina. *J. Comp. Neurol.* 300: 5–25.

Curcio, C. A., Sloan, K. R., Packer, O., Hendrickson, A. E., and Kalina, R. E. (1987). Distribution of cones in human and monkey retina: Individual variability and radial asymmetry. *Science* 236: 579–581.

Danckert, J., and Goodale, M. A. (2000a). Real and imagined movements in the upper and lower visual fields. *Cogn. Neurosci. Soc. Abstr.* 67.

Danckert, J., and Goodale, M. A. (2000b). Blindsight: A conscious route to unconscious vision. *Curr. Biol.* 10: R64–R67.

Danckert, J., and Goodale, M. A. (2001). Superior performance for visually guided pointing in the lower visual field. *Exp. Brain Res.* 137: 303–308.

Danckert, J., Maruff, P., Kinsella, G., de Graaff, S., and Currie, J. (1998). Investigating form and colour perception in blindsight using an interference task. *NeuroReport* 9: 2919–2925.

Danckert, J., Sharif, N., and Goodale, M. A. (2001). Intercepting moving targets in the upper and lower visual fields. *J. Vision* 1: 319a.

Decety, J., Jeannerod, M., and Prablanc, C. (1989). The timing of mentally represented actions. *Behav. Brain Res.* 34: 35–42.

Decety, J., Perani, D., Jeannerod, M., Bettinardi, V., Tadary, B., Woods, R., Mazziotta, J. C., and Fazio, F. (1994). Mapping motor representations with positron emission tomography. *Nature* 371: 600–602.

de Gelder, B., Pourtois, G., Raamsdonk, M., Vroomen, J., and Weiskrantz, L. (2001). Unseen stimuli modulate conscious visual experience: Evidence from inter-hemispheric summation. *NeuroReport* 12: 385–391.

Driver, J., and Mattingley, J. B. (1998). Parietal neglect and visual awareness. *Nature Neurosci.* 1: 17–22.

Driver, J., Baylis, G. C., Goodrich, S. J., and Rafal, R. D. (1994). Axis-based neglect of visual shapes. *Neuropsychologia* 32: 1353–1365.

Edgar, G. K., and Smith, A. T. (1990). Hemifield differences in perceived spatial frequency. *Perception* 19: 759–766.

Efron, R. (1990). *The Decline and Fall of Hemispheric Specialization*. Hillsdale, N.J.: Lawrence Erlbaum.

Ellison, A., and Walsh, V. (2000). Visual field asymmetries in attention and learning. *Spat. Vis.* 14: 3–9.

Farah, M. J. (1984). The neurological basis of mental imagery: A componential analysis. *Cognition* 18: 245–272.

Fecteau, J. H., Enns, J. T., and Kingstone, A. (2000). Competition-induced visual field differences in search. *Psychol. Sci.* 11: 386–393.

Ferber, S., and Karnath, H.-O. (2001). How to assess spatial neglect—line bisection or cancellation tasks? *J. Clin. Exp. Neuropsychol.* 23: 599–607.

Fioretto, M., Gandolfo, E., Orione, C., Fatone, M., Rela, S., and Sannita, W. G. (1995). Automatic perimetry and visual P300: Differences between upper and lower visual fields stimulation in healthy subjects. *J. Med. Eng. Technol.* 19: 80–83.

Fitts, P. M. (1954). The information capacity of the human motor system in controlling the amplitude of movement. *J. Exp. Psychol.* 47: 381–391.

Galletti, C., Battaglini, P. P., and Fattori, P. (1993). Parietal neurons encoding spatial locations in craniotopic coordinates. *Exp. Brain Res.* 96: 221–229.

Galletti, C., Fattori, P., Kutz, D. F., and Battaglini, P. P. (1997). Arm-movement-related neurons in the visual area V6A of the macaque superior parietal lobule. *Eur. J. Neurosci.* 9: 410–414.

Galletti, C., Fattori, P., Kutz, D. F., and Gamberini, M. (1999). Brain location and visual topography of cortical area V6A in the macaque monkey. *Exp. Brain Res.* 124: 287–294.

Goodale, M. A., and Milner, A. D. (1992). Separate visual pathways for perception and action. *Trends Neurosci.* 15: 20–25.

Goodale, M. A., and Murphy, K. J. (1997). Action and perception in the visual periphery. In *Parietal Lobe Contributions to Orientation in 3D Space,* P. Their and H.-O. Karnath (eds.). Heidelberg: Springer-Verlag, pp. 447–461.

Goodale, M. A., and Servos, P. (1996). The visual control of prehension. In *Advances in Motor Learning and Control,* H. Zelaznik (ed.). Champaign, Ill.: Human Kinetics, pp. 87–121.

Grafton, S. T., Fagg, A. H., Woods, R. P., and Arbib, M. A. (1996). Functional anatomy of pointing and grasping in humans. *Cereb. Cortex* 6: 226–237.

Gross, C. G., Rocha-Miranda, C. E., and Bender, D. B. (1971). Visual properties of neurons in inferotemporal cortex of the macaque. *J. Neurophysiol.* 35: 96–111.

Hadjikhani, N., Liu, A. K., Dale, A. M., Cavanagh, P., and Tootell, R. B. H. (1998). Retinotopy and colour sensitivity in human visual cortical area V8. *Nature Neurosci.* 1: 235–241.

He, S., Cavanagh, P., and Intrilligator, J. (1996). Attentional resolution and the locus of visual awareness. *Nature* 383: 334–337.

Heron, W. (1957). Perception as a function of retinal locus and attention. *Am. J. Psychol.* 70: 38–48.

Hussain, M., Mattingley, J. B., Rorden, C., Kennard, C., and Driver, J. (2000). Distinguishing sensory and motor biases in parietal and frontal neglect. *Brain* 123: 1643–1659.

Jeannerod, M. (1994). The representing brain: Neural correlates of motor intention and imagery. *Behav. Brain Sci.* 17: 187–245.

Jeannerod, M. (1997). *The Cognitive Neuroscience of Action.* Cambridge, Mass.: Blackwell.

Jones, D. C., and Blume, W. T. (2000). Pattern-evoked potential latencies from central and peripheral visual fields. *J. Clin. Neurophysiol.* 17: 68–76.

Kajii, N., and Osaka, N. (2000). Optimal viewing position in vertically and horizontally presented Japanese words. *Percept. Psychophys.* 62: 1634–1644.

Karnath, H.-O., Ferber, S., and Himmelbach, M. (2001). Spatial awareness is a function of the temporal not the posterior parietal lobe. *Nature* 411: 950–953.

Kentridge, R. W., Heywood, C. A., and Weiskrantz, L. (1997). Residual vision in multiple retinal locations within a scotoma: Implications for blindsight. *J. Cogn. Neurosci.* 9: 191–202.

Kerkhoff, G. (1993). Displacement of the egocentric visual midline in altitudinal postchiasmatic scotomata. *Neuropsychologia* 31: 261–265.

Kitajima, M., Korogi, Y., Kido, T., Ikeda, O., Morishita, S., and Takahashi, M. (1998). *Neuroradiology* 40: 710–715.

Kleiser, R., Wittsack, J., Niedeggen, M., Goebel, R., and Stoerig, P. (2001). Is V1 necessary for conscious vision in areas of relative cortical blindness? *NeuroImage* 13: 654–661.

Li, C. S., and Andersen, R. A. (1994). Up-down asymmetry of saccade related and fixation activity in area LIP. *Soc. Neurosci. Abs.* 20: 773.

Lotze, M., Montoya, P., Erb, M., Hulsmann, E., Flor, H., Klose, U., Birbaumer, N., and Grodd, W. (1999). Activation of cortical and cerebellar motor areas during executed and imagined hand movements: An fMRI study. *J. Cogn. Neurosci.* 11: 491–501.

Lyon, D. C., and Kaas, J. H. (2001). Connectional and architectonic evidence for dorsal and ventral V3, and dorsomedial area in marmoset monkeys. *J. Neurosci.* 21: 249–261.

MacKenzie, C. L., Marteniuk, R. G., Dugas, C., Liske, D., and Eickmeier, B. (1987). Three-dimensional movement trajectories in Fitts' task: Implications for control. *Q. J. Exp. Psychol.* 39A: 629–647.

Maruff, P., Wilson, P. H., DeFazio, J., Cerritelli, B., Hedt, A., and Currie, J. (1999a). Asymmetries between dominant and nondominant hands in real and imagined motor task performance. *Neuropsychologia* 37: 379–384.

Maruff, P., Wilson, P., Trebilcock, M., and Currie, J. (1999b). Abnormalities of imagined motor sequences in children with developmental coordination disorder. *Neuropsychologia* 37: 1317–1324.

Marzi, C. A., Tassinari, G., Aglioti, S., and Lutzemberger, L. (1986). Spatial summation across the vertical meridian in hemianopics: A test of blindsight. *Neuropsychologia* 24: 749–758.

Maunsell, J. H. R., and Newsome, W. T. (1987). Visual processing in monkey extrastriate cortex. *Annu. Rev. Neurosci.* 10: 363–401.

Maunsell, J. H. R., and Van Essen, D. C. (1987). Topographical organization of the middle temporal visual area in the macaque monkey: Representational biases and the relationship to callosal connections and myeloarchitectonic boundaries. *J. Comp. Neurol.* 266: 535–555.

Mennemeier, M., Wertman, E., and Heilman, K. M. (1992). Neglect of near peripersonal space: Evidence for multidirectional attentional systems in humans. *Brain* 115: 37–50.

Milner, A. D., and Goodale, M. A. (1995). *The Visual Brain in Action*. New York: Oxford University Press.

Miniussi, C., Girelli, M., and Marzi, C. A. (1998). Neural site of the redundant target effect: electrophysiological evidence. *J. Cogn. Neurosci.* 10: 216–230.

Mishkin, M., and Forgays, D. G. (1952). Word recognition as a function of retinal locus. *J. Exp. Psychol.* 43: 43–48.

Mohr, J. P., and Pessin, M. S. (1992). Posterior cerebral disease. In *Stroke*, 2d ed., H. M. J. Barnett, B. M. Stein, J. P. Mohr, and F. M. Yatsu (eds.). New York: Churchill Livingstone, pp. 419–442.

Murphy, K. J., and Goodale, M. A. (1997). Manual prehension is superior in the lower visual hemifield. *Soc. Neurosci. Abstr.* 23: 178.

O'Craven, K. M., and Kanwisher, N. (2000). Mental imagery of faces and places activates corresponding stimulus-specific brain regions. *J. Cogn. Neurosci.* 12: 1013–1023.

Perenin, M. T., and Rossetti, Y. (1996). Grasping without form discrimination in a hemianopic field. *NeuroReport* 7: 793–797.

Pitzalis, S., Di Russo, F., Spinelli, D., and Zuccolotti, P. (2001). Influence of the radial and vertical dimensions on lateral neglect. *Exp. Brain Res.* 136: 281–294.

Portin, K., Vanni, S., Virsu, V., and Hari, R. (1999). Stronger occipital cortical activation to lower than upper visual field stimuli: Neuromagnetic recordings. *Exp. Brain Res.* 124: 287–294.

Posner, M. I., and Dehaene, S. (1994). Attentional networks. *Trends Neurosci.* 17: 75–79.

Prablanc, C., Echallier, J. E., Jeannerod, M., and Komlis, E. (1979). Optimal response of eye and hand motor systems in pointing at a visual target: 2. Static and dynamic visual cues in the control of hand movement. *Biol. Cybern.* 35: 183–187.

Previc, F. H. (1990). Functional specialisation in the lower and upper visual fields in humans: Its ecological origins and neurophysiological implications. *Behav. Brain Sci.* 13: 519–575.

Previc, F. H. (1998). The neuropsychology of 3-D space. *Psychol. Bull.* 124: 123–164.

Previc, F. H., and Blume, J. L. (1993). Visual search asymmetries in three-dimensional space. *Vision Res.* 33: 2697–2704.

Previc, F. H., and Murphy, S. J. (1997). Vertical eye movements during mental tasks: A re-examination and hypothesis. *Percept. Mot. Skills* 84: 835–847.

Previc, F. H., and Naegele, P. D. (2001). Target-tilt and vertical-hemifield asymmetries in free-scan search for 3-D targets. *Percept. Psychophys.* 63: 445–457.

Pylyshyn, Z. W., and Storm, R. W. (1988). Tracking multiple independent targets: Evidence for a parallel tracking mechanism. *Spat. Vis.* 3: 179–197.

Rafal, R. D. (1998). Neglect. In *The Attentive Brain*, R. Parasuraman (ed.). Cambridge, Mass.: MIT Press, pp. 489–525.

Rapcsak, S. Z., Cimino, C. R., and Heilman, K. M. (1988). Altitudinal neglect. *Neurology* 38: 277–281.

Rezec, A., and Dobkins, K. R. (2001). Sensory and attention based visual field asymmetries for motion and orientation discrimination. *J. Vision* 1: 89a.

Rubin, N., Nakayama, K., and Shapley, R. (1996). Enhanced perception of illusory contours in the lower versus upper visual hemifields. *Science* 271: 651–653.

Schein, S. J., and de Monasterio, F. M. (1987). Mapping of retinal and geniculate neurons onto striate cortex of macaque. *J. Neurosci.* 7: 996–1009.

Schlykowa, L., Koffman, K. P., Bremmer, F., Thiele, A., and Ehrenstein, W. H. (1996). Monkey saccadic latency and pursuit velocity show a preference for upward directions of target motion. *Neuroreport* 7: 409–412.

Shelliga, B. M., Craighero, L., Riggio, L., and Rizzolatti, G. (1997). Effects of spatial attention on directional manual and ocular responses. *Exp. Brain Res.* 114: 339–351.

Shelton, P. A., Bowers, D., and Heilman, K. M. (1990). Peripersonal and vertical neglect. *Brain* 113: 191–205.

Sirigu, A., Duhamel, J.-R., Cohen, L., Pillon, B., Dubois, B., and Agid, Y. (1996). The mental representation of hand movements after parietal cortex damage. *Science* 273: 1564–1568.

Skrandies, W. (1987). The upper and lower visual fields of man: Electrophysiological and functional differences. In H. Autrum et al. (eds.). *Progress in Sensory Physiology* Vol 8. Springer-Verlag.

Smith, C. G., and Richardson, W. G. F. (1966). The course and distribution of the arteries supplying the visual (striate) cortex. *Am. J. Ophthalmol.* 61: 1391–1396.

Snyder, L. H., Batista, A. P., and Andersen, R. A. (1997). Coding of intention in the posterior parietal cortex. *Nature* 386: 167–170.

Stoerig, P. (1996). Varieties of vision: From blind responses to conscious recognition. *Trends Neurosci.* 19: 401–406.

Stoerig, P., and Cowey, A. (1997). Blindsight in man and monkey. *Brain* 120: 535–559.

Talgar, C. P., and Carrasco, M. (2001). The effects of attention in texture segmentation in the lower and upper visual fields. *J. Vision* 1: 76a.

Tootell, R. B. H., Dale, A. M., Sereno, M. I., and Malach, R. (1996). New images from human visual cortex. *Trends Neurosci.* 19: 481–489.

Tootell, R. B. H., Hadjikhani, N. K., Vanduffel, W., Liu, A. K., Mendola, J. D., Sereno, M. I., and Dale, A. M. (1998a). Functional analysis of primary visual cortex (V1) in humans. *Proc. Natl. Acad. Sci. U. S. A.* 95: 811–817.

Tootell, R. B. H., Hadjikhani, N., Hall, E. K., Marrett, S., Vanduffel, W., Vaughan, J. T., and Dale, A. M. (1998b). The retinotopy of visual spatial attention. *Neuron* 21: 1409–1422.

Tweed, D., and Vilis, T. (1987). Implications of rotational kinematics for the oculomotor system in three dimensions. *J. Neurophysiol.* 58: 832–849.

Tzelepi, A., Ioannides, A. A., and Poghosyan, V. (2001). Early (N70m) neuromagnetic signal topography and striate and extrastriate generators following pattern onset quadrant stimulation. *NeuroImage* 13: 702–718.

Ungerleider, L. G., and Mishkin, M. (1982). Two cortical visual systems. In *Analysis of Visual Behavior*, D. J. Ingle, M. A. Goodale, and R. J. W. Mansfield (eds.). Cambridge, Mass.: MIT Press, pp. 549–586.

Weiskrantz, L. (1986). *Blindsight: A Case Study and Implications*. Oxford: Oxford University Press.

Weiskrantz, L. (1987). Residual vision in a scotoma: A follow-up study of "form" discrimination. *Brain* 110: 77–92.

Weiskrantz, L., Warrington, E. K., Sanders, M. D., and Marshall, J. (1974). Visual capacity in the hemianopic field following a restricted occipital ablation. *Brain* 97: 709–728.

Weiss, P. H., Marshall, J. C., Wunderlich, G., Tellman, L., Halligan, P. W., Freund, H.-J., Zilles, K., and Fink, G. R. (2000). Neural consequences of acting in near versus far space: a physiological basis for clinical dissociations. *Brain* 123: 2531–2541.

Zhou, W., and King, W. M. (2002). Attentional sensitivity and asymmetries of vertical saccade generation in monkeys. *Vis. Res.* 42: 771–779.

Zihl, J., and Werth, R. (1984a). Contributions to the study of "blindsight": 1. Can stray light account for saccadic localisation in patients with postgeniculate field defects? *Neuropsychologia* 22: 1–11.

Zihl, J., and Werth, R. (1984b). Contributions to the study of "blindsight": 2. The role of specific practice for saccadic localisation in patients with postgeniculate visual field defects. *Neuropsychologia* 22: 13–22.

II

Intention and Simulation

Some have described the functional distinction between ventral and dorsal streams in terms of consciousness, with the dorsal stream involved in automatic actions and the ventral stream involved in more intentional acts. Rosetti and Pisella (chapter 3) argue instead for a rostrocaudal gradient of automaticity. At one end are automatic, on-line actions; at the other are deliberate, intentional actions. Drawing on evidence from tasks that involve inhibiting direct responses to specific stimuli, they show that intentional actions draw more heavily on frontal mechanisms, whereas automatic actions rely more on parietal mechanisms.

In considering intention and the neural basis of observational learning and imitation, Iacoboni (chapter 4) investigates the "common code hypothesis": We understand others' acts through activating our own internal action representations. Consistent with this hypothesis, Iacoboni presents a large body of original research indicating that observing others' actions evokes many of the same mechanisms evoked by active imitation. He suggests that this "mirror" system not only forms the neural basis of observational learning but may be critical for deciphering others' intentions in social settings.

The enticing possibility that we internally simulate the actions of others in order to decipher their meaning is also taken up by Jeannerod (chapter 5). According to his model, such simulation is but one of several types of internal simulations or "S-states." In organizing the rapidly growing literature on internally simulated actions into a coherent theoretical framework, Jeannerod provides a taxonomy that will serve to guide future investigations of the role of S-states in action planning and comprehension.

3

Mediate Responses as Direct Evidence for Intention: Neuropsychology of Not-To, Not-Now, and Not-There Tasks

Yves Rossetti and Laure Pisella

Les mouvements volontaires sont donc des réactions aussi nécessaires que les mouvements réflexes simples; seulement ces derniers sont les réactions immédiates des impressions périphériques directes, les autres sont les réactions médiates des sensations centrales indirectes, c'est à dire des images ou idées parmi lesquelles doivent nécessairement se trouver celles du mouvement même. . . .
—Alexander Herzen, 1874, pp. 96–97

3.1 Introduction

Intention is a concept frequently referred to in everyday neuroscience. Because consciousness studies are mostly concerned with "consciousness of" (awareness), the aspect of intention that is usually studied is "intention to" (intentional behavior). Intention is thus most often contrasted with reflexive and automatic activities, that is, negatively defined. A well-known formulation of the dissociation between consciousness (admittedly a prerequisite for intention; see Revonsuo and Rossetti, 2000) and automatism has been provided by Penfield (1975, p. 39) in his analysis of complex behavior observed during epileptic seizures:

In an attack of automatism the patient becomes suddenly unconscious, but, since other mechanisms in the brain continue to function, he changes into an automaton. He may wander about, confused and aimless. Or he may continue to carry out whatever purpose his mind was in the act of handing on to his automatic sensory-motor mechanism when the highest brain mechanism went out of action. Or he follows a stereotyped, habitual pattern of behavior. In every case, however, the automaton can make few, if any, decisions for which there has been no precedent.

Although Penfield's "confused" may refer to an altered conscious state and his "aimless," "automatic," and "stereotyped" to altered intentional control of action, he is clearly contrasting his automaton with intentional behavior, at least implicitly. Penfield (1975, p. 47) goes on to define what the automaton cannot do: "The human automaton, which replaces the man when the highest brain mechanism is inactivated, is a thing without the capacity to make completely new decisions. . . . The automaton is incapable of thrilling to the beauty of a sunset or of experiencing contentment, happiness, love, compassion. These like all awarenesses, are functions of the mind." Penfield's automaton exhibits the "inability to make new decisions," which, among other features, is described as a mind property and implicitly contrasted with the automatic properties of brain matter. Without naming intention, Penfield (1975, p. 47) also proposes a positive definition of the automaton, which can in turn serve as a negative definition of intention: "The automaton is a thing that makes use of the reflexes and the skills, inborn and acquired, that are housed in the computer. . . . This automatic coordinator . . . is ever active within each of us. . . ."

Thus automatic behavior can be opposed to and dissociated from both consciousness (see Revonsuo et al., 2000) and intention (table 3.1). Revonsuo and colleagues (2000, p. 335), distinguish between "weak zombiehood," where a person is "not conscious but can only carry out routine action programs" and "strong zombiehood," where a person "can carry out nonroutine tasks involving new decisions and the processing of the meaning of the task and surrounding objects." Although these two types of zombiehood both refer to states where consciousness would be absent, it is questionable whether strong zombiehood could imply intention. That complex behavior may be expressed in the absence of consciousness does not imply that such behavior is intentional. Indeed, as their review of the literature shows, Revonsuo and colleagues (2000) conclude that, although weak zombiehood can be observed during epileptic seizures or sleep-related motor disorders, there is no evidence for strong zombiehood, nor is there evidence that a proper judgment could be exercised or new decisions be made during either state.

If we admit that nonautomatic behavior is by nature intentional, then intentional or voluntary actions should include most of our daily activities, such as grasping objects, moving around, or driving a car. There is no doubt that some of these activities are at least initiated intentionally and occasionally performed under voluntary control. The main purpose of intention, however, is to deal with the higher-order organization of our lives, such as long-term planning or strategies. On the other hand, the vast majority of the processes participating in simple actions are unconscious and nonintentional. When you grasp a single object in front of you, a cup, say, the

Table 3.1
Main characteristics of automatisms

Automatisms	Behavior initiation	On-line control	Sensory awareness	Self-consciousness
Visuomotor reactions	No	Elementary	Dissociated or delayed	Normal
Habits	No (only subsequences)	Elementary and sequence control	Unattended	Normal
Environmental dependency syndrome	Yes	Elementary and sequence control	Full	Normal?
Sleep related motor disorders and epileptic seizures	Yes	?	None or misinterpreted	Altered
Psychoses	Yes	Distorted	Distorted	Altered

Note: "On-line control" may range from elementary on-line control (e.g., parietal automatic pilot; Pisella et al., 2000) to complex sequences (e.g., following an itinerary, walking to an object and throwing it, and social interaction). "Sensory awareness" refers to the ability of the subject to process relevant sensory information during the automatic behavior. "Self-consciousness" refers to reflexive consciousness. "Environmental dependency syndrome" refers to what appears to be the most complex case of automatism, where behavior can be initiated and controlled on the basis of on-line sensory inputs without obvious self-consciousness alteration.

only intentional aspect here is to trigger the action. Existence of an intention becomes more obvious if you decide to grasp the cup in an unusual way, for example, if you guide your hand throughout a complicated trajectory, if you use two middle fingers to form the grip, or grasp the cup upside down. Alternatively, it may be expressed by the selection processes that precedes the action when several potential goals are present. Along this line, you may wonder how intention might be approached under experimental laboratory conditions.

Can we seriously refer to intention in overtrained animals that perform a simple task such as looking and pointing at a stimulus when this task has been practiced hundreds or thousands of times daily over months and years? Are not these experimental conditions closer to pavlovian conditioning than to anything related to intention at all? Is the animal's intention to perform the task or to get a reward? Even in the more complex case of problem solving, because the number of possible solutions is usually extremely limited with regard to the huge number of practice and reinforcement trials performed by the animal, the task of the animal may consist of recognizing a situation and a solution more through automated association processes than through intentional strategic processes. As colleagues working with monkeys often say: "This monkey is too clever to comply with the instructions and perform the task." Indeed, under such experimental conditions, the best manifestation of the animal's intention would be to *stop* performing the task. Such a conclusion is consistent with the fact that intention is most often incorrectly referred to as "preparatory activity" before an action is initiated (e.g., Boussaoud, 2001; Synder et al., 1997), whereas, in point of fact, a preparatory activity takes place even when an action is produced reflexively. As pointed out by Toni and colleagues (2001), the brain activity recorded during the delay introduced between stimulus and response does not necessarily correspond to intention-related activity.

In human studies as well, most experimental conditions designed to explore voluntary actions rely on reactions to a stimulus as a clue to intention. These reactions are most often overlearned in everyday life (e.g., pointing or grasping, key pressing) or are investigated after a learning session in the case of more complex tasks. Therefore the intention of the subject may be restricted to the will to perform the task or to comply with the instructions. Reaction time tasks by definition test the subject's ability to *react* to a stimulus rather than to intentionally respond to it. Clinical examination may provide a less constrained way to explore intentional aspects of behavior. "Intentional" is often used to describe the tremor observed during cerebellar ataxia, for example. But here it refers only to the fact that the tremor appears during the performance of an action rather than at rest, as is the case in Parkinson's disease. The best manifestation of a deficit of intention per se is the inability to comply with simple instructions. Such deficits are observed chiefly in patients with damage in the frontal lobes. Presented with a comb or a toothbrush and asked to ignore it, or even specifically instructed not to grasp it, a typical frontal patient will grasp and use it immediately (see Lhermitte, 1983). In the case of "anarchic hand," observed following frontocallosal lesion (Della Salla et al., 1994), the patient reports that the affected hand moves of its own accord, for example, grasping the pencil being used by the other hand. So strong is the deficit in intentional control that patients neither criticize their reactions nor express any frustration at not succeeding in the task. This symptom has led Marchetti and Della Salla (1998) to distinguish between "anarchic hand" and "alien hand," where the patient is aware of the inappropriate behavior of the affected hand and spontaneously complains about it. As these examples clearly illustrate, the expression of intention may be more obvious in a not-to-respond task than in a classical response task. The phrase "mediated reaction of indirect central sensations" used by Herzen in 1874 (as cited in Starobinski, 1999, pp. 139–140; see chapter epigraph) clearly means that an intermediate stage of processing has to be involved—that such a reaction must be distinguished from "immediate reactions of direct peripheral impressions." As we will see, in complex behavior expressed during epileptic seizures or sleep-related motor disorders (see Revonsuo et al., 2000), where an altered state of consciousness is responsible for a disconnection between the inner and the outer world, the illusion of intention may reflect the subjects' following an internal goal rather than their reacting to external stimuli.

Intention is best expressed when subjects are not forced to submit to the stimuli presented in the environment, as they are under most experimental conditions. The aim of the present chapter is to review some of the tasks used to explore intentional behavior, focusing on indirect responses rather than on the overlearned direct responses subjects perform hundreds of times daily.

3.2 A Clinical Aspect of Frontal Lobe Functions

Because pathologies of intention are all expressed by negative symptoms (i.e., a deficit in intentional control) rather than by positive symptoms (what would hyper-intention stand for?), it is difficult, if not impossible, to provide a positive definition of intention. It is therefore useful to examine the functional deficits associated with intention disorders. To emphasize the point made in section 3.1, let us briefly review the example of patients with frontal damage. Patients with a dysinhibition syndrome provide us with a characteristic negative image of intention. It is their lack of intentional control that releases automatisms, both simple (e.g., perseveration) and even complex. Behaving in a reactive mode to the environment, typical patients grasp any object (e.g., a comb) presented to them, even when instructed not to do so, and automatically perform the action normally appropriate for the object grasped (e.g., they comb their hair). In the case of complex actions, such as grasping a toothbrush and using it, the patients' "purposeful" behavior may well appear to be intentional. However, such automatic "utilization behavior" (Lhermitte, 1983; Lhermitte et al., 1986) in fact represents a loss of autonomy and is characteristic of the "environmental dependency syndrome" (Lhermitte, 1986) that accompanies frontal lobe lesion (Lhermitte, 1983). It is observed both for social stimuli (imitation behavior) and for physical stimuli (utilization behavior; Lhermitte et al., 1986). The ability to perform a goal-oriented action, even complex, should not therefore be considered as evidence for intention. Rather, patients behave "as though implicit in the environment was an order to respond to the situation" in which they find themselves (Lhermitte, 1986, p. 342). This environmental dependency syndrome can be observed in a home setting such as a bedroom (the patient preparing to go to bed) or in a doctor's office (the patient taking the doctor's blood pressure). A clear and simple experimental demonstration of this idea has been also provided by Riddoch and colleagues (2000), who asked patients with frontal lobe damage (with an "anarchic hand syndrome") to reach to and grasp a cup of tea presented to them. When instructed simply to grasp the cup with the hand on the side of the handle, patients performed the task accurately. But when instructed to use the given hand, patients made numerous errors, where the handle of the cup "triggered" an action from the wrong hand. Also, when patients were reaching to the target cup, their hand might be "captured in flight" by a distracter cup presented close to the hand's trajectory (Humphreys and Riddoch, 2000). Their environmental dependency is thus clearly the result of a deficit in intentional control of action. According to Heckhausen and Beckmann (1990), this dependency corresponds to the expression of habits or overlearned stimulus-response transformations. The following sections will therefore consider tasks in which independence from the experimental stimulus is expressed, that is, where an *indirect* response has to be performed.

3.3   Stop Tasks

A deficit in inhibitory control just as exhibited by patients with frontal lobe lesion represents a pathology of intention, so subservience to external stimulus exhibited by normal subjects in most experimental conditions represents an attenuated equivalent of the frontal patient's "utilization behavior," hence a nonintentional behavior. Thus the "stop task" paradigm is the most obvious paradigm to consider when the issue of intention is raised.

Blocking the Initiation of Action

When Slater-Hammel (1960) asked normal subjects presented with a dot running around a circle to respond synchronously to a particular dot position on the circle, they were able to easily anticipate the course of the dot so as to lift their finger with the appropriate timing. This result suggests that the motor response had to be triggered by the central command before the dot actually reached the crucial position. When, however, the dot stopped for a time before reaching this position, subjects could inhibit their response only if the delay between the dot immobilization and the expected time to reach the position was longer than about 200 ms. This result suggests that, once a simple movement has been triggered, even if not overtly initiated, the intention to stop it cannot block its expression.

In the "stop signal" paradigm developed by Logan and coworkers (see Logan, 1981), participants in a typical experiment perform a speeded reaction time task (e.g., visual discrimination) and are occasionally presented with a stop signal (e.g., a tone) that instruct them to withhold their response. The stop signal paradigm has been applied to both hand and eye responses (most often, withholding key presses and countermanding saccades). The stop signal is usually triggered at different delays after presentation of the stimulus. Depending on the length of the delay, subjects are more or less successful in withholding their response. One of the most notable findings with this paradigm is that the stop signal reaction time (SSRT), that is, the latency for interrupting a response, is usually shorter than the classical reaction time. Ranging around 200 ms, SSRTs tend to be shorter for the eye than for the hand (usually shorter than 200 ms; e.g., De Jong et al., 1995; Logan and Irwin, 2000), and shorter in monkey than in human subjects (Hanes and Shall, 1995). As might be expected, the modality in which the stop signal is provided also modulates the latency for interrupting a response (Cabel et al., 2000). The difference found between the response reaction time and the stop signal reaction time suggests that different mechanisms are at work in stop signal tasks, as does differential modification of the two responses by experimental manipulation (e.g., Logan and Irwin, 2000). Consistently, reaction times to go and stop signals follow different time courses over the life span (Williams et al., 1999) and inhibitory control of behavior is impaired by a moderate dose of alcohol that does not affect response reaction time (Mulvihill et al., 1997). Let us now consider how these two responses are produced.

As the delay of the stop signal increases, humans and monkeys increasingly fail to withhold the response. The hypothesis is that the generation of the response is determined by a race between a go and a stop process (e.g., De Jong et al., 1995; Hanes and Shall, 1995). This race model predicts and describes the probability of inhibition as a function of stop signal delay and response reaction time, although comparison of various versions of the stop signal paradigm suggests that several stop signal processing mechanisms may be involved. When the stop signal required subjects to inhibit any response (stop-all) or only one response (selective stop), inhibition was found to be effected by a peripheral mechanism (De Jong et al., 1995). Moreover, analysis of agonist-antagonist electromyographic (EMG) activity during fast elbow extension movements showed that the EMG response to response inhibition may correspond to an adapted reflex activity (Kudo and Ohtsuki, 1998). By contrast, when subjects had to produce a fixed alternative response to the stop signal (stop-change), the lateralized readiness potential suggested that a selective, central inhibition mechanism was involved (De Jong et al., 1995). For eye movement, there is good evidence that the monkey frontal eye field (FEF) is critically involved in the inhibition of saccades (Hanes et al., 1998).

The brain areas chiefly involved in stop tasks are found in the frontal cortex. Recent brain imaging studies have shown that the inferior frontal cortex plays an important role in the inhibition of inappropriate responses: They consistently report that the inferior frontal cortex is activated together with either the left prefrontal cortex (Collette et al., 2001); the premotor cortex, right anterior cingulate, and inferior parietal lobule (Menon et al., 2001; Rubia et al., 2001); or the bilateral dorsolateral prefrontal cortex (Rubia et al., 2001).

Blocking the Execution of Action

Because the stop signal paradigm, as generally applied, requires that subjects inhibit initiation of their main response, no response is produced during critical trials. Another experimental approach, motor psychophysics, analyzes movement kinematics in various conditions (e.g., Prablanc, 1979), focusing instead on fast reactions to a stimulus change. Its findings are worth comparing with those of stop signal studies. Motor psychophysics studies of the control of simple goal-directed actions have shown that movements, even of short duration, can be corrected on-line (see Rossetti et al., 2000; Pisella and Rossetti, 2000; Rossetti and Pisella, 2002). For instance, fast modifications of motor components were observed during grasping movements in response to changes in object orientation or location (Desmurget et al., 1995, 1996; Gréa et al., 2000, forthcoming). Similarly, after a fast pointing movement has been programmed and initiated toward a visual target, it can be corrected without a significant increase in movement time (Pélisson et al., 1986; Goodale et al., 1986), that is, without reprogramming a new motor output. Interestingly, the latency for updating an ongoing movement is usually found to be around 100 ms, which is much faster than the reaction time observed with the stop signal paradigm. In addition, such on-line corrections can be observed whether or not the target displacement is consciously perceived (Pélisson et al., 1986; Prablanc and Martin, 1992). If the corrective system can bypass the conscious decision level, to what extent can such an automatic system resist intentional control? Could corrective movements be considered the equivalent, in normal subjects, of unwilled movements toward objects (e.g., anarchic hand syndrome; Della Sala et al., 1994) in frontal patients? What explains the apparent slow stop signal reactions with regard to these fast movement corrections? The stop signal and the motor psychophysics approaches have not been combined to answer these questions until recently. We have conducted a series of experiments in which subjects had to point at a visual target (Pisella et al., 1998, 1999, 2000). During the pointing movement execution, the visual target could be altered on a fraction of trials. This target change could be used as a go signal to perform an in-flight correction to a new target location or as a stop signal to interrupt the ongoing movement. Therefore the two types of response had to interfere with an already ongoing pointing action. In contrast to previous researchers, we investigated whether the hand would perform a correction or be interrupted, rather than whether a movement would be initiated. Accordingly, our stop signal did not appear before movement initiation but was triggered by the movement onset. Two types of perturbations were designed to test whether automatic corrective processes can be triggered in response to a chromatic change as well as to a target jump; they were also used as stop signals to create a conflict between the automatic correction system and voluntary motor control.

In a "location-stop" pointing experiment, subjects were first presented with one green target and asked to point at it at specified rates. This target remained stationary on 80% of the trials and unexpectedly jumped to the right or left at movement onset on the remaining 20%. Subjects were asked to systematically interrupt their ongoing movement to touch the target when it jumped. The direction of the target jump was thus irrelevant for this task. Strict compliance with the "Stop" instruction would imply that subjects would either succeed in stopping their movement or fail to interrupt their action and therefore touch the primary position of the target (Pisella et al., 2000). In striking contrast to this prediction, however, a significant percentage of corrective movement were performed in the direction of the target jump despite the "Stop" instruction. Because these corrections were produced spontaneously by naive subjects and against their own intention to stop their movement in accordance with the instruction, they must be considered automatic. After touching the displaced target, subjects were fully aware of their mistakes and spontaneously expressed a strong frustration.

We explored whether the ongoing hand movement was corrected or interrupted with respect to movement times. Sampled movement times ranged from about 100 ms to 450 ms with a Gaussian distribution, corresponding to movement speeds because the distance between targets and starting point was constant in the experiment. In figures 3.1A–C, fast automatic movement corrections with respect to stimulus and instruction are shown in green, and slow intentional movement corrections in red. Four conditions combined two types of instruction—correction (go) or interruption (stop). In the two location conditions (left column), subjects were instructed to point, under different time constraints, to one target first presented on the tactile screen (see Pisella et al., 2000). At movement onset, a target jump could be triggered unexpectedly, in response to which subjects were instructed either to correct (location-go condition) or to stop (location-stop condition) their ongoing pointing movement to the target. In the two color conditions (right column), subjects were first presented with one green and one red target on the tactile screen and instructed to point to the green target. At movement onset, the two targets could exchange colors unexpectedly (see Pisella et al., 2000), in response to which subjects were instructed either to correct (color-go condition) or to stop (color-stop condition) their ongoing pointing movement to the green target. For each condition, the horizontal bars indicate 95% confidence intervals of movement time computed for all unperturbed trials. Figure 3.1a shows the number of corrected movements made by three control subjects with respect to movement duration. Because they occurred in a restricted temporal window, escaping the slower processes of voluntary interruption, the involuntary corrections resulted from a failure to inhibit an automatic process of on-line visuomotor guidance. This "automatic pilot" (see also Place, 2000), which was systematically activated during movement execution, led subjects to produce disallowed corrective movements over a narrow range of movement times, between about 150 ms and 300 ms. Over a range of about 200–240 ms, the same rate of correction was found in this (location-stop) condition and in a control (location-go) condition where subjects had to correct the action in response to the target jump. Only movements slower than 300 ms could be fully controlled by voluntary processes. In contrast to this normal pattern, patient I.G. with a bilateral lesion of the posterior parietal cortex showed a lack of on-line automatic corrective processes, whereas intentional motor processes were preserved (figure 3.1b; Pisella et al., 2000, experiment 3). From this finding, we concluded that fast movements are controlled by a (posterior) parietal "automatic pilot" (PAP) located in the dorsal stream, whereas slow movements are controlled by intentional motor processes that remain largely independent of the posterior parietal cortex. Thus the notion of automatic pilot extended that of "hand sight" (Rossetti et al., 2000) in the sense that it refers not only to unconscious visual processing by the action system, but also to an autonomous use of visual information, which bypasses and even counteracts intention. Following Lhermitte's hypothesis (Lhermitte et al., 1986), the automatic activity observed in this experimental situation seems to result from the "release of parietal lobe activities."

Thus the automatic behavior shown here by normals may be related to the dysfunction of executive skills in patients with a frontal lobe lesion. Indeed, that normal subjects make disallowed corrections even when target jumps signal them to stop their movements is reminiscent of the weakness of intentional control over ongoing activity described in frontal patients, in which "the ongoing activity exerts a more powerful influence than the encoded intention-action" (Cockburn, 1995, p. 95). The parietal automatic pilot observed in normal subjects may thus be one possible substrate of the environment dependency syndrome. Accordingly, frontal patients

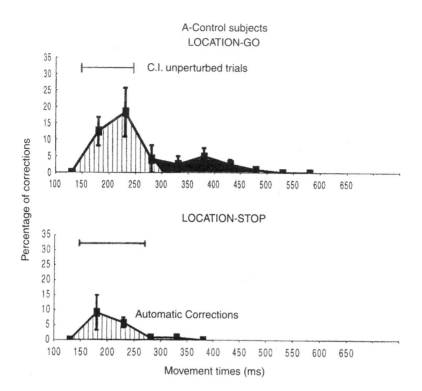

Figure 3.1

(A) Parietal automatic pilot. Three control subjects performed corrections instead of stopping their ongoing movement in response to target jump in the location-stop condition. These corrections were performed with movement times comparable to unperturbed trials (horizontal bar) and against the subjects' intention to stop the movement. We identified them as fast automatic corrections (in green). In the location-go condition, when subjects were explicitly instructed to correct their movement, we observed an additional pool of corrections performed with a substantial increase of movement duration as compared to unperturbed trials (horizontal bar). We identified them as slow intentional corrections (in red). In response to the color change (right column), only slow intentional corrections were performed. The automatic pilot guiding the fast automatic corrections could not be triggered by this "ventral" feature.

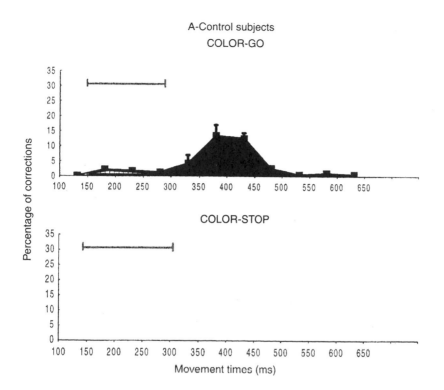

Figure 3.1 (*continued*)

tested on the same tasks should exhibit a complete loss of intentional inhibition of their automatic corrections. In support of this hypothesis, a recent experiment showed that patient G.C. with a unilateral lesion of the dorsolateral convexity of the frontal lobe performed 100% corrections, when the target jump was associated with a stop instruction (location-stop condition; figure 3.1c), even though she was able to orally repeat the instruction throughout the experiment (see Pisella et al., 2000). However, the frustration expressed by our normal subjects over corrections despite themselves stands in contrast with the usual lack of concern displayed by frontal patients or even with the patients' report that "they had to do it" (e.g., Lhermitte, 1986). This main difference may involve a time factor. On the one hand, the impairment in frontal patients has been described for the execution of the serial tasks lasting several seconds (e.g., Lhermitte, 1986; Cockburn, 1995). On the other, the normal subjects' automatic corrections for simple aiming movements fall only within a narrow time window, representing

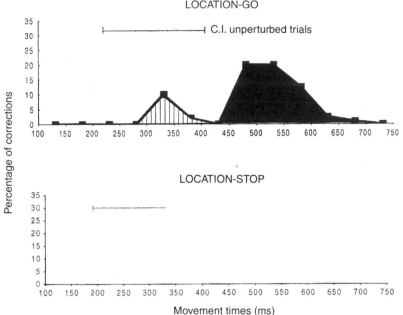

Figure 3.1 (*continued*)
(*B*) Parietal automatic pilot. Patient I.G., with a bilateral lesion of the posterior parietal cortex (PPC), showed a specific impairment for producing the fast automatic corrections. In the go conditions, she performed only slow intentional corrections in response to both the target jump and the color change. In the stop conditions, she could always follow the instruction of interrupting the ongoing movement. This lack of fast automatic corrections cannot be explained by a general slowing of visual or motor processing (see Pisella et al., 2000). We concluded that the PPC is necessary for the processes of the automatic pilot.

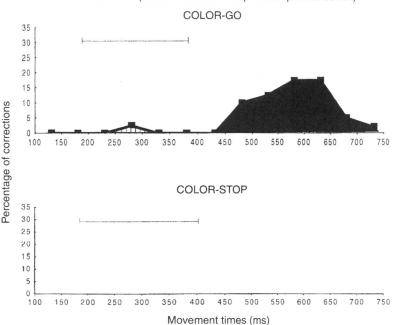

Figure 3.1 (*continued*)

only a temporary lack of voluntary control. It may be hypothesized that normal subjects behave in the same way as frontal patients because the speed constraints of our paradigm do not give the frontal lobe enough time to inhibit automatic corrective processes.

It is clear that intention can be overtly expressed in tasks where a reaction to a stimulus has to be repressed. It is interesting to note that most of the simple direct tasks performed in experimental conditions would be performed at least as well by frontal patients as by normals. Although not to respond to a stimulus may appear simpler than actually responding to it, this is obviously not the case in frontal and normal subjects, especially under time constraints, when the control of an ongoing action is concerned. On the other hand, it would be misleading to assume that intention can be expressed specifically through the inhibition of action, as has been claimed (e.g., Libet, 1993). The following sections present a variety of tasks involving not only the repression of the most direct response to a stimulus but the more complex use of the stimulus in a process evocative of intentional response organization.

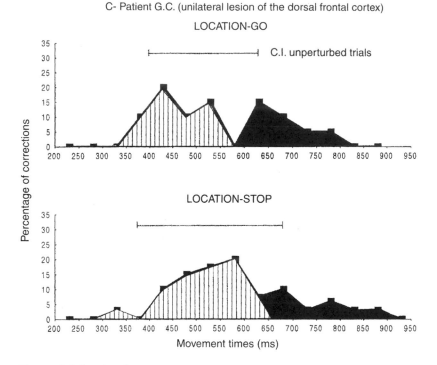

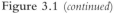

Figure 3.1 (*continued*)

(C) Parietal automatic pilot. The pointing performance of patient G.C., with a unilateral lesion of the dorsal prefrontal cortex, reveals a lack of inhibition of both fast automatic corrections (as in control subjects) and slow intentional corrections (contrary to control subjects), although she was able to orally repeat the instruction throughout the experiment. The lack of concern displayed by patient G.C. stands in contrast with the frustration expressed by the control subjects over the corrections that escaped them. This main difference may be linked to a time factor. The control subjects' automatic guidance was released only for simple aiming movements falling within a narrow time window. Their automatic corrections resulted from only a temporary lack of voluntary control.

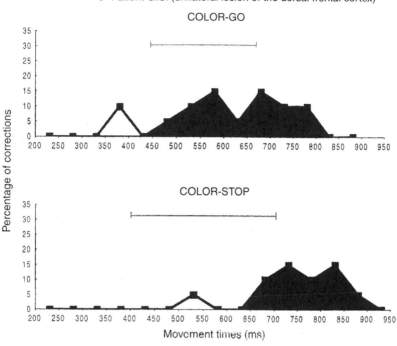

Figure 3.1 *(continued)*

3.4 Delayed Tasks

To achieve a distant goal, self-control is a necessary aspect of intelligent behavior. Delaying an action is obviously a difficult task to perform for a patient with frontal lobe damage. As we have seen, one of the aspects of the environmental dependency syndrome is the deficit in inhibiting immediate responses. When patients with a prefrontal lesion are compared to patients with a posterior lesion or to healthy controls, they exhibit a profound deficit in delayed response tasks (Verin et al., 1993). If immediate and delayed responses can be dissociated in these patients, then different functional organization may be responsible for the two types of response.

Differences between immediate and delayed responses have been reported for both eye and hand movements. There is a general decrease in performance when the delay introduced between stimulus and response increases, chiefly manifested as an increase in response variability. The interesting aspect of these results is that the time course of the change does not

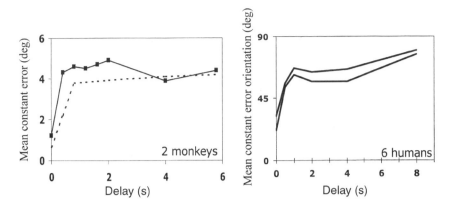

Figure 3.2
(*A*) Effect of delay on distribution of errors. Constant errors are plotted as a function
of the delays; plotted points are the errors averaged across all target locations. When
delay intervals between the target extinction and the go signal were increased,
similar effects on accuracy and precision were observed in two studies of ocular
(left) and manual (right) motor responses. The left panel, which depicts constant
saccadic errors in two monkeys, shows a sharp increase between 0 s and 1 s and
stabilization at longer delays (White et al., 1994). The right panel, which depicts
constant pointing errors toward visual targets in human subjects, also shows a sharp
increase between 0 s and 1 s, followed by a plateau at longer delays. (Adapted with
permission from Rossetti et al., 1994.)

follow a smooth curve. For example, it was shown that the amount of error
observed for delayed saccade in monkeys increased sharply when the delay
increased from 0 ms to 400 ms and then reached a nearly horizontal plateau
(figure 3.2A). In the same way, immediate and delayed grasping movements
performed by human subjects exhibit different kinematic patterns, irrespective of the duration of delay (2 s or 30 s) introduced between stimulus and
response (figure 3.2B, Goodale et al., 1994; see also Hu et al., 1999). In
particular, delayed movements exhibit an altered opening and closure of
the finger grip and a reduced maximal grip size as compared to normal
movements. Strikingly, pantomimed movements performed beside the object are similar to movements delayed by 2 s or 30 s.

Beyond these structural changes, it is interesting to explore the nature
of the representation subserving immediate versus delayed actions. Using
a simple experimental design, Rossetti and colleagues (see Rossetti and Pisella, 2002) had normal subjects point with various delays to visual targets
flashed on a monitor. Nine target locations were used, and organized along
an arc centered on the starting position (see Rossetti, 1998). Several accu-

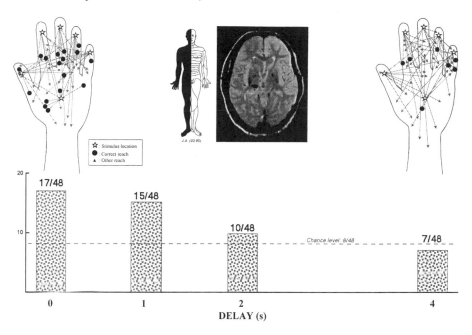

Figure 3.2 *(continued)*
(B) Effect of delayed tasks on action-numbsense. Patient J.A., with a thalamic lesion (areas VL and VPL) producing complete insensitivity of the right half of his body, was tested for tactile stimuli delivered to the hand. Four different sessions tested the effect of four delays introduced between the stimulus delivery and the go signal: 0 s, 1 s, 2 s, and 4 s. In each session, 48 stimuli were randomly delivered to six possible locations (stars). The number of correct responses (black dots) decreased abruptly from an above-chance (immediate and 1 s) to a near-chance level (2 s and 4 s). This result suggests that the residual somatosensory information used to direct J.A.'s response was available only for a brief period (about 1 s). (Reprinted with permission from Rossetti, 1998.)

racy parameters were investigated (see Rossetti and Pisella, 2002). First, the global variability, as assessed by the surface of the confidence ellipse fitting the movement endpoints, was found to increase continuously with the delay. Second, the orientation of the main axis of the confidence ellipses was found to follow a two-slope function: It tended to be aligned with movement direction in the absence of delay and then rapidly increased for 500 ms delay (see Rossetti and Pisella, 2002, figure 3.2C). With a delay of between 500 ms and 8 s, a fairly horizontal plateau was reached, with an ellipse orientation tending to be aligned with the target array, that is, orthogonal to movement direction (see Rossetti et al., 2000, figure 10). Third, the orientation of the constant error vector in space was also found to follow

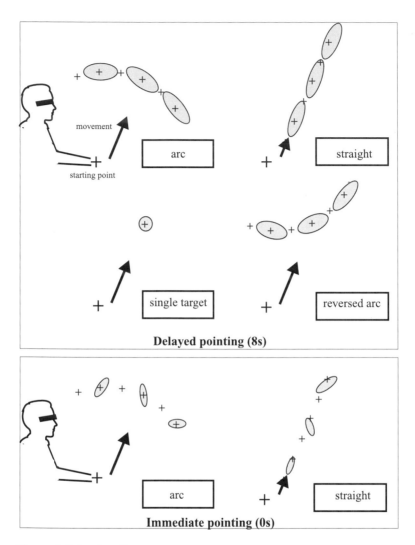

Figure 3.2 (*continued*)

(C) Effect of delay on the distribution of pointing scatters. Schematic drawing of pointing scatters observed for immediate (delay = 0 s) and delayed movements (delay = 8 s) when a unique proprioceptive target or six targets were presented on an arc array, a line array, or an inverted arc array. Whereas no specific orientation of the pointing scatter is observed when an immediate response is produced (in the case of proprioceptive targets), after the delay, the scatter main axis tends to align with the target arrays, revealing an allocentric coding of the target location: In the case of the arc array, it tends to reach 90° for delayed pointing movements. On the contrary, in the case of a line array aligned with the direction of the movement, the scatter orientation tends to be about 180°. Although the two types of responses can be considered as voluntary actions, the reactive mode and the controlled mode clearly exhibit different properties. (See also Rossetti, 1998, and Rossetti and Pisella, 2002.)

a similar two-slope trend. These results indicate that a different type of sensorimotor process is at work in the immediate and in the delayed condition. A short-lived *egocentric* representation of the target location seems to be used to guide immediate actions, whereas *allocentric* coding of the visual target seems to participate in the delayed action, which is affected by the global spatial context of the experiment extracted by a trial-to-trial integration over time. Similar results have been observed for delayed pointing to proprioceptively defined targets (Rossetti and Régnier, 1995; Rossetti et al., 1996; for review, see Rossetti and Pisella, 2002). This contextual integration confirms the hypothesis that the indirect responses produced in delayed tasks rely on complex spatial representations that are compatible with intentional rather than automatic control.

Delayed tasks have also been given to neurological patients with a lesion of the dorsal or ventral stream. The visual agnosia patient D.F. could correctly reach to and grasp objects she could not describe, but lost this preserved motor ability when her action was delayed by only 2 s (Goodale et al., 1994). Conversely, optic ataxia patient A.T., described by Milner and colleagues (1999), performed imprecise reach and grasp movements when instructed to act immediately to objects, but (paradoxically) improved when a delay was introduced between stimulus and pointing response (see also Milner and Dijkerman, 2001; Dijkerman et al., 2001; McIntosh et al., 2001). These results further support the idea that immediate and delayed actions rely on two different processes; furthermore, they suggest that these two different processes rely on the dorsal and the ventral streams. Indeed, a lesion of the dorsal stream (optic ataxia) affects the system underlying immediate actions, whereas a lesion of the ventral stream (visual agnosia) affects the system underlying delayed and pantomimed actions. "Action-blindsight" and "action-numbsense" have also been shown to be disrupted when a delay is introduced between stimulus and response (see Rossetti, 1998; Rossetti and Pisella, 2002).

Our recent series of experiments to further explore the control of action in optic ataxia (Dijkerman et al., 2001; McIntosh et al., 2001; Rossetti and Pisella, 2002) gave a striking demonstration of the link between delayed tasks and intentional control. In trials with optic ataxia patient I.G., we first confirmed that delayed pointing improves performance, which suggests that optic ataxia involves a deficit of on-line sensorimotor processing, but that a temporal delay allows a cognitive representation of the target to emerge that can be used by the intentional action system. If this interpretation is correct, it should be possible to generate conflict between intentional and reflexive action control. Visual target was presented to optic ataxia patients A.T. and I.G. for 2 s, hidden for 5 s, then presented again. These subjects were required to point toward the target as soon as it was presented for the second time. In a minority of trials, however, the target was displaced between first and second presentations. In these critical trials, A.T. and I.G. both tended to respond to the remembered location of the first presentation rather than to the actual location of the target at second presentation (figure 3.3A; a closely similar result was obtained for grasping simple objects of different sizes; Milner et al., 2001). This behavior contrasts with that of control subjects, who responded exclusively to the actual location of the target at second presentation. These results confirm that sensorimotor and cognitive representations have different time constraints (see Rossetti, 1998). Whereas sensorimotor representations can be elaborated in real time but are extremely short-lived, the cognitive representation needs more time to emerge but can be evoked off-line in the intentional organization of action. We also observed an interesting difference between the two patients. When I.G. became aware that the target was sometimes displaced during the delay period, she began to produce correction-like modifications of her ongoing movements toward stationary targets, which would drive her hand away from them (figure 3.3B). At the end of the testing, she explained that sometimes she was not sure whether the target had been displaced, and therefore modified her trajectory when she thought so. Her hand movements were (slowly) corrected according to her belief, irrespective of the actual target location and of a change in target location. By contrast, A.T. was never aware of our covert target displacements and did not produce this intentional correction-like behavior. Presumably, in the absence of the dorsal stream responsible for automatically controlling the action, the prefrontal cortex can elaborate predictions about external events and generate appropriate responses. Because of associated problems in peripheral vision such as simultanagnosia, these predictions appear to be defective.

All these results converge to support the conclusion that when action is delayed and the object has disappeared, the parameters of object position and characteristics used by the action system can only be accessed from a sustained cognitive representation compatible with perceptual awareness and intention. This type of representation and the immediate action system obviously rely on different frames of reference. Furthermore, the neuropsy-

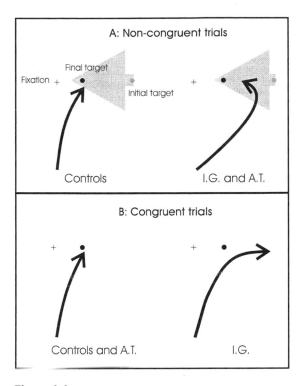

Figure 3.3
Conflict between intention and automatism. Patients A.T. and I.G. having a bilateral posterior parietal cortex lesion were presented with a visual target for 2 s, which was hidden for 5 s, then shown again; they were required to respond as soon as it was uncovered. In a minority of trials, however, the target was displaced between first and second presentations. (*A*) In these critical, noncongruent trials, A.T. and I.G. both tended to respond to the remembered location of the first target rather than to the physically present "second" target. (*B*) Interestingly, in the congruent trials, the two patients exhibited different behaviors: A.T. did not become aware that the target could change location during the delay and behaved just like a normal subject; I.G. became aware of the change and consequently performed some anti-corrective corrections, as if the object had jumped during the delay. This striking effect shows that I.G.'s belief that the object had changed location could not be checked by on-line input about the real position of the target and therefore contaminated the action by generating intentional changes of goal. (Adapted with permission from McIntosh et al., 2001.)

chological data suggest that the dorsal stream is able to build a short-lived sensorimotor representation of the target that is only available for immediate, reactive actions rather than for intentionally controlled actions.

3.5   Mirror Tasks

Tasks requiring the motor response to be produced in a direction opposite to the stimulus have been investigated with two main types of effectors: the eye and the hand. In such indirect "mirror tasks," subjects are typically asked, in effect, to inhibit "utilization behavior" in their response to the stimulus, thus generating a more sophisticated stimulus-response translation.

Antisaccade

Every day, we perform thousands of reflexive eye movements to visual stimuli appearing or moving within our peripheral visual field. In a much more pronounced way than for hand movements, a vast majority of our eye movements cannot be considered voluntary. To investigate the voluntary control of eye movements, a novel task was therefore introduced: the antisaccade task (Hallet, 1978), in which the subject is asked to perform a saccade to a virtual point that matches the mirror location of the stimulus with respect to the fixation point (for review, see Everling and Fisher, 1998). The antisaccade task requires subjects to inhibit their "reflexive" prosaccade to a flashed visual stimulus and to generate the opposite movement, namely, an antisaccade. Earlier latency studies (e.g., Fisher and Weber, 1992) suggested that the coordinates that specify the location of the visual stimulus are simply mirror reflected rather than rotated through 180°. Thus a deficit in voluntary control would be manifested as a significant number of prosaccades performed in the place of antisaccades. The main difference between immediate prosaccades and antisaccades is that antisaccades have longer latencies, which suggests that this task generates a conflict between the two responses, one that appears to be more pronounced for targets presented in the peripheral than in the central visual field (Logan and Irwin, 2000), which in turn suggests that peripheral eye movements are more reflexive than central movements. The pattern of errors observed for visually guided antisaccades, unlike the pattern for prosaccades, resembles that of the memory-guided antisaccades (Krappmann, 1998). Thus the nature of the difference between pro- and antisaccades should resemble that of the difference between immediate and delayed saccades.

Antisaccade tasks have been used with many groups of patients (for review, see Everling and Fisher, 1998). Direct evidence for a frontal lobe involvement in antisaccade generation was obtained from several studies showing that patients with unilateral lesion of the frontal lobe had greater difficulty producing antisaccades, although focal lesion of the frontal eye field (FEF) or the supplementary eye field (SEF) do not increase the error rate in this task. As for the stop signal paradigm, it is rather odd that more studies investigated antisaccades in psychiatric disorders than in neurological disorders. The common assumption in these studies remains that the frontal cortex, basal ganglia, or both participate in antisaccades.

To address the issue of dorsal versus ventral stream within this framework, Dijkerman and colleagues (1997) investigated antisaccades in the visual agnosia patient D.F. They demonstrated that her bilateral occipitotemporal lesion did not impair her ability to perform immediate prosaccades, as had been the case for pointing (Goodale et al., 1994). But their most interesting finding was that D.F.'s ability to perform antisaccades was severely impaired, which suggests that the human ventral stream is necessary to the voluntary control of eye movements, whereas the dorsal stream would only allow direct prosaccades. The anatomical correlates of human "antimovements" will be further addressed in the next section.

Antipointing

Day and Lyon (2000) used a pointing task in which the target could be displaced during the hand movement. Subjects were asked to produce either a corrective movement toward the new target location (direct pointing) or to redirect their hand movement in a direction opposite to the actual target jump (antipointing). As in Pisella et al., 2000, fast movements were shown to be under the control of automatic processes, which could participate in the direct pointing performance, but not in the antipointing task derived from the antisaccade paradigm, which they even counteracted. The incompatibility between automatic processes and antimovement tasks is also apparent when the orientation of attention is investigated. The automatic anticipatory orientation of attention that is observed during a saccade preparation around the final position of the saccade being prepared is not observed in the case of antisaccades (see Schneider and Deubel, 2002).

A recent fMRI investigation (Connolly et al., 2000) found that the neural network participating in direct pointing in humans was activated during antipointing as well, although areas that were prefrontal eye field and presupplementary motor area (lying anterior to areas activated during both direct pointing and antipointing) were selectively activated during antipointing, which confirms that more anterior frontal areas are implicated in the inhibition of automatic responses. Interestingly, a few areas were activated only during direct pointing and direct saccades, and not during antisaccades and antipointing. All three of these areas are located along the medial wall of the frontoparietal cortex, that is, in the most dorsal position within the visuomotor network, a result consistent with the view that the dorsal end of the visuomotor network is mainly involved in the automatic on-line control that we called the parietal automatic pilot (Pisella et al., 2000; Rossetti and Pisella, 2002).

3.6   Other Indirect Tasks

Matching and Pantomimed Tasks

If one considers the motor abilities left intact in optic ataxia patients to be intentionally controlled, then matching tasks are good candidates for exploring intention. As mentioned earlier, patients with optic ataxia exhibit difficulties in reaching to or adjusting their finger grip to an object. In contrast, they seem to remain able to indicate the size of a stimulus with their finger grip while the hand remained away from the stimulus (see Jeannerod et al., 1994). As pointed out by several authors (e.g., Milner and Dijkerman, 2001), the boundary between matching tasks and pantomime tasks can be rather fuzzy. In Goodale et al., 1994, the kinematic structure of pantomimed movements was found to be similar to that of movements delayed by 2 s or 30 s, underscoring the necessity for motor representations to have on-line access to target parameters. The effect of subtle changes in the type of motor output requested from subjects can also strongly affect the type of processing involved. A rather clear example has been provided by Bridgeman (2002), who compared communicative pointing to instrumental pointing. Subjects were asked either to point at an object or to act on it by pushing it down. The latter response provided a stronger difference from the perceptual tasks used in the same experiment, suggesting that the former response could be considered an imitation of the actual action.

Sequential Tasks

Also included among simple tasks where intention can be obviously, though indirectly, expressed are sequential tasks. It has long been known that performing a movement to grasp an object can be strongly influenced by the planned use of this object. Thus we do not grasp a pen in the same way when we intend to write as when we intend to pass it to someone else. Experiments have shown that the reach-to-grasp movements performed toward an object to be placed on a platform exhibit different duration and different kinematic patterns depending on whether the platform is tiny or large (Marteniuk et al., 1987). In the same way, the first stroke of sequential pointing to a first (standard) target and a second target varying in size is affected by the ultimate goal of the whole action, that is, by the target of the second stroke. This pattern of results is quite robust and seems to be observed even in schizophrenic patients (Saoud et al., 2000).

The sequential task paradigm can inform us of pathological alterations of intention. For many years, it was thought that hemispatial neglect might consist at least partly of a deficit in intention directed to the left side of space. Several experiments using various types of manipulandum have nicely shown that the direction of the final effector (e.g., a cursor) is less relevant than the direction of the real arm action performed by the patient (for review, see Heilman, forthcoming), although whether the direction of the movement being *programmed* or the movement *intended* is the crucial parameter is difficult to determine under experimental conditions. When neglect patients are asked to first reach to and grasp a ball placed in front of them and then to throw it to the left or right, the initial reach-to-grasp movement is modulated by the final direction of the whole action. Reaching movements before a throwing movement to the left are slower than those before a throwing movement to the right (figure 3.4). This pattern of results is fully consistent with the hypothesis that there is an intentional component in the deficit exhibited by neglect patients. Interestingly, this pattern can be reversed by a short session of adaptation to right-deviating wedge prisms, which demonstrates that confounding factors such as biomechanical constraints are not responsible for the difference found before neglect was improved by the adaptation (as shown on various neglect tests: Rossetti et al., 1998, 1999; Rode et al., 1999, 2001; Pisella et al., 2002; Farnè et al., 2002). The chief advantage of sequential tasks is that they allow researchers to observe intention in an altogether indirect way, at a stage of the action that is remote from its actual final goal, though strictly dependent on this goal. Their chief disadvantage, however, is that, relying on low-level kinematic parameters to indicate intentional

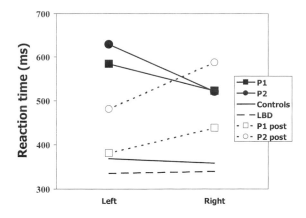

Figure 3.4
Indirect task demonstrating an intentional modulation of action in hemispatial neglect. We investigated whether the left hypokinesia found in hemispatial neglect
would be observed in a grasping action when the subsequent movement was directed to the left. Subjects had to reach and grasp a tennis ball placed on their
sagittal axis and then throw it into a left or a right basket; neglect patients were
slower to initiate their movements ending to the left as compared to right (solid
symbols). No comparable effect was found in the control group. This result suggests
that the preparation of a movement sequence ending to the left is subjected to
unilateral neglect. Anticipation of the ultimate goal of an action may lead to a
retrograde transfer of the neglect bias onto action elements which have no left-
right component by themselves. Unexpectedly, this trend was reversed after a short
wedge-prism adaptation session (open symbols). (Adapted from Rode et al., 2000.)

modulation, sequential tasks can explore only a limited range of action
qualities.

Distractor Avoidance Tasks

Sequential and distractor avoidance tasks may be considered mirror images:
In the first, stimulus must be reached, whereas, in the second, it must be
avoided, before the ultimate goal of the action can be achieved. The main
difference between the two types of tasks would be that, in distractor avoidance tasks, this stimulus has to resemble the action goal (Humphreys and
Riddoch, 2000), whereas, in sequential tasks, it does not. The distinction
between positive and negative effects of distractors (see Tipper, 2001)
would provide an efficient way to discriminate between environment dependency and its intentional inhibition.

Still another good way to ensure that a movement is controlled by
intention is to require subjects to *imagine* preparing and performing an ac-

tion (see Frith et al., 2000). Imagined movements seem to share several properties with actual movements (see Jeannerod 2001; Danckert and Goodale, chapter 2; Jeannerod, chapter 5; and Sirigu et al., chapter 6, all this volume), and the inhibition of overt action is a good marker that subjects are intentionally performing the task. Although we have long known that the duration of a mental action is proportional to that of the real one, it is obviously difficult to control for the correctness of the execution of such an action, which may explain why relatively few patient categories have been investigated using such tasks. In particular, it would be interesting to investigate how patients with prefrontal lobe lesion would perform imaginary actions without producing covert movements (see Jeannerod, 2001).

The above list of indirect tasks to explore the intentional control of action is by no means exhaustive. At this stage, however, too few neuropsychological studies have made use of even these tasks to accurately assess their efficiency and practical relevance.

3.7   Intention Is Slower than Reaction

Several authors have proposed that conscious awareness is slower than reactions to many sensory stimuli (for review, see Rossetti, 1998). If intention is dependent on consciousness, then at least the same temporal dissociation should apply to intention and these reactions. Some of the experiments reviewed above suggest that some sensorimotor reactions can be produced even before the intention to react to the stimulus has time to take charge of the response. This is particularly clear when intention and the sensorimotor reaction to a target are in conflict for the control of an ongoing movement (as in Pisella et al., 2000).

As we noted above for pointing, when I.G. was asked to delay her grasping action, she improved her poor ability to perform accurate actions (for review, see Milner and Dijkerman, 2001). Knowing that the effect of a memory delay is different from that of a long presentation of a stimulus in normals (see Rossetti and Pisella, 2002), we investigated this possibility with I.G. She exhibited a better performance in both tasks, suggesting that the long presentation and the delay enabled her to form a representation of the object that could be used by the action system. Given her bilateral lesion of the posterior parietal cortex, this representation was postulated to be formed via the ventral stream (see also Milner et al., 1999). An interesting question arises whether it is possible to generate a conflict between this sustained cognitive representation necessary for intention and the more automatic short-lived representations. Together with David Milner and Chris Dijkerman, we designed an experiment in which an object was presented for 2 s, then hidden behind a panel for 8 s, then presented again. Under these conditions, I.G. improved her grip scaling with respect to an immediate action condition. When, however, the object was unexpectedly replaced by a larger or smaller one, she initially scaled her grip to her internal representation rather than to the actual object she was reaching to (see Rossetti and Pisella, 2002: figure 19). Control subjects tested under the same conditions exhibited an on-line grip formation that was adapted to the object actually in front of them at the time of the grasp (see also Milner and Dijkerman, 2001). In addition to the effect found on grip size, the time to maximal grip aperture was reached earlier in the "large→small" condition with respect to the large condition for each of the six control subjects, whereas I.G. exhibited a similar value in the two conditions. In the particular trials where she "correctly" opened her hand widely on "small→large" catch trials, the wide grip aperture actually occurred abnormally late in the movement. This result strongly suggests that I.G. could not process the change in size that had occurred during the delay fast enough to early update her ongoing movement.

These results clearly confirm that sensorimotor and cognitive representation have different time constraints. They also suggest that responses produced by normal subjects in serial experimental conditions can be triggered even before the intention to control the action has been formed.

3.8   Intention: Parietal-Frontal versus Dorsal-Ventral

As predicted by Lhermitte et al. (1986), the environmental dependency syndrome described in patients with a frontal lesion appears to result from the release of parietal lobe activities. The main brain areas where a lesion may induce a dysinhibition syndrome lie in the orbitofrontal and basotemporal cortex, predominantly in the right hemisphere (for review, see Starkstein and Robinson, 1997), as was already indicated in the case of epileptic seizures by Penfield (1975). After reviewing studies on patients with closed head injuries, brain tumors, stroke lesions, and focal epilepsy, Starkstein and Robinson (1997, p. 112) concluded: "Based on the phylogenetic origin of these cortical areas and their main connections with dorsal regions related to visuospatial functions, somatosensation, and spatial memory, the orbitofrontal and basotemporal cortices may selectively inhibit or release motor, instinctive, affective, and intellectual behaviors elaborated in the dorsal cortex." Although some (e.g., Rolls, 1999) have claimed that the automatisms released following a frontal lesion may be linked to a basal ganglia activity, others (e.g., Pisella et al., 2000; Rossetti and Pisella, 2002) propose that the posterior parietal cortex is a key structure for the automatic control of action.

The findings that automatic corrections in response to a change in target location are disrupted in optic ataxia whereas these corrections are fully released following a lesion of the frontal cortex suggest the existence of a double dissociation between parietal and frontal patients for the control of very simple visual pointing (Pisella et al., 2000). Frith and colleagues (2000) also describe optic ataxia and anarchic hand syndrome as involving mirror deficits. Whereas optic ataxia patients cannot form representations of objects needed to make the appropriate movements to reach to and grasp them, anarchic hand patients cannot prevent the sight of the objects from eliciting those movements.

That the posterior parietal cortex is involved in the release of automatic behavior is consistent with the most recent versions of the dorsal-ventral distinction (e.g., Rossetti et al., 2000; Pisella et al., 2000). Indeed, we have proposed that a specific activation of the dorsal stream, at least of the superior parietal cortex, would occur only in the case of automatic on-line control of an ongoing action, whereas tasks such as movement initiation would involve the inferior parietal cortex, and more indirect tasks (e.g., identification) would depend on the ventral stream (for review, see Rossetti and Pisella, 2002). (It should be remembered here that complex behavior can be initiated by frontal patients or during epileptic seizures and sleep, but by contrast to normal conditions, this initiation is strongly linked to an alteration of consciousness that is obvious at least during seizures and sleep related motor disorders [see Revonsuo et al., 2000].) In the postulated gradient of activity ranging from on-line action control to action initiation to action planning to cognitive tasks, the precise distribution of frontal projections of the various pathways remains unclear. Nevertheless, analysis of the visuomotor networks involved in action control (see Burnod, 1999; Rossetti et al., 2000; Pisella and Rossetti, 2000; Marconi et al., 2001; Rossetti and Pisella, 2002) shows that several frontal areas may be involved separately. In particular, because projections from the ventral stream extend into the more anterior frontal areas, the indirect tasks left intact in optic ataxia may share some neurological substrate with the frontal areas involved in intentional aspects of behavior. On the other hand, the frontal projections from the posterior parietal cortex involved in the hand automatic pilot seem to be directly connected to the premotor areas, which may not primarily participate in intentional action.

Thus the dissociation proposed between dorsal and ventral streams may not be the most relevant distinction to the issue of intention. Rather, the processes governing automatic and intentional behavior appear to be associated with posterior parietal and prefrontal areas respectively.

3.9   Conclusion

Intention lies at the intersection of several approaches. To experimentally explore intention, we need to arrive at a pragmatic definition and operating criteria. This task becomes very difficult when global functions are concerned, as is the case with neuropsychology or clinical neurology. Although there is no unified framework in which we might describe a specific "pathology of intention," and, in particular, no positive symptomatology of intention disorders, neuroscientists seem less reluctant to refer to "intention" than to "consciousness," perhaps because intention is attached to behavior—to overt phenomena—whereas consciousness remains largely a covert phenomenon. Thus it seems easier to distinguish between automatic and intentional than between conscious and nonconscious processes. Nevertheless, there is a strong link between intention and consciousness. Even though consciousness does not imply intention, intention implies consciousness (cf. Revonsuo and Rossetti, 2000). Indeed, it is only when a subject has conscious knowledge of the elements of a given situation that an intentional project can emerge. This functional property is consistent with the thesis that lesion of both orbitofrontal and basotemporal areas may result in dysinhibited behavior (Starkstein and Robinson, 1997).

Intentional behavior can be characterized by two main features: (1) the ability to inhibit immediate reactions to external stimuli; and (2) the ability to plan a goal-oriented organized sequence of actions. Indirect tasks, because they better express the freedom of the individual to respond or not to respond to a given stimulus, seem to be more relevant to the issue of intention than most classical motor psychophysics tasks, all of which allow investigators to specifically activate the temporoprefrontal network rather than the dorsal stream (cf. Rossetti and Pisella, 2002).

One should carefully consider the theoretical distinction between intention and automatism. Although they are less direct responses to stimuli than immediate responses, delayed tasks may be well conditioned, as can be seen in animal experiments. And although no-go tasks may appear to be typical intentional tasks, in the case of overtraining, the boundary between intentional and automatic responses becomes fuzzier. Indeed, intense training may transform an intentional response of an automatic conditioned reaction into a stimulus. This aspect of the relationship between intentional and automatic control of behavior is worth keeping in mind before making firm conclusions about the neurobiology of intention.

Because particular aspects of sensory processing for the purpose of action, and especially for movement guidance, remain fully independent of conscious perception (Pélisson et al., 1986), action can be directed to unconsciously perceived stimuli, even though conscious awareness allows for a perceptual control of action (Pisella et al., 2000). Specifically, conscious visual perception and intention select the goal for the action, but the triggering and the realization of the action may escape their control.

We have proposed elsewhere (Rossetti et al., 2000; Pisella and Rossetti, 2000; Rossetti and Pisella, 2002) that the temporal dimension is a key to understanding complex interconnected networks such as the visual brain. Because the relationship between perception and action and that between conscious awareness and intention are linked, we submit that temporal factors may be relevant to the latter as well. As proposed by Milner and Dijkerman (2001), the primary role of consciousness may be to delay action in order to gain behavioral efficiency, just as an animal's ability to slow, delay, or inhibit immediate actions may also help it achieve a more useful (hidden external or internal) goal (Rossetti and Pisella, 2002). The prospective memory paradigm may offer an optimal tool to explore the ability to plan—and hold an intention toward—future behavior. In this regard, it is interesting that patients with frontal lobe lesion may exhibit a deficit in prospective memory without a corresponding deficit in retrospective memory (Cockburn, 1995).

References

Boussaoud, D. (2001). Attention vs. intention in the primate premotor cortex. *Neuro-Image* 14: S40–S45.

Bridgeman, B. (2002). The Roelofs effect. In *Attention and Performance XIX: Common Mehanisms in Perception and Action*, W. Prinz and B. Hommel (eds.). OXFORD: Oxford University Press, pp. 120–135.

Burnod, Y., Baraduc, P., Battaglia-Mayer, A., Guigon, E., Koechlin, E., Ferraina, S., Lacquaniti, F., and Caminiti, R. (1999). Parieto-frontal coding of reaching: An integrated framework. *Exp. Brain Res.* 129: 325–346.

Cabel, D. W., Armstrong I. T., Reingold E., and Munoz D. P. (2000). Control of saccade initiation in a countermanding task using visual and auditory stop signals. *Exp. Brain Res.* 133: 431–441.

Cockburn J. (1995). Task interruption in prospective memory: A frontal lobe function? *Cortex* 31: 87–97.

Collette, F., Van der Linden, M., Delfiore, G., Degueldre, C., Luxen, A., and Salmon, E. (2001). The functional anatomy of inhibition processes investigated with the Hayling task. *NeuroImage* 14: 258–267.

Connolly, J. D., Goodale, M. A., DeSouza, J. F. X., Menon, R., and Vilis, T. (2000). A comparison of frontoparietal fMRI activation during anti-saccades and anti-pointing. *J. Neurophysiol.* 84: 1645–1655.

Day, B. L., and Lyon, I. N. (2000). Voluntary modification of automatic arm movements evoked by motion of a visual target. *Exp. Brain Res.* 130: 159–168.

De Jong, R., Coles, M. G., and Logan, G. D. (1995). Strategies and mechanisms in nonselective and selective inhibitory motor control. *J. Exp. Psychol. Hum. Percept. Perform.* 21: 498–511.

Della Sala, S., Marchetti, C., and Spinnler, H. (1994). The anarchic hand: A fronto-mesial sign. In *Handbook of Neuropsychology*, F. Boller and J. Grafman (eds.). Amsterdam: Elsevier, pp. 233–255.

Desmurget, M., Prablanc, C., Rossetti, Y., Arzi, M., Paulignan, Y., Urquizar, C., and Mignot, J. C. (1995). Postural and synergic control for three-dimensional movements of grasping. *J. Neurophysiol.* 74: 905–910.

Desmurget, M., Prablanc, C., Arzi, M., Rossetti, Y., Paulignan, Y., and Urquizar, C. (1996). Integrated control of hand transport and orientation during prehension movements. *Exp. Brain Res.* 110: 265–278.

Dijkerman, H. C., Milner, A. D., and Carey, D. P. (1997). Impaired delayed and anti-saccades in a visual form agnosic. *Exp. Brain Res. Supp.* 117: S66.

Dijkerman, H. C., Rossetti, Y., Pisella, L., McIntosh, R. D., Tilikete, C., Vighetto, A., and Milner A. D. (2001). A conflict between present and represented object size in optic ataxia. Poster presented at the international symposium, Neural Control of Space Coding and Action Production, Lyon. March 24–26.

Everling, S., and Fisher, B. (1998). The antisaccade: A review of basic research and clinical studies. *Neuropsychologia* 36: 885–899.

Farnè, A., Rossetti, Y., Toniolo, S., and Làdavas, E. (2002). Ameliorating neglect with prism adaptation: Visuo-manual vs. visuo-verbal measures. *Neuropsychologia* 40: 718–729.

Fisher, B., and Weber, H. (1992). Characteristics of "anti" saccades in man. *Exp. Brain Res.* 89: 415–424.

Frith, C., Blakemore, S.-J., and Wolpert, D. M. (2000). Abnormalities in the awareness and control of action. *Philos. Trans. R. Soc. Lond. B Biol. Sci.* 355: 1771–1788.

Goodale, M. A., Pélisson, D., and Prablanc, C. (1986). Large adjustments in visually guided reaching do not depend on vision of the hand or perception of target displacement. *Nature* 320: 748–750.

Goodale, M. A., Jakobson, L. S., and Keillor, J. M. (1994). Differences in the visual control of pantomimed and natural grasping movements. *Neuropsychologia* 32: 1159–1178.

Gréa, H., Desmurget, M., and Prablanc, M. (2000). Postural invariance in three-dimensional reaching and grasping movements. *Exp. Brain Res.* 134: 155–162.

Gréa, H., Pisella, L., Desmurget, M., Tilikete, C., Vighetto, A., Grafton, S., Prablanc, C., and Rossetti, Y. (Forthcoming). The posterior parietal cortex mediates on-line adjustments during aiming movements. *Neuropsychologia*.

Hallet, P. (1978). Primary and secondary saccades to goals defined by instructions. *Vision Res.* 18: 1279–1296.

Hanes, D. P., Patterson II, W. F., and Schall, J. D. (1998). Role of frontal eye fields in countermanding saccades: Visual, movement, and fixation activity. *J. Neurophysiol.* 79: 817–834.

Hanes, D. P., and Schall, J. D. (1995). Countermanding saccades in macaque. *Vis. Neurosci.* 12: 929–937.

Heckhausen, H., and Beckmann, J. (1990). Intentional action and action slips. *Psychol. Rev.* 97: 36–48.

Heilman, K. (Forthcoming). Intentional neglect. In *The Cognitive and Neural Bases of Spatial Neglect*, H. O. Karnath, A. D. Milner, and G. Vallar (eds.). Oxford: Oxford University Press.

Hu, Y., Eagleson, R., and Goodale, M. A. (1999). The effects of delay on the kinematics of grasping. *Exp. Brain Res.* 126: 109–116.

Humphreys, G. W., and Riddoch, J. (2000). One more cup of coffee for the road: Object-action assemblies, response blocking and response capture after frontal damage. *Exp. Brain Res.* 133: 8193.

Jeannerod, M. (2001). Neural simulation of action: A unifying mechanism for motor cognition. *NeuroImage* 14: S103–S109.

Jeannerod, M., Decety, J., and Michel, F. (1994). Impairment of grasping movements following a bilateral posterior parietal lesion. *Neuropsychologia* 32: 369–380.

Krappmann, P. (1998). Accuracy of visually directed and memory-guided antisaccades in man. *Vision Res.* 38: 2979–2985.

Kudo, K., and Ohtsuki, T. (1998). Functional modification of agonist-antagonist electromyographic activity for rapid movement inhibition. *Exp. Brain Res.* 122: 23–30.

Lahav, R. (1993). What neuropsychology tells us about consciousness. *Philos. Sci.* 60: 67–85.

Lhermitte, F. "Utilization behavior" and its relation to lesions of the frontal lobes. *Brain* 106: 237–255.

Lhermitte, F., Pillon, B., and Serdaru, M. (1986). Human autonomy and the frontal lobes: 1. Imitation and utilization behavior: A neuropsychological study of 75 patients. *Ann. Neurol.* 19: 326–334.

Lhermitte, F. Human autonomy and the frontal lobes: 2. Patient behavior in complex and social situations: The "environmental dependency syndrome." *Ann. Neurol.* 19: 335–343.

Libet, B. (1993). The neural time factor in conscious and unconscious events. In *Experimental and Theoretical Studies of Consciousness*. Chichester, England: pp. 123–146.

Logan, G. D. (1981). Attention. automaticity, and the ability to stop a speeded choice response. In *Attention and Performance IX*, J. Long and A. D. Baddeley (eds.). Hillsdale, N.J.: Erlbaum, pp. 205–222.

Logan, G. D., and Irwin, D. E. (2000). Don't look! Don't touch! Inhibitory control of eye and hand movements. *Psychonom. Bull. Rev.* 7: 107–112.

Marchetti, C., and Della Sala, S. (1998). Disentangling the alien and anarchic hand. *Cogn. Neuropsychiat.* 3: 191–208.

Marconi, B., Genovesio, A., Battaglia-Mayer, A., Ferraina, S., Squatrito, S., Molinari, M., and Caminiti, R. (2001). Eye-hand coordination during reaching: 1. Anatomical relationships between parietal and frontal cortex. *Cereb. Cortex* 11: 513–527.

Marteniuk, R. G., MacKenzie, C. L., Jeannerod, M., Athenes, S., and Dugas, C. (1987). Constraints on human arm movement trajectories. *Can. J. Psychol.* 41: 365–378.

McIntosh, R. M., Pisella, L., Danckert, J., Tilikete, C., Dijkerman, C., Vighetto, A., Michel, F., Milner, A. D., and Rossetti, Y. (2001). A conflict between present and represented object position in optic ataxia. Poster presented at International symposium, Neural Control of Space Coding and Action Production, Lyon. March 22–24.

Menon, V., Adleman, N. E., White, C. D., Glover, G. H., and Reiss, A. L. (2001). Error-related brain activation during a go/no-go response inhibition task. *Hum. Brain Mapp.* 12: 131–143.

Milner, A. D., and Dijkerman, C. (2001). Direct and indirect visual routes to action. In *Varieties of Unconscious Processing: New Findings and New Comparisons*, B. de Gelder, E. H. F. de Haan, and C. A. Heywood (eds.). Oxford: Oxford University Press. pp 241–264.

Milner, A. D., Paulignan, Y., Dijkerman, H. C., Michel, F., and Jeannerod, M. (1999). A paradoxical improvement of misreaching in optic ataxia: New evidence for two separate neural systems for visual localization. *Proc. R. Soc. Lond. B Biol. Sci.* 266: 2225–2229.

Milner, D., Dijkerman, C., Pisella, L., Tilikete, C., McIntosh, R., Vighetto, A., and Rossetti, Y. (2001). Grasping the past: Delay can improve visuomotor performance. *Curr. Biol.* 11: 1896–1901.

Mulvihill, L. E., Skilling, T. A., and Vogel-Sprott, M. (1997). Alcohol and the ability to inhibit behavior in men and women. *J. Stud. Alcohol* 58: 600–605.

Pélisson, D., Prablanc, C., Goodale, M. A., and Jeannerod, M. (1986). Visual control of reaching movements without vision of the limb: 2. Evidence of fast unconscious process correcting the trajectory of the hand to the final position of a double-step stimulus. *Exp. Brain Res.* 62: 303–311.

Penfield, W. (1975). *The Mystery of the Mind.* Princeton, N.J.: Princeton University Press.

Pisella, L., and Rossetti, Y. (2000). Interaction between conscious identification and non-conscious sensorimotor processing: temporal constraints. In *Beyond Dissociation: Interaction between Dissociated Implicit and Explicit Processing,* Y. Rossetti and A. Revonsuo (eds.). Amsterdam: Benjamins, pp. 129–151.

Pisella, L., Rossetti, Y., and Arzi, M. (1998). The timing of color and location processing in the motor context. *Exp. Brain Res.* 121: 270–276.

Pisella, L., Tilikete, C., Rode, G., Boisson, D., Vighetto, A., and Rossetti, Y. (1999). Automatic corrections prevail in spite of an instructed stopping response. In *Studies in Perception and Action V.* M. A. Grealy and J. A. Thomson (eds.). Mahwah, N.J.: Erlbaum, pp. 275–279.

Pisella, L., Gréa, H., Tiliket, C., Vighetto, A., Desmurget, M., Rode, G., Boisson, D., and Rossetti, Y. (2000). An automatic pilot for the hand in the human posterior parietal cortex: Toward a reinterpretation of optic ataxia. *Nat. Neurosci.* 3: 729–736.

Pisella, L., Rode, G., Farnè, A., Boisson, D., and Rosetti, Y. (2002). Dissociated long-lasting improvements of straight-ahead pointing and line bisection tasks in two hemineglect patients. *Neuropsychologia.* 40: 327–334.

Place, U. T. (2000). The zombie-within. In Beyond Dissociation: Interaction between Dissociated Implicit and Explicit Processing, Y. Rossetti and A. Revonsuo (eds.). Amsterdam: Benjamins.

Prablanc, C., Echallier, J. E., Jeannerod, M., and Komilis, E. (1979). Optimal responses of eye and hand motor systems in pointing at visual target: 2. Static and dynamic visual cues in the control of hand movement. *Biol. Cybern.* 35: 183–187.

Prablanc, C., and Martin, O. (1992). Automatic control during hand reaching at undetected two-dimensional target displacements. *J. Neurophysiol.* 67: 455–469.

Revonsuo, A., and Rosetti, Y. (2000). Dissociation and interaction: Windows to the hidden mechanisms of consciousness. In *Beyond Dissociation: Interaction between Dissociated Implicit and Explicit Processing,* Y. Rossetti and A. Revonsuo (eds.). Amsterdam: Benjamins, pp. 351–366.

Revonsuo, A., Johanson, M., Wedlund, J.-E., and Chaplin, J. (2000). The zombies among us: Consciousness and automatic behaviour. In *Beyond Dissociation: Interaction between Dissociated Implicit and Explicit Processing,* Y. Rossetti and A. Revonsuo (eds.). Amsterdam: Benjamins, pp. 331–351.

Riddoch, J., Humphreys, G. W., and Edwards, M. G. (2000). Visual affordance and object selection. In *Attention and Performance XVIII: Control of Cognitive Processes,* S. Monsell and J. Driver (eds.). Cambridge, Mass.: MIT Press, pp. 603–625.

Rode, G., Rossetti, Y., Li, L., and Boisson, D. (1999). The effect of prism adaptation on neglect for visual imagery. *Behav. Neurol.* 11: 251–258.

Rode, G., Rossetti, Y., Farnè, A., Boisson, D., and Bisiach, E. (2000). The motor control of a movement sequence ending to the left is altered in unilateral neglect. Poster presented at the Euroconference, Cognitive and Neural Bases of Spatial Neglect, Como. September.

Rode, G., Rossetti Y., and Boisson, D. (2001). Prism adaptation improves representational neglect. *Neuropsychologia* 39: 1250–1254.

Rolls, E. T. (1999). A theory of consciousness and its application to understanding emotion and pleasure. In *The Brain and Emotion,* Oxford: Oxford University Press, pp. 244–265.

Rossetti, Y. (1998). Implicit short-lived motor representation of space in brain-damaged and healthy subjects. *Conscious. Cognit.* 7: 520–558.

Rossetti, Y., and Pisella, L. (2002). Several "vision for action" systems: A guide to dissociating and integrating dorsal and ventral functions. In *Attention and Performance XIX: Common Mechanisms in Perception and Action,* W. Prinz and B. Hommel (eds.). Oxford: Oxford University Press. pp. 62–119

Rossetti, Y., and Régnier, C. (1995). Representations in action: pointing to a target with various representations. In *Studies in Perception and Action III,* B. G. Bardy, R. J. Bootsma, and Y. Guiard (eds.). Mahwah, N.J.: Erlbaum, pp. 233–236.

Rossetti, Y., Lacquaniti, F., Carrozzo, M., and Borghese, A. (1994). Errors of pointing toward memorized visual targets indicate a change in reference frame with memory delay.

Rossetti, Y., Gaunet, F., and Thinus-Blanc, C. (1996). Early visual experience affects memorization and spatial representation of proprioceptive targets. *NeuroReport* 7: 1219–1223.

Rossetti, Y., Rode, G., Pisella, L., Farnè, A., Ling, L., Boisson, D., and Perenin, M. T. (1998). Prism adaptation to a rightward optical deviation rehabilitates left hemispatial neglect. *Nature* 395: 166–169.

Rossetti, Y., Rode, G., Pisella, L., Farnè, A., Ling, L., and Boisson, D. (1999). Sensorimotor plasticity and cognition: Prism adaptation can affect various levels of space representation. In *Studies in Perception and Action,* M. Grealy and J. A. Thomson (eds.). Mahwah, N.J.: Erlbaum, pp. 265–269.

Rossetti, Y., Pisella, L., and Pélisson, D. (2000). Eye blindness and hand sight: temporal aspects of visuo-motor processing. *Vis. Cognit.* 7: 785–808.

Rubia, K., Russell, T., Overmeyer, S., Brammer, M. J., Bullmore, E. T., Sharma, T. Simmons, A., Williams, S. C., Giampietro, V., Andrew, C. M., and Taylor, E. (2001). Mapping motor inhibition: Conjunctive brain activations across different versions of go/no-go and stop tasks. *NeuroImage* 13: 250–261.

Saoud, M. (2000). Context processing and action in schizophrenia. Presented to first joint meeting of the Institute for Cognitive Science and the Institute of Cognitive Neuroscience, From Perception to Action Representation: Neural Bases and Disorders, Lyon. September 25–26.

Schneider, W., and Deubel, H. (2002). In *Attention and Performance XIX:* Common Mechanisms in Perception and Action. W. Prinz and B. Hommel (eds.). Oxford: Oxford University Press. pp. 609–627.

Slater-Hammel, A. T. (1960). Reliability, accuracy, and refractoriness of a transit reaction. *Res. Q.* 31: 217-228.

Snyder, L. H., Batista, A. P., and Andersen, R. A. (1997). Coding of intention in the posterior parietal cortex. *Nature* 386: 167–170.

Starkstein, S. E., and Robinson, R. G. (1997). Mechanism of disinhibition after brain lesions. *J. Nerv. Ment. Dis.* 185: 108–114.

Starobinski, J. (1999). *Action et réaction: Vie et aventures d'un couple.* Paris: Editions du Seuil.

Stuphorn, V., Taylor, T. L., and Schall, J. D. (2000). Performance monitoring by the supplementary eye field. *Nature* 408: 857–860.

Tipper, S. P. (2001). In *Attention and Performance XVIII: Control of Cognitive Processes.* S. Monsell and J. Driver (eds.). Cambridge, Mass.: MIT Press.

Toni, I., Thoenissen, D., and Zilles, K. (2001). Movement preparation and motor intention. *NeuroImage* 14: S110–S117.

Verin, M., Patriot, A., Pillon, B., Malapani, C., Agid, Y., and Dubois, B. (1993). Delayed response tasks and prefrontal lesions in man: Evidence for self-generated patterns of behaviour with poor environmental modulation. *Neuropsychologia* 31: 1379–1396.

White, J. M., Sparks, D. L., and Standford, T. R. (1994). Saccades to remembered target locations: An analysis of systematic and variable errors. *Vision Res.* 34: 79–92.

Williams, B. R., Ponesse, J. S., Shachar, R. J., Logan, G. D., and Tannock, R. (1999). Development of inhibitory control across the life span. *Dev. Psychol.* 35: 205–213.

Understanding Intentions through Imitation

Marco Iacoboni

4.1   Why Imitation?

A fundamental behavior during development, imitation facilitates the acquisition of motor skills and of cognitive abilities critical to social cognition, such as understanding the intentions and the emotions of others and mapping these intentions and emotions onto one's own intentions and emotions. By means of this mapping mechanism, the developing mind understands other people as "like me" (Meltzoff and Brooks, 2001). This chapter summarizes the first results of research into the neural basis of imitative behavior.

A large body of behavioral science literature, based mostly on developmental psychology, comparative psychology, and ethology, is focused on imitation (Bekkering et al., 2000; Byrne, 1995; Byrne and Russon, 1998; Tomasello et al., 1993; Whiten, 2000; Whiten and Brown, 1999; Whiten et al., 1999). Despite their long-standing interest in imitation, however, behavioral and brain scientists have, until recently, spent almost no time studying its neural basis. Indeed, the only available study attempting to correlate neural and imitative functions had been undertaken by behavioral neurologists and neuropsychologists on patients with apraxia following left-hemisphere lesions (Heilman and Valenstein, 1993). Although the neurological findings were often conflicting and based on theoretical frameworks that would now be considered insufficient, they converged on two main features that had been replicated over and over again. First, imitative disorders were associated with lesions located anteriorly in the inferior part of the lateral wall of the frontal lobe and posteriorly in temporoparietal areas. Second, imitative disorders were often associated with language disorders (Heilman and Valenstein, 1993). As we will see, these two features are critical to understanding the evolution of the anatomical and functional phylogenetic changes in the primate brain pertinent to imitation.

Definitions of imitation range from the very broad, as Baldwin's suggestion (1895, p. 278) that "all organic adaptation in a changing environment is a phenomenon of biological or organic imitation," to the very narrow, accepting imitation only when other factors are ruled out. For instance, "stimulus enhancement" is invoked when the observing animal, having directed its attention to a given object that happens to be the goal of the imitated behavior, might then acquire the new behavior by trial and error (Byrne and Russon, 1998).

The neurophysiological studies reviewed here, some of which used functional magnetic resonance imaging (fMRI), positron-emission tomography (PET), or transcranial magnetic stimulation (TMS), did not attempt to study imitation as a form of motor learning, in that, as we will see, the observed and copied actions were simple actions already present in the motor repertoire of the subjects. There are two main reasons why this approach was used. First, neuroimaging and neurophysiology pose experimental constraints that often make it difficult to study complex integrative behaviors such as imitation as they unfold in real life. Second, some fundamental neural structures and neural mechanisms may well be invoked both when we observe and copy actions we already know how to perform and when we observe and copy actions we are learning to perform through imitation.

4.2   The Role of Frontoparietal Mirror Areas in Imitation and Their Relationship to Language

The Common Code Hypothesis: Mirror Neurons and Early Studies on Grasping

In principle, motor actions can be recognized—and replicated—if there is a common code between the observed motor events and an internally produced motor activity. Until recently, however, neurophysiological evidence in support of this putative common code was lacking. A breakthrough in this field was the discovery in the monkey of a surprising set of neurons, called "mirror neurons," in the ventral premotor cortex and in the anterior part of the posterior parietal cortex, which discharge both when the monkey makes an action directed toward an object and when the monkey *observes* another individual making a similar action. Typically, the effective observed and executed actions are very similar. This finding suggests that an individual can recognize an action made by others because the observed action evokes a discharge in the same neurons that fire when the individual performs that action. This same neural mechanism may be the evolutionary precursor of neural mechanisms that form the basis of imitative behavior.

Even though imitation is a complex behavior requiring the integration of a multitude of sensory stimuli and a variety of movements, at birth, humans and other primates are able to imitate facial and some manual gestures (Meltzoff and Moore, 1977). This built-in behavior must therefore be based on a relatively simple neural mechanism, such as a direct matching of a description of the observed action, either kinematic or pictorial, onto the internal mental representation of the same action. The "mirror neurons" described in frontal and parietal areas of the macaque brain seem the perfect neural substrate for this functional matching mechanism. Some evidence for mirror neurons in the human brain was provided in the mid-1990s by a series of PET and TMS studies on action execution and observation. In one PET study (Rizzolatti et al., 1996b), normal subjects were asked to perform reaching and grasping movements to common three-dimensional objects. In two additional tasks, they were asked to observe others perform grasping movements or simply to observe graspable objects. Observing others reach to and grasp the objects activated Brodmann area (BA) 45, whereas simply observing the objects did not. On the other hand, simply observing the objects activated BA 44, whereas actually reaching to and grasping the objects failed to do so. In a subsequent PET study (Grafton et al., 1996), subjects were again asked to observe others reach to and grasp three-dimensional objects and simply to observe the objects. The grasping execution task was replaced in this second PET study with a grasping imagination task, in which subjects were asked to mentally rehearse a reaching and grasping action on three-dimensional objects. The rationale for doing so was provided by a series of studies suggesting that motor execution and motor imagery share similar neural substrates (Jeannerod, 1994, 1999). Again, observing others grasp objects activated BA 45, whereas imagining the grasping of objects activated BA 44. Taken together, these PET findings failed to confirm the mirror neuron hypothesis, which would have predicted a complete overlap of neural activity between observing action and executing or imagining it. On the other hand, some of the findings suggested the existence of neural mechanisms in the human brain that may have evolved from mirror neurons in the macaque brain. Both studies demonstrated that observing action activated BA 45, which belongs to a functionally larger region, known as "Broca's area" (Heilman and Valenstein, 1993). Encompassing both BAs 44 and 45, this region is critical to the production and comprehension of language; moreover, lesions to it are associated with apraxia and imitation deficits (Heilman and Valenstein, 1993). Further, several considerations support the hypothesis that area F5 of the macaque brain, where mirror neurons were first identified, and Broca's area share anatomical and functional homologies, although the anatomical and functional homologies seem especially valid for BA 44 in the human brain (Petrides and Pandya, 1994; Preuss et al., 1996; Rizzolatti et al., 1996a). Thus, in light of the evolutionary and comparative neurology considerations just mentioned, the PET findings were somewhat encouraging, even though they did not confirm the hypothesis of "mirror neurons" in the human inferior frontal cortex. Evidence in support of this hypothesis would be provided by several other studies. Using different techniques and different activation paradigms, three studies (Parsons et al., 1995; Krams et al., 1998; Nishitani and Hari, 2000) suggested that Brodmann area 44 may play a critical role in copying, observing, and imagining actions. A combined fMRI and cytoarchitectonic study (Binkofski et al., 2000) did so more precisely in terms of spatial localization than the previous PET studies: Cytoarchitectonic maps of human brains were coregistered with the activation maps.

In their meta-analysis of some imaging studies, however, Grezes and Decety (2001) have questioned whether Brodmann area 44 is indeed activated when action is observed and whether an action observation/execution matching system even exists in Broca's area. There are three major problems with this meta-analysis. First, there is a problem with its selectivity. Grezes and Decety did not include some studies, even some cited in the meta-analysis, despite their meeting the criteria for inclusion, such as the imitation study of finger movements undertaken by my colleagues and me (Iacoboni et al., 1999). Second, there is a problem with its logic. Evidence abounds that BA 44 is activated during the execution of hand movements (Rizzolatti et al., 1996b; Krams et al., 1998; Iacoboni et al., 1999; Nishitani and Hari, 2000), for the representation of which this area can thus be considered one of the premotor areas. The meta-analysis showed no activity in BA 44 during hand movement observation but did show activity during such observation in all other premotor areas representing hand movements. How is it possible that only BA 44, which looks like any other premotor area when one observes motor execution tasks involving hand movements, behaves so differently from all other premotor areas when it comes to observation of hand movements? Third, there is a problem with its methodology. Given that the meta-analysis did not involve reanalysis of a large number of subjects observing hand movements, it could not resolve statistical power issues. That is, if one looks at a series of studies all having a small number of subjects, as did Grezes and Decety, it may so happen that these studies consistently fail to show activation due to lack of statistical power. Looking at the outcome of all of them, however, does not improve the likelihood of determining whether a given area is activated when there is a common statistical power problem. To overcome this problem, we reanalyzed the fMRI data from 58 subjects observing hand movements in various experiments performed in our laboratory. If BA 44 were activated during hand action observation, this reanalysis of 58 subjects should well show it. And, indeed, it did. We observed, a bilateral activation of the pars opercularis of the left inferior frontal gyrus, where Brodmann area 44 is more likely to be located (Amunts et al., 1999), during hand action observation (figure 4.1). Thus we answered the question of whether BA 44 is activated by hand action observation with a resounding yes (Molnar-Szakacs et al., 2002).

Interestingly, some of the studies reviewed here also show activation of the anterior part of the posterior parietal cortex, especially BA 40, during action execution, imagination, and observation (Parsons et al., 1995; Grafton et al., 1996; Krams et al., 1998), although these parietal activations are not emphasized in the discussion of findings. This may be because parietal mirror neurons were described some years after the description of frontal mirror neurons in the macaque brain (Fogassi et al., 1998, versus diPellegrino et al., 1992; Gallese et al., 1996), and because, as of this writing, a full report on their properties is still lacking.

Imaging Human Imitation: The Role of Broca's Area

My colleagues and I recently performed a brain imaging study of imitation (Iacoboni et al., 1999) using fMRI to test the hypothesis that mirror neurons and a functional direct matching mechanism constitute the basis of our capacity to imitate the actions of others. We asked subjects to imitate finger movements, and we compared brain activity during imitation with brain activity during two control motor tasks in which subjects were required to perform the same finger movements as in the imitation task, but in response to symbolic or spatial cues. We reasoned that, if some human

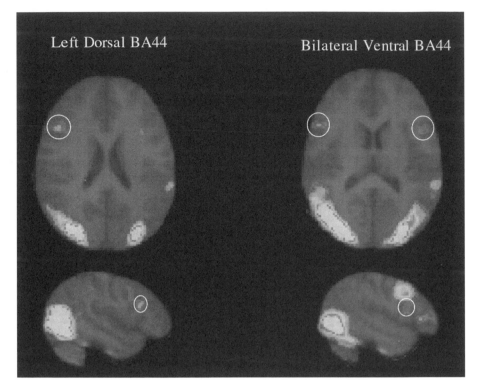

Figure 4.1
Bilateral activation of the pars opercularis of the inferior frontal gyrus, resulting
from a reanalysis of 58 fMRI sessions on normal subjects watching hand actions.

brain areas had mirror properties during imitation, then these areas should
become active during action execution regardless of how the action was
elicited, and should also become more active during imitation: Because the
action to be performed is also observed during imitation, brain areas with
mirror properties would be simultaneously activated by the motor command to be executed and by the visual input representing the observed
action. Moreover, these areas should become more active during action
observation than at rest. We found two areas with these properties: one in
the inferior frontal cortex of the left hemisphere, corresponding to BA 44
(figure 4.2); and a second in the rostral posterior parietal cortex in the right
hemisphere. The anatomical location of these areas closely parallels that of
mirror neurons in the macaque brain. This finding suggests an evolutionary
continuity that implicitly supports the hypothesis that the activations observed in our study, are due to some kind of neuronal mirror activity

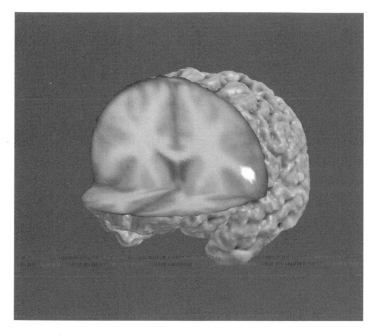

Figure 4.2
Three-dimensional rendering of the activation in Brodmann area 44 (in white) that demonstrated mirror properties during imitation of finger movements.

in the human brain. After considering the characteristics of neurons located in the inferior frontal and the most rostral posterior parietal cortex in the primate brain, and based on data showing that F5 neurons code the general goal of a movement (Gallese et al., 1996), whereas parietal neurons code a proprioceptive storage of limb position (Mountcastle et al., 1975), we proposed that the left inferior frontal cortex codes the observed action in terms of its motor goal, whereas the right posterior parietal area codes the precise kinesthetic aspect of the movement (Iacoboni et al., 1999).

The demonstration of mirror properties in Broca's area during imitation supports the hypothesis that language evolved from a basic mechanism originally related to nonlinguistic communication: the observation/execution matching "mirror" system, with its ability to generate and recognize actions (Rizzolatti et al., 1996a). Further evidence in support of this hypothesis is provided by magnetoencephalography (MEG) of action observation, execution, and imitation, showing the activation of BA 44 in all these tasks (Nishitani and Hari, 2000). During imitation, the activation in BA 44 was stronger than in the other two tasks, as was the case for our fMRI findings. Developmental and evolutionary considerations regarding language, tool use, and their relationships to brain activity had already predicted that Broca's area might play a central role in linking language and manual action (Greenfield, 1991). These more recent imaging findings seem to point to BA 44, within Broca's area, as the site having neural properties associated with imitation, action observation, and language alike, which is also in accord with the comparative anatomy homologies between BA 44 and area F5 in the macaque brain (Petrides and Pandya, 1994).

It has been suggested, however, that the activation of BA 44 during imitation might actually be due to some kind of covert naming of the action to be imitated (Heyes, 2001), which predicts that activation of BA 44 during action observation and imitation should be greater for meaningful than for meaningless gestures. An earlier PET study (Grezes et al., 1998) during which subjects observed meaningful and meaningless actions with the intent to imitate them or without any purpose (actual imitation did not occur in the scanner) found this not to be the case. Activity in the inferior frontal cortex was higher when subjects observed meaningful movements without any purpose, than when they observed them with the intent to imitate, whereas the covert naming hypothesis would have predicted higher activity for observation of meaningful movements both with the intent to imitate and without any purpose.

A way of further testing this hypothesis is to look at imitative behaviors that share several features. If one continues to detect differential activity between imitative conditions despite their increasing similarity, then the more similar the imitation and action observation conditions are, the more unlikely the covert naming hypothesis is. We recently performed an fMRI study of imitation and action observation (Koski et al., 2003) with the intent to better understand the neural correlates of "specular" (mirror-symmetrical) versus "anatomic" imitation. It turns out that there is a strong tendency to imitate others in mirror-symmetrical fashion such that when the actor moves the left hand the imitator moves the right hand (Kephart, 1971; Schofield, 1976; Bekkering et al., 2000). This preference may be due to a natural tendency to interact with other people by using a common sector of space. We tested the hypothesis that frontoparietal mirror areas relevant to imitation would show a modulation of activity from "specular" to "anatomic" imitation, with greater activity for the type of imitation for which there is a strong natural tendency, that is, "specular" imitation. Using the

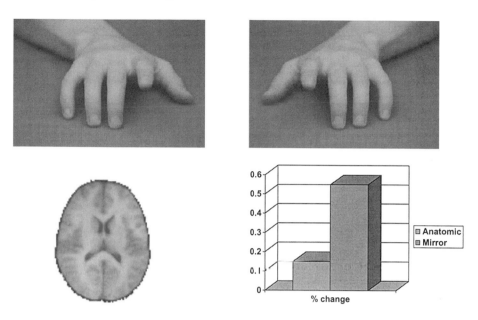

Figure 4.3
Area (marked "⊦," lower left panel) located in the left Brodmann area 44 and showing differential activity for "specular" imitation (*upper right*) versus "anatomic" imitation (*upper left*). Subjects were imitating left- and right-hand actions with their right hand. "Specular" (mirror) imitation produces a fourfold increase from baseline in blood oxygen level–dependent (BOLD) response signal, compared to "anatomic" imitation.

same finger movements we adopted in our previous study on human imitation, we asked subjects to imitate both left-hand and right-hand actions, with their right hand in other words, to perform "specular" imitation and "anatomic" imitation, respectively. We observed greater activity for "specular" imitation than for "anatomic" imitation in the two previously identified frontoparietal mirror areas, that is, inferior frontal cortex (BA 44; figure 4.3) and posterior parietal cortex (BAs 40–7). We also observed greater activity for "specular" imitation than for "anatomic" imitation, in the supplementary motor area (SMA) proper, the complex MT-V5, and an area in parieto-occipital cortex. (Two other regions demonstrating the same pattern of activity will be discussed in separate sections.) These findings suggest three things: First, there is a clear brain-behavior relationship between frontoparietal mirror areas and different types of imitative behavior. The form of imitation for which people seem to have a strong tendency is also associated with greater activity in frontoparietal mirror areas. Second, imitation is a complex phenomenon and its neural correlates are not simply confined to the frontoparietal mirror area. Regions upstream and downstream in the network of areas relevant to the sensorimotor transformations required by imitation seem to show activity tightly coupled with the activity in fronto-parietal mirror areas. Future studies will face the task of better defining the differential role of frontoparietal mirror areas and of other cortical regions during imitation. Third, the hypothesis that the activation of Broca's area during imitation is due to some form of covert naming seems very unlikely. To reconcile our data on "specular" versus "anatomic" imitation with the covert naming hypothesis, one would have to somehow account for why imitating a left-hand action invokes more silent naming than imitating a right-hand action.

Further evidence against the covert naming hypothesis was recently provided by an fMRI study (Buccino et al., 2001), which demonstrated a somatotopic pattern of activity extending from ventral to more dorsal regions of premotor cortex during the observation of mouth, arm/hand, and foot actions, respectively. In contrast, the covert naming hypothesis would have predicted similar pattern of activity in Broca's area across all observation tasks.

The most compelling evidence against the thesis that the activation of the pars opercularis of the inferior frontal gyrus during imitation is epiphenomenal has been recently provided by a "virtual lesion" study (Heiser et al., 2003) performed in our laboratory using transcranial magnetic stimulation (rTMS). Subjects were asked to imitate sequences of key presses. As a control visuomotor task, they performed similar sequences of key presses in response to visual cues. While they were performing these tasks, three cortical sites were stimulated, the left pars opercularis, the right pars opercularis, and a control site, the occipital lobe. The results demonstrated a selective impairment of performance at the imitation task only for stimulation of the two pars opercularis sites (figure 4.4), complementing well the results of our reanalysis of 58 subjects observing hand actions and showing bilateral activation of the pars opercularis of the inferior frontal gyrus (see figure 4.1). Thirty-nine of those subjects also performed a hand action imitation task. An analysis of their neural activity confirmed that, during hand action imitation, the pars opercularis of the inferior frontal gyrus was bilaterally activated. This is in keeping with our first study on imitation (Iacoboni et al., 1999), in which we observed a bilateral pattern of activation at sub-threshold statistical level, although we reported threshold-reaching activation in the left pars opercularis only.

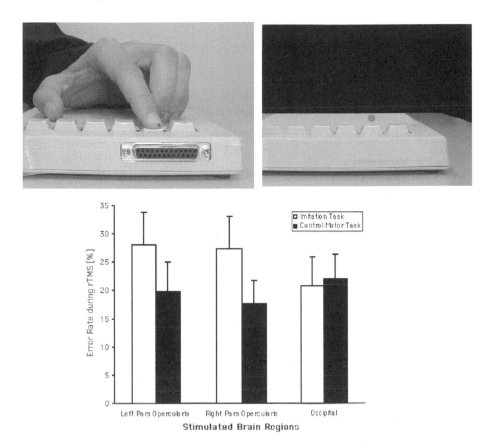

Figure 4.4
Percentage errors in an imitation task (*upper left*) and a visuomotor control task (*upper right*) while repetitive transcranial magnetic stimulation (rTMS) was applied to the left pars opercularis, the right pars opercularis, and a control site in the occipital lobe. A significant increase in percentage errors is observed when rTMS is applied to the left and right pars opercularis.

The main implication of the hypothesized homologies between area F5 and Brodmann area 44 and of the mirror system as a precursor of the language system is that the language function is not encapsulated, with dedicated neural machinery. Rather, language and motor control functions, even those clearly requiring no form of symbolic processing, are functionally linked and influence each other. Indeed, recent studies (Gentilucci and Gangitano, 1998; Gentilucci et al., 2000) have shown that, even in tasks requiring no explicit processing of printed words describing objects to be grasped, the kinematics of reaching-grasping were influenced by the meaning and grammar of those words.

4.3   Learning Novel Actions: The Role of the Superior Temporal Cortex

Reafferent Copies of Imitated Actions in the Superior Temporal Cortex

The mechanism matching the observed action with (mapping it onto) an internal motor representation of that action provided by the frontoparietal mirror areas, though sufficient at least in principle, for individuals when they have to imitate actions already present in their motor repertoire, does not seem, sufficient when they have to copy a new action or to adjust an action present in their motor repertoire to a different observed action. Here an additional mechanism seems to be needed, one that would allow the imitator to compare the visual description of the action to be imitated with the sensory consequences of the action planned to imitate it. The idea of an internal sensory copy of an action to be performed has been recently elaborated in detail in the motor control literature as forward internal models (Wolpert and Kawato, 1998; Kawato, 1999) and in the psychological literature as the ideomotor theory of learning (Brass et al., 2000). If planned actions indeed evoke an internal sensory representation of their consequences, then imitation of an action that does not belong to the motor repertoire of the imitator can be easily achieved by a mechanism matching this sensory representation with the visual representation of the movement to be imitated; activation of the relevant motor representation necessary to execute the imitated action will lead to successful imitation. An open question is whether there is a visual area that codes the observed actions as well as the remote effects of voluntary movements. The cortical region around the superior temporal sulcus (STS), whose visual neurons respond to the observation of biological actions (Perrett et al., 1989, 1990; Perrett and Emery, 1994) is reciprocally connected with prefrontal (PF) cortex (and indirectly with area F5) in the macaque brain. Thus both functional properties and anatomical considerations make the STS region a likely site for matching the predicted sensory consequences of planned actions with the visual description of observed actions. Moreover, imaging studies in which volunteers observed actions, such as hand or eye movements, also supported the thesis that biological moving stimuli activate the human superior temporal region (Grafton et al., 1996; Puce et al., 1998; Frith and Frith, 1999).

In our study on imitation of finger movements, my colleagues and I (Iacoboni et al., 2000) reported that an area located in the superior temporal sulcus showed a pattern of activity compatible with the hypothesized mechanism to match the sensory consequences of a planned action with the visual description of an observed action. This area showed greater activity for imitation than for the control motor tasks, for action observation than for the control visual tasks, and for imitation than for action observation, although the differences in activity were only marginally significant. Additional empirical evidence on the functional properties of the STS area in the human brain is thus needed.

We therefore, performed, a region-of-interest analysis on ten subjects performing "specular" versus "anatomic" imitation reported in section 4.2 (Koski et al., 2003), an ideal paradigm to test the hypothesis of reafferent information on the predicted sensory consequences of motor actions. It is likely indeed that the phenomenon of imitating others as if in front of a mirror (observed left-hand actions imitated by right hand actions) reflects a natural tendency to interact with other people by using a common sector of space. There is no reason for this tendency to be present, however, when the observer simply looks at another individual *without* the intent to imitate. Thus we predicted that if the hypothesized mechanism of comparing a visual description of an action with the sensory consequence of the planned copy of that action was actually located in the STS area, a clear-cut pattern should emerge. During imitation, neural activity in the STS area should be greater when the imitators observed the hand mirror image of the hand they used (left hand as visual stimulus and right hand as motor effector), whereas, during observation, activity in the STS area need not be greater for the left hand as visual stimulus. We obtained exactly this pattern of activity in the STS area as depicted in figure 4.5 and plate 1, most likely reflecting the modulation of the STS areas visual activity by the imitative behavior (Iacoboni et al., 2001).

Topography in the Superior Temporal Sulcus and "Minimal Neural Architecture" for Imitation

The imaging data described above, together with neurophysiological and neuroanatomical features observed in nonhuman primates, led my colleagues and me to propose the following model of a "minimal neural architecture" necessary to implement information processing during imitation (Iacoboni et al., 2001). The STS area would provide an early visual description of the action to parietal mirror neurons, which would add additional somatosensory information to the movement to be imitated. This more com-

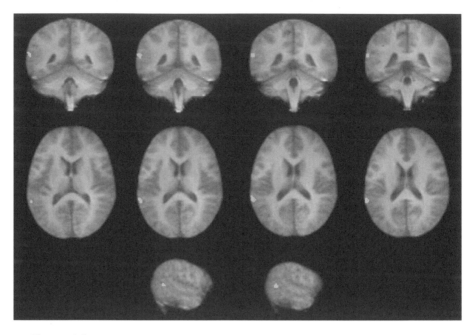

Figure 4.5
Area (red) in the superior temporal cortex region that seems to be matching a visual description of the action to be imitated with the predicted sensory consequences of a planned imitative action. In this picture, the right hemisphere is on the left side. See plate 1 for color version.

plex multimodal information would be transmitted to the inferior frontal cortex (Broca's area), which in turn would code the goal of the action to be imitated. Sensory copies of the imitated actions would then be sent back to the STS area for monitoring ("My actions are like the ones I have seen").

Based on this model and on a well-documented somatotopy in parietal and premotor regions (Buccino et al., 2001), topographically organized regions that have strong functional communication with the STS area, two predictions can be immediately made: (1) that Broca's area should respond to the presence of visible goals in actions to be imitated; and (2) that the STS area should have topography for observed actions performed with different body parts. We have collected data supporting both predictions. The first will be discussed in section 4.2; we tested the second prediction with fMRI by studying normal subjects observing eye, hand, and mouth movements. In the eye movement condition, subjects watched a face making saccadic eye movements and, in the control condition, the same face with moving arrows in lieu of eyes. In hand and mouth conditions, subjects watched a hand lifting the index or middle finger and a mouth speaking syllables silently; in the control conditions, boxes or bars, moving with the same speed as the finger and the lips (Dubeau et al., 2001a). Observing eye, hand, and mouth movements produced peaks of neural activity with a clear topography, In the STS area, the peak for hand movements was the most dorsal, whereas the peak for mouth movements was located more anteriorly than the peak for eyes movements. We believe that this topography reflects functional intercommunication between premotor and parietal regions (where a somatotopy of body parts is known) and the STS region. In line with our model, we posit that this intercommunication is the expression of functional integration between a visual description of an action and the sensory consequences of a motor plan necessary to replicate it.

4.4   Modulation of Primary Motor Activity during Action Observation and Imitation

Primary Motor Activity during Action Observation and Imitation

Sections 4.2 and 4.3 discussed the role of inferior frontal cortex, the most rostral posterior parietal cortex, and the most caudal superior temporal cortex in imitation. This section discusses the role of primary motor cortex in building motor representations relevant to action observation, imitation, and learning.

In the first study to directly address this question, Fadiga and colleagues (1995) compared corticospinal excitability over the primary motor cortex while subjects observed actions and performed visual control tasks. As argued above if human premotor neurons are activated by the observation of action, this activation should in turn facilitate primary motor cortex excitability, given that premotor areas are directly connected to primary motor cortex. Fadiga and colleagues did indeed observe such facilitation, whose cortical nature was subsequently demonstrated by Strafella and Paus (2000) with the paired-pulse technique. Using magnetoencephalography (MEG), Hari and colleagues (1998) had also demonstrated that action observation activated the human primary motor cortex (M1), although PET and fMRI have had generally little success in observing the activation of M1 during action observation. A possible reason for this apparent inconsistency in results between techniques that rely more directly on neural changes, such as TMS and MEG, and techniques that rely on blood flow changes secondary to neural activity, such as PET and fMRI, may have been provided by a recent report (Logothetis et al., 2001) on simultaneous recordings of neural activity and blood oxygen level–dependent (BOLD) fMRI signal change in primary visual cortex of nonhuman primates during visual stimulation. Indeed, these simultaneous recordings of neural activity and BOLD fMRI signal change have shown that the signal-to-noise ratio of the neural signal is of about 25 orders of magnitude higher than that of the BOLD signal. Thus image statistics applied to BOLD fMRI (and probably also PET) data are *not* likely to detect activation of brain regions despite robust underlying changes in neural activity (Logothetis et al., 2001).

As noted in section 4.2, we also performed an fMRI study on "specular" versus "anatomic" imitation (Koski et al., 2003). The natural question to ask here is whether "specular" and "anatomic" imitation, and action observation, affect the activity in M1 differently. We indeed observed greater neural activity for in M1 "specular" imitation than for "anatomic" imitation, and for imitative than for control motor tasks, as shown in figure 4.6, but no change in activity as detected by BOLD fMRI during action observation only. Thus imitation seems to modulate primary motor cortex activity as detected by BOLD fMRI signal change,whereas action observation does not. Thus, even within imitative tasks, one can observe differences in signal change in M1. In contrast, the neural changes detected by TMS and MEG during action observation seem too small to determine detectable blood flow changes with fMRI.

Imitation as Goal–Oriented Behavior: Its Effect on Primary Motor and Inferior Frontal Cortex

The frontoparietal mirror system presumably orchestrates the various components involved in the complex sensorimotor transformations required by imitation and its properties may spread to other cortical areas, as we have seen in the experiment on mirror versus anatomic imitation described in section 4.2. Behaviors, especially ones as complex as imitation, are not simply learned and replicated as unified, nondecomposed patterns. In terms of neural control, the two key features of interest here are "internal models" and "primitives." "Internal models" are neural mechanisms that can mimic the input-output characteristics of the learning system (Wolpert and Kawato, 1998; Kawato 1999). To learn, a system must be able to generalize beyond the sensory stimuli and movements experienced in the past. This generalization is possible only through the internal repre-

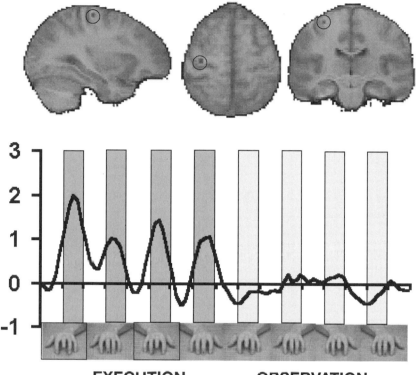

EXECUTION   **OBSERVATION**

Figure 4.6

Modulation of activity in primary motor cortex (M1) during "specular" and "anatomic" imitation (the activated area appears as a darkened square in the top three panels). The darker bands represent task periods and the pictures of hands at the bottom of the graph indicate which stimuli subjects were watching. The hands with the lifted finger indicate that subjects were watching an action in the corresponding block. The hands with the cross on middle finger indicate that subjects were watching static hands with a symbolic cue in the corresponding block. The first four blocks correspond to execution tasks and the last four blocks to observation only tasks. The order of tasks was counterbalanced in the actual experiment. The two imitation tasks are marked with a box around the picture of the hand. The activity is expressed in normalized percent change.

sentation of sensory consequences of motor commands (the forward model) or, inversely, through the extrapolation of motor commands from the observation of motor behavior (the inverse model). "Primitives" are the building blocks of a given complex behavior (Bizzi et al., 1991). For instance, motor primitives are simple, meaningful behaviors (wiping, reaching) that can be evoked through the stimulation of single points of the spinal cord. Few motor primitives can be combined to obtain a large motor repertoire (Tresch et al., 1999). Higher-order primitives may exist in the cerebral cortex, perhaps reflected in the activity observed in the mirror system of the monkey and of the human brain. That is, the representation of action supported by mirror neurons seems to be more a representation of action goals than of motor outputs (Gallese et al., 1996). If there is a system that codes for goals, then it remains to be established how these goals may be combined to form a repertoire of purposeful and adaptive behavior.

Action goals are hierarchically organized in human imitative behavior (Bekkering et al., 2000), a feature also observed in motor primitives. For instance, when two fields corresponding to two motor primitives are stimulated simultaneously, the resulting behavior may be dominated by one of the two primitives (Mussa-Ivaldi et al., 1994). Studies on imitation in children show that preschoolers represent the most salient goal of the action to be imitated, but often ignore lower goals (Bekkering et al., 2000). Goals are easily embodied by an object (Mary grasps a *cup*). Thus the role of objects in action observation and learning by imitation seems to be crucial and needs to be clarified. In, the macaque brain, mirror neurons are chiefly associated with object-oriented actions: They show a narrow tuning with respect to the type of object and the way it is treated, but quite a broad tuning for the trajectory of the movement or the motor effector involved (Gallese et al., 1996). The presence of real objects, however, alters the motor component of the task and makes it more difficult to interpret imaging data. Thus, inspired by developmental and chronometric studies, my colleagues and I used features that can be easily conceptualized as objects and salient action goals, even though they do not alter the characteristics of the movement to be observed and imitated. For instance, experimental data, in the form of both developmental studies in children (Bekkering et al., 2000) and chronometric studies in adults (Wolschläger and Bekkering, 2002) suggest that dots or marks on a table can be used as end points of imitated actions. Because these dots or marks are known to alter the imitative behavior of preschoolers and adults, they are useful stimuli for an imaging study. In Bekkering et al., 2000, the model initiated ipsilateral and contralateral hand movements to one of two dots on a table and asked the children to imitate his actions. In another condition, the same movements were performed and were imitated, except that this time the movements were directed to the same places on the table but no dots were visible. In the latter condition, children imitated well the movements of the model, whereas when dots were visible children would often reach for the correct dot with the ipsilateral hand, even when the correct motor response required the use of the contralateral hand. This is because when observing object-oriented actions, the object activates a "direct" motor program, one that leads most directly to the effect the action has on the object. In this case, the ipsilateral motor response was the fastest way to cover the dot previously covered by the experimenter. Similar results were obtained in adults (Wolschläger and Bekkering, 2002) in a paradigm derived by the paradigm used by Bekkering and colleagues in children. Obviously, the effect observed in adults was restricted to reaction times, and did not extend to accuracy. Adults were able to suppress the incorrect motor response for imitation of contralateral actions directed to the dot, but this suppression required time and was expressed by reaction time costs.

Without objects, the relative positions of the fingers became the goal of the action. These goals also evoked the "direct" motor program, but now the "direct" motor program matched the observed non-object-oriented action. This result led us to make two predictions. First, that Broca's area, as a goal-oriented area, should be more active during the imitation of object-oriented than of non-object-oriented movements: If it is the homologue of the monkey's mirror neuron system (tuned for object-oriented actions), then Broca's area should also be better tuned for object-oriented than for non-object-oriented actions. Second, the parietal mirror neuron area should be more active during the imitation of non-object-oriented than of object-oriented movements: For imitating non-object-oriented actions, it is necessary to precisely encode the detailed description of the movement, whereas, for imitating object-oriented actions, it is only necessary to encode which object was involved and what was done to it.

To understand the mechanisms underlying the hierarchical organization of action goals, we performed an fMRI study in 14 normal adults using the same paradigm adopted by Wolschläger and Bekkering (Koski et al., 2002). Our data support our first prediction. An area in the inferior frontal cortex, but not one in the posterior parietal cortex, responded to the presence of the dots and to the interaction between the presence of the dots and the type of action to be imitated (ipsilateral, contralateral). Interestingly, the pattern of activity observed in primary motor cortex was slightly different. There was a main effect of the type of action, with greater activity for crossed movements and an interaction between the presence of the dots and the type of action to be imitated (figure 4.7).

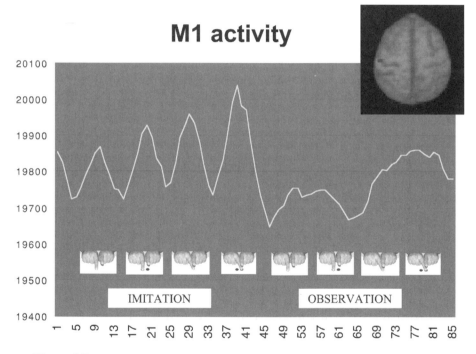

Figure 4.7
Modulation of activity in primary motor cortex (M1) during goal-oriented and non-goal-oriented imitation. The activated area appears as a darkened rectangle within circle (upper right). Activity is expressed in raw signal rescaled by the smoothing process. During imitation, there is an effect of type of movement (crossed movements yielding greater activity than uncrossed movements), of visible goals (finger movements covering the dots yielding greater activity than finger movements not covering the dots) and an interaction between type of imitated movements and presence of visible goals. As in other studies, there is no evident task-related activity during observation of action.

4.5 Understanding Other People: Gaze Following, Empathy, Intentionality

Understanding Where Others Direct Their Attention

Understanding where other individuals direct their attention is a fundamental component of social behavior. In humans, the ability to follow the gaze of others is normally expressed around 12 months of age and the ability to direct attention with another individual on the same object, around 18 months (Butterworth, 1991). Recent studies (Allison et al., 2000; George et al., 2001; Hoffman and Haxby, 2000; Puce et al., 1998) have pointed to the superior temporal sulcus, fusiform gyrus, intraparietal sulcus, and amygdala as critical structures for processing gaze. When one follows the gaze of others in real life, however, one moves one's eyes in the same direction as theirs. To the best of our knowledge, in none of the studies reported in the literature thus far were subjects asked to move their eyes following the gaze of another individual. In a preliminary fMRI study (Dubeau et al., 2001b),we asked our subjects to do just that, based on reasoning similar to that of our initial study on imitation of finger movements. Subjects shown the face of an individual looking from the center to the left or from the center to the right were asked to imitate that individual's leftward or rightward gaze (gaze following). In a first control condition, they were asked to perform the same eye movements as in the previous condition, but this time in response to an image of the same face, with eyes digitally removed and replaced by arrows to cue gaze direction. In a second control condition, subjects were presented only with arrows on the screen and again asked to perform the same eye movements as in the previous conditions. Subjects thus performed the same action in response to three different stimuli: the face of an individual looking at different space sectors, (full action), an image of that face with eyes replaced by a symbolic representation, and finally only spatial cues without any biological significance. Additionally, subjects were asked to simply observe, in three other conditions, these three types of stimuli. We predicted that, if there was a mirror mechanism for gaze following, then the first condition should show greater activity than the other two conditions because of the visual encoding of the act of looking at somewhere from somebody. Our failure to find an area with such a pattern of activity should not be considered as evidence that no mirror mechanism exists. We may have failed to detect such a mechanism simply because of lack of sensitivity (see Logothetis et al., 2001).

What we did find, however, was that a region in the anterior and lateral right cerebellum responded strongly to both gaze following and execution of eye movements in response to the face with the arrows, but did not respond at all to execution of eye movements in response to simple spatial cues. This pattern of activity during eye movements was also replicated during simple observation of the stimuli. The overall activity in this cerebellar area was the same for execution of eye movements as for simple observation.

Two possible explanations for these findings come immediately to mind: First, the cerebellar region encodes the sensory aspect of the stimuli it responds to. This possibility is unlikely, given the region's anatomical location (but see Bower, 1997). Second, the cerebellar region expresses the ability to predict the sensory consequences of an intended act. This possibility, in light of the recent wave of studies on internal models in the cerebellum (Wolpert et al., 1998; Kawato, 1999; Imamizu et al., 2000; Iacoboni, 2001) is far more likely. But what kind of "intended act" are we talking about here? We believe that subjects are invoking the idea of somebody looking at something, even during simple observation, and even when they are watching a face with arrows embedded in it, and cannot help but generate the representation of a similar movement. The lack of neural activity when subjects were presented only with spatial cues indicates that the intended act is not simply looking leftward or rightward, but rather looking at some sector of space *jointly with somebody else*. It is a *social*, not a cognitive, act. Our interpretation of the findings is thus consistent with Courchesne's hypothesis, (1997) of a cerebellar dysfunction in autistic patients.

Feeling the Emotions of Others

The perception-action model (PAM; Brass et al., 2000) suggests that perceiving an action of another, generates a representation of that action, which, in turn, activates brain regions responsible for the preparation and execution of that same action in the observer. We have seen that single-unit studies and functional neuroimaging experiments of imitation have supported the PAM and suggested the existence of a "mirror system" of brain areas critical in building representations of motor actions. The mirror neuron system seems to serve as a mechanism for understanding the actions and intentions of others. It has been hypothesized that a similar system in the domain of emotion might serve as a mechanism for empathy (Preston and deWaal, 2002), albeit in different areas of the brain. The areas thus far identified with mirror properties, belong to a frontoparietal circuit, generally associated, not with emotions, but with sensorimotor functions. How then does the limbic system get information from the frontoparietal mirror system when empathy takes place? If one looks at available anatomical connectivity data, the dysgranular field of the primate insula, which connects limbic areas with inferior frontal, anterior posterior parietal, and superior temporal cortex, fulfills all the requisites for relay station between a system matching observation and execution of action and one involved with emotional processing. My colleagues and I tested this hypothesis in a recently performed fMRI study (Carr et al., under revision). We asked subjects to observe and imitate emotional facial expressions or simply to observe them. Our prediction was that, during imitation of facial expression, the insula would be activated due to its hypothesized relay function from the frontoparietal mirror system to the limbic system. As control conditions, we asked our subjects to observe and imitate only the eyes or only the mouth extracted from the same faces expressing emotions as in the previous conditions or simply to observe them. We did so because the single-unit data in the macaque brain suggest that in frontoparietal mirror areas there are representations of hand and mouth movements, but not of eye movements. We hypothesized that the imitation of eye movements having emotional valence might not activate the frontoparietal mirror system and, consequently, not require that the insula be activated as relay station to the limbic system. Our results clearly demonstrated the activation of the insula during all imitation tasks, supporting our hypothesis that the insula plays a key role in affect generation and serves as relay station between frontal cortices and limbic structures, thus representing a possible pathway for empathy (figure 4.8 and plate 2). That the insula was activated even during imitation of emotional eye movement can be readily explained: Imitating a facial expression is a holistic act, one that can scarcely be decomposed. Indeed: we obtained substantially identical maps of activation for all three imitation tasks, with no reliable differences between them.

Moreover, we obtained a complete spatial overlap of neural activation between imitation and observation of facial emotional expression, which supports the main claim of the perception-action model, suggesting that the model's functional mechanism could apply to the realm of emotion and form the basis of empathy (Preston and deWaal, 2002).

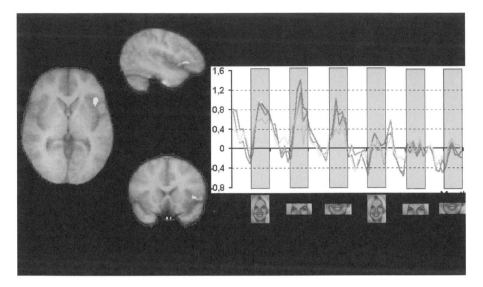

Figure 4.8
Insula as relay? During imitation of facial emotional expressions, activation occurs in the left frontal operculum (red), in the right frontal operculum (blue), and in the anterior insula (green). Corresponding time series expressed as normalized percentage change are shown with corresponding colors. See plate 2 for color version.

Understanding the Intentions of Others

Despite its fundamental role in intentional relations and social behavior, little is known about how individuals recognize the intentions underlying the actions of others. Intention can be conceptualized as the highest goal of an action; understanding it may serve as a powerful mechanism of learning by imitation and "mind reading." How do individuals recognize and understand the intentions of others? Although I believe that the observation/execution matching system is the perfect neural system for understanding the actions of others, understanding those actions has two meanings. The first is to understand what others have done; the second is to understand what they *intended* by doing it. Is it sufficient to observe someone's body movement to produce mirror activation, or does the mirror system become active because it reflects a voluntary action and the intention that is disclosed by that movement? These two possibilities can be disentangled experimentally.

Let us imagine someone grasping a cup. In normal life, not only do we understand that someone is grasping the cup, but we also guess (hypothesize) why: because that individual wants to drink, or say, plans to clean the table. When we observe someone grasping a cup and guess why, we take what philosophers call an "intentional stance" (Dennett, 1987). In a preliminary fMRI study on the neural bases of understanding the intentions of others while observing their actions, my colleagues and I asked subjects to observe grasping a cup under four different conditions. In the CONTROL condition, the action was displayed against a plain black background; in the DRINK condition, against a background image of breakfast on a table; and in the CLEAN condition, against a background image of empty dishes piled up on a table. In these three conditions, subjects were told to attend to the type of grip. In a fourth, CONTENT condition, the background image randomly alternated between those used for the DRINK and CLEAN conditions; here subjects were told to attend to the purpose of the action according to the context.

There are three main views on the nature of intentionality. One view is that intentionality is based on internal symbols, and derived intentionality requires the mediation of a symbol-based system (Fodor, 1975; Pylishin, 1984). The second maintains the opposite: Intentionality is essentially nonlinguistic, based on acting competently in the world, and expressed by predictable patterns of interactions between the intentional system and the environment (Dennett, 1987). And the third view maintains that intentionality is essentially normative, thus determined by social practices (Heidegger, 1927; Merleau-Ponty, 1945; Dreyfus, 1982, 1992; Haugeland, 1997).

We assumed that the patterns of brain activity we detected would lead us to discover how intentionality actually works: If language- or math-related areas were activated in the critical experimental comparisons, the first view would be correct and intentionality would probably be symbol based. If sensorimotor and prefrontal areas were activated in the critical experimental comparisons, then the second view would be correct. Finally, if the "social brain" (limbic system, orbitofrontal cortex) and sensorimotor areas were mostly activated in the critical experimental comparisons, then the third view would be correct.

In all four conditions, both visual areas and the frontoparietal areas associated with grasping execution were activated—with the exception of M1. The anterior cingulate (BA 32) (figure 4.9 and plate 3), middle temporal gyrus (BA 21), posterior parietal cortex (BA 7), medial temporal area, and orbitofrontal cortex were more active when subjects observed the grasping action in a specific context than in the CONTROL condition (no

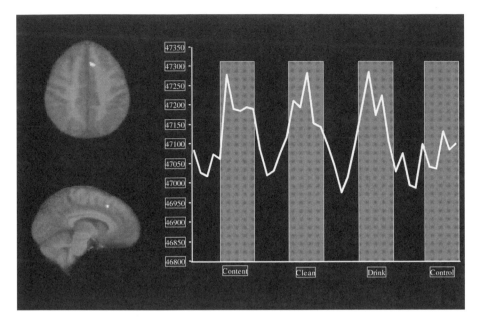

Figure 4.9
Activity (white) in a caudal area of the anterior cingulate (BA 32) that responds to the presence of the context but not to the explicit request of processing the purpose of the action according to the context. Activity is expressed in raw signal rescaled by the smoothing process. See plate 3 for color version.

context). These regions were not differentially activated in the DRINK, CLEAN, or CONTENT conditions.

Thus, from our fMRI data, humans understand the intentions of others through processing the visual context (BA 21) and invoking the motor representations of the actions we used in that context (premotor, BA 7, and BA 32). Our data on the activation of the neural circuitry associated with motivation and reward and with sensorimotor behavior clearly support the third or "normative" view of intentionality. The first or symbol-based view seems ruled out by the absence of neural activity in the language-related or even math-related areas, especially in the alternating context (CONTENT) condition, when subjects were explicitly instructed to pay attention to the purpose of the action. The second view seems ruled out both by the absence of neural activity in prefrontal areas and by the presence of activity in limbic areas.

The frontoparietal grasping circuit, which partly overlaps with the frontoparietal mirror system, was activated equally in all conditions, even the CONTROL (no-context) condition. This could be interpreted as suggesting that the frontoparietal mirror system is a system for recognition of preintentional basic acts that become intentional only against a background of a meaningfully ordered world (Dreyfus, 1992).

4.6   Conclusion: The Way Ahead

This chapter has summarized the first results of a research program on the basic mechanisms underlying our social behavior through the observation and imitation of the actions of others. Recent breakthroughs in neurophysiology, advances in technology, and the emergence of interdisciplinary fields such as cognitive neuroscience and computational neuroscience have paved the way for this line of research, which had been confined to the social sciences and philosophy until a few years ago.

The tentative conclusion of this research is that a general mechanism for understanding the actions, intentions, and emotions of others involves "mirroring." That is, witnessing and imitating the actions, intentions, and emotions of others triggers the same neural activity associated with our own actions, intentions, and emotions.

My colleagues and I believe that a useful way of asking what it is like to be a human is by looking at the neural and functional mechanisms underlying our actions, at how they are learned and disseminated among other individuals, how they relate to the world of communication and symbols, and how they are woven into the social context in which they emerge. Our next step will be to apply some of the knowledge we have gained through this research to better understand how the mechanisms for action observation and imitation in the adult brain map onto the developing brain, as a key to understanding the basic principles of human development.

Acknowledgments

The research described in this chapter has been supported in part by Brain Mapping Medical Research Organization, Brain Mapping Support Foundation, Pierson-Lovelace Foundation, the Ahmanson Foundation, Tamkin Foundation, Jennifer Jones-Simon Foundation, Capital Group Companies Charitable Foundation, Robson Family, Northstar Fund, and by grants from the National Center for Research Resources, National Science Foundation, and Human Frontier Science Program.

References

Adolphs, R. (1999). Social cognition and the human brain. *Trends Cogn. Sci.* 3: 469–479.

Adolphs, R., Damasio, H., Tranel, D., Cooper, G., and Damasio, A. R. (2000). A role for somatosensory cortices in the visual recognition of emotion as revealed by three-dimensional lesion mapping. *J. Neurosci.* 20: 2683–2690.

Allison, T., Puce, A., and McCarthy, G. (2000). Social perception from visual cues: Role of the STS region. *Trends Cogn. Sci.* 4: 267–278.

Amunts, K., Schleicher, A., Burgel, U., Mohlberg, H., Uylings, H. B. M., and Zilles, K. (1999). Broca's region revisited: Cytoarchitecture and intersubject variability. *J. Comp. Neurol.* 412: 319–341.

Arbib, M. A., Billard, A., Iacoboni, M., and Oztop, E. (2000). Synthetic brain imaging: Grasping, mirror neurons and imitation. *Neural Networks* 13: 975–997.

Baldwin, J. M. (1895). Mental development in the child and the race. New York: Macmillan.

Bekkering, H., Wohlschläger, A., and Gattis, M. (2000). Imitation of gestures in children is goal-directed. *Q. J. Exp. Psychol.* 53A: 153–164.

Binkofski, F., Amunts, K., Stephan, K. M., Posse, S., Schormann, T., Freund, H. J., et al. (2000). Broca's region subserves imagery of motion: A combined cytoarchitectonic and fMRI study. *Hum. Brain Mapp.* 11: 273–285.

Bizzi, E., Mussa-Ivaldi, F. A., and Giszter, S. (1991). Computations underlying the execution of movement: A biological perspective. *Science* 253: 287–291.

Bower, J. M. (1997). Is the cerebellum sensory for motor's sake, or motor for sensory's sake: The view from the whiskers of a rat? *Progr. Brain Res.* 114: 463–496.

Brass, M., Bekkering, H., Wohlschläger, A., and Prinz, W. (2000). Compatibility between observed and executed finger movements: Comparing symbolic, spatial and imitative cues. *Brain Cogn.* 44: 129–154.

Buccino, G., Binkofski, F., Fink, G. R., Fadiga, L., Fogassi, L., Gallese, V., et al. (2001). Action observation activates premotor and parietal areas in a somatotopic manner: An fMRI study. *Eur. J. Neurosci.* 13: 400–404.

Butterworth, G. (1991). The ontogeny and phylogeny of joint visual attention. In *Natural Theories of Mind: Evolution, Development and Simulation of Everyday Mindreading*, A. Whiten (ed.). Cambridge, Mass.: Basil Blackwell, pp. 223–232.

Byrne, R. (1995). *The Thinking Ape: Evolutionary Origins of Intelligence*. Oxford: Oxford University Press.

Byrne, R. W., and Russon, A. E. (1998). Learning by imitation: A hierarchical approach. *Behav. Brain Sci.* 21: 667–712.

Carr, L., Iacoboni, M., Dubeau, M.-C., Mazziotta, J. C., and Lenzi, G. L. (under revision). Neural mechanisms of empathy in humans: A relay from neural systems for imitation to limbic areas. *Proc. Natl. Acad. Sci. USA.*

Courchesne, E. (1997). Brainstem, cerebellar and limbic neuroanatomical abnormalities in autism. *Curr. Opin. Neurobiol.* 7: 269–278.

Dennett, D. C. (1987). *The Intentional Stance.* Cambridge, Mass.: MIT Press.

diPellegrino, G., Fadiga, L., Fogassi, L., Gallese, V., and Rizzolatti, G. (1992). Understanding motor events: A neurophysiological study. *Exp. Brain Res.* 91: 176–180.

Dreyfus, H. L. (1982). *Husserl, Intentionality, and Cognitive Science.* Cambridge, Mass.: MIT Press.

Dreyfus, H. L. (1992). *What Computers Still Can't Do: A Critique of Artificial Reason.* Cambridge, Mass.: MIT Press.

Dubeau, M. C., Iacoboni, M., Koski, L., Markovac, J., and Mazziotta, J. C. (2001a). Topography for body parts motion in the STS region. *Soc. Neurosci. Abstr.* 27.

Dubeau, M. C., Iacoboni, M., Koski, L., and Mazziotta, J. C. (2001b). Gaze and joint attention: The role of the cerebellum. *NeuroImage* 13: S1157.

Elman, J., et al. (1996). *Rethinking Innateness: A Connectionist Perspective on Development.* Cambridge, Mass.: MIT Press.

Fadiga, L., Fogassi, L., Pavesi, G., and Rizzolatti, G. (1995). Motor facilitation during action observation: A magnetic stimulation study. *J. Neurophysiol.* 73: 2608–2611.

Fodor, J. A. (1975). The Language of Thought. New York: Crowell.

Fogassi, L., Gallese, V., Fadiga, L., and Rizzolatti, G. (1998). Neurons responding to the sight of goal-directed hand/arm actions in the parietal area PF (7b) of the macaque monkey. *Soc. Neurosci. Abstr.* 24: 654.

Frith, C. D., and Frith, U. (1999). Interacting minds: A biological basis. *Science* 286: 1692–1695.

Gallese, V., Fadiga, L., Fogassi, L., and Rizzolatti, G. (1996). Action recognition in the premotor cortex. *Brain* 119: 593–609.

Gentilucci, M., and Gangitano, M. (1998). Influence of automatic word reading on motor control. *Eur. J. Neurosci.* 10: 752–756.

Gentilucci, M., Benuzzi, F., Bertolani, L., Daprati, E., and Gangitano, M. (2000). Language and motor control. *Exp. Brain Res.* 133: 468–490.

George, N., Driver, J., and Dolan, R. J. (2001). Seen gaze-direction modulates fusiform activity and its coupling with other brain areas during face processing. *NeuroImage* 13: 1102–1112.

Grafton, S. T., Arbib, M. A., Fadiga, L., and Rizzolatti, G. (1996). Localization of grasp representation in humans by positron emission tomography: 2. Observation compared with imagination. *Exp. Brain Res.* 112: 103–111.

Greenfield, P. M. (1991). Language, tools and brain: The ontogeny and phylogeny of hierarchically organized sequential behavior. *Behav. Brain Sci.* 14: 531–595.

Grezes, J., and Decety, J. (2001). Functional anatomy of execution, mental simulation, observation, and verb generation of actions: A meta-analysis. *Hum. Brain Mapp.* 12: 1–19.

Grezes, J., Costes, N., and Decety, J. (1998). Top-down effect of strategy on the perception of human biological motion: A PET investigation. *Cogn. Neuropsychol.* 15: 553–582.

Hari, R., Forss, N., Avikainen, S., Kirveskari, E., Salenius, S., and Rizzolatti, G. (1998). Activation of human primary motor cortex during action observation: a neuromagnetic study. *Proc. Natl. Acad. Sci. U. S. A.* 95: 15061–15065.

Haugeland, J. (1997). What is mind design? In *Mind Design II*, J. Haugeland (ed.). Cambridge, Mass.: MIT Press, pp. 1–28.

Heidegger, M. (1927). *Being and Time*. New York: Harper and Row.

Heilman, K. M., and Valenstein, E. (1993). *Clinical Neuropsychology*. New York: Oxford University Press.

Heiser, M., Iacoboni, M., Maeda, F., Marcus, J., and Mazziotta, J. C. (2003). The essential role of Broca's area in imitation. *Eur. J. Neurosci.*, in press.

Heyes, C. (2001). Causes and consequences of imitation. *Trends Cogn. Sci.* 5: 253–261.

Hoffman, E. A., and Haxby, J. (2000). Distinct representations of eye gaze and identity in the distributed human neural system for face perception. *Nat. Neurosci.* 3: 80–84.

Iacoboni, M. (2001). Playing tennis with the cerebellum. *Nat. Neurosci.* 4: 555–556.

Iacoboni, M., Woods, R. P., Brass, M., Bekkering, H., Mazziotta, J. C., and Rizzolatti, G. (1999). Cortical mechanisms of human imitation. *Science* 286: 2526–2528.

Iacoboni, M., Woods, R. P., Brass, M., Bekkering, H., Mazziotta, J. C., and Rizzolatti, G. (2000). Mirror properties in a sulcus angularis area. *NeuroImage* 5: S821.

Iacoboni, M., Koski, L., Brass, M., Bekkering, H., Woods, R. P., Dubea, M.-C., Mazziotta, J. C., and Rizzolatti, G. (2001). Re-afferent copies of imitated actions in the right superior temporal cortex. *Proc. Natl. Acad. Sci. U. S. A.* 98: 13995–13999.

Imamizu, H., Miyauchi, S., Tamada, T., Sasaki, Y., Takino, R., Putz, B. et al. (2000). Human cerebellar activity reflecting an acquired internal model of a new tool. *Nature* 403: 192–195.

Jeannerod, M. (1994). The representing brain: Neural correlates of motor intention and imagery. *Behav. Brain Sci.* 17: 187–245.

Jeannerod, M. (1999). To act or not to act: Perspectives on the representation of actions. *Q. J. Exp. Psychol.* 52A: 1–29.

Kawato, M. (1999). Internal models for motor control and trajectory planning. *Curr. Opin. Neurobiol.* 9: 718–727.

Kephart, N. C. (1971). The slow learner in the classroom. Columbus, Oh.: Merrill.

Koski, L., Wohlschläger, A., Bekkering, H., Woods, R. P., Dubeau M.-C., Mazziotta, J. C., and Iacoboni, M. (2002). Modulation of motor and premotor activity during imitation of target-directed actions. *Cereb. Cortex* 12: 847–855.

Koski, L. M., Iacoboni, M., Dubeau, M.-C., Woods, R. P., and Mazziotta, J. C. (2003). Modulation of cortical activity during different imitative behaviors. *J. Neurophysiol.* 89: 460–471.

Krams, M., Rushworth, M. F. S., Deiber, M.-P., Frackowiak, R. S. J., and Passingham, R. E. (1998). The preparation, execution, and suppression of copied movements in the human brain. *Exp. Brain Res.* 120: 386–398.

Logothetis, N. K., Pauls, J., Augath, M., Trinath, T., and Oeltermann, A. (2001). Neurophysiological investigation of the basis of the fMRI signal. *Nature* 12: 150–157.

Meltzoff, A. N., and Brooks, R. (2001). "Like me" as a building block for understanding other minds: Bodily acts, attention, and intention. In *Intentions and Intentionality: Foundations of Social Cognition*, B. F. Malle, L. J. Moses, and D. A. Baldwin (eds.). Cambridge, Mass.: MIT Press.

Meltzoff, A. N., and Moore, M. K. (1977). Imitation of facial and manual gestures by human neonates. *Science* 198: 74–78.

Merleau-Ponty, M. (1945). *Phenomenology of Perception*. London: Routledge.

Molnar-Szakacs, I., Iacoboni, M., Koski, L. M., Maeda, F., Dubeau, M.-C., Aziz-Zadeh, L., and Mazziotta, J. C. (2002). Action observation in the pars opercularis: Evidence from 58 subjects studied with fMRI. *J. Cog. Neurosci. Suppl.* S: F118.

Mountcastle, V., Lynch, J., Georgopoulos, A., Sakata, H., and Acuna, C. (1975). Posterior parietal association cortex of the monkey: Command functions for operations within extrapersonal space. *J. Neurophysiol.* 38: 871–908.

Mussa-Ivaldi, F. A., Giszter, S., and Bizzi, E. (1994). Linear combinations of primitives in vertebrate motor control. *Proc. Natl. Acad. Sci. U. S. A.* 91: 7534–7538.

Nishitani, N., and Hari, R. (2000). Temporal dynamics of cortical representation for action. *Proc. Natl. Acad. Sci. U. S. A.* 97: 913–918.

Parsons, L. M., Fox, P. T., Downs, J. H., Glass, T., Hirsch, T. B., Martin, C. C., et al. (1995). Use of implicit motor imagery for visual shape discrimination as revealed by PET. *Nature* 375: 54–58.

Passingham, R. E. (1993). *The Frontal Lobes and Voluntary Action*. New York: Oxford University Press.

Perrett, D. I., and Emery, N. J. (1994). Understanding the intentions of others from visual signals: Neurophysiological evidence. *Curr. Psychol. Cogn.* 13: 683–694.

Perrett, D. I., Harries, M. H., Bevan, R., Thomas, S., Benson, P. J., Mistlin, A. J., et al. (1989). Frameworks of analysis for the neural representation of animate objects and actions. *J. Exp. Biol.* 146: 87–113.

Perrett, D. I., Harries, M. H., Mistlin, A. J., Hietanen, J. K., Benson, P. J., Bevan, R., et al. (1990). Social signals analyzed at the single cell level: Someone is looking at me, something touched me, something moved! *Int. J. Comp. Psychol.* 4: 25–55.

Petrides, M., and Pandya, D. N. (1994). Comparative architectonic analysis of the human and the macaque frontal cortex. In *Handbook of Neuropsychology*, Vol. 9, F. Boller and J. Grafman (eds.). Amsterdam: Elsevier, pp. 17–58.

Preston, S. D., and deWaal, F. B. M. (2002). Empathy: Its ultimate and proximate bases. *Behav. Brain Sci.* 25: 1–72.

Preuss, T., Stepniewska, I., and Kaas, J. (1996). Movement representation in the dorsal and ventral premotor areas of owl monkeys: A microstimulation study. *J. Comp. Neurol.* 371: 649–676.

Puce, A., Allison, T., Bentin, S., Gore, J. C., and McCarthy, G. (1998). Temporal cortex activation in humans viewing eye and mouth movements. *J. Neurosci.* 18: 2188–2199.

Pylishin, Z. W. (1984). *Computation and Cognition: Toward a Foundation for Cognitive Science.* Cambridge, Mass.: MIT Press.

Rizzolatti, G., Fadiga, L., Gallese, V., and Fogassi, L. (1996a). Premotor cortex and the recognition of motor actions. *Cogn. Brain Res.* 3: 131–141.

Rizzolatti, G., Fadiga, L., Matelli, M., Bettinardi, V., Paulesu, E., Perani, D., et al. (1996b). Localization of grasp representations in humans by PET: 1. Observation versus execution. *Exp. Brain Res.* 111: 246–252.

Schofield, W. N. (1976). Do children find movements which cross the body midline difficult? *Q. J. Exp. Psychol.* 28: 571–582.

Strafella, A. P., and Paus, T.(2000). Modulation of cortical excitability during action observation: A transcranial magnetic stimulation study. *NeuroReport* 11: 2289–2292.

Tomasello, M., Kruger, A. C., and Ratner, H. H. (1993). Cultural learning. *Behav. Brain Sci.* 16: 495–552.

Tresch, M. C., Saltiel, P., and Bizzi, E. (1999). The construction of movement by the spinal cord. *Nat. Neurosci.* 2: 162–167.

Whiten, A. (2000). Primate culture and social learning. *Cogn. Sci.* 24: 477–508.

Whiten, A., and Brown, J. D. (1999). Imitation and the reading of other minds: Perspectives from the study of autism, normal children and non-human primates. In *Intersubjective Communication and Emotion in Early Ontogeny*, S. Braten (ed.). Cambridge: Cambridge University Press, pp. 260–280.

Whiten, A., Goodall, J., McGrew, W. C., Nishida, T., Reynolds, V., Sugiyama, Y., et al. (1999). Cultures in chimpanzees. *Nature* 399: 682–685.

Wohlschläger, A., and Bekkering, H. (2002). Is human imitation based on a mirror-neuron system? Some behavioural evidence. *Exp. Brain Res.* 143: 335–341.

Wolpert, D. M., and Kawato, M. (1998). Multiple paired forward and inverse models for motor control. *Neural Networks* 11: 1317–1329.

Wolpert, D. M., Miall, R. C., and Kawato, M. (1998). Internal models in the cerebellum. *Trends Cogn. Sci.* 2: 338–347.

5

Simulation of Action as a Unifying Concept for Motor Cognition

Marc Jeannerod

5.1 Action as a Goal-Directed Process

In the last decade, the methodology for studying mental states having no overt behavioral correlates has become firmly established. Combining introspection with brain mapping techniques has given neuroscientists experimental access to how the brain represents itself to itself (see Jeannerod, 1994).

To conceive of an action without the overt behavior attached to it, and without the interactions with the external environment that such behavior normally produces, presents special difficulties: One must have recourse to concepts beyond the realm of physiology. One must realize that actions are also autonomous constructs, that they may have no immediate relationship to external events, and that they cannot be considered as mere reactions to stimuli and responses to external events. Only then does it become possible to define covert actions and bring them under experimental scrutiny.

A major improvement in this regard was the introduction of "goal-directedness" as a primary constituent of action. To consider the generation of an action to be goal directed implies that the responsible mechanism must represent, not only the present state of the action generation system, but also its future state after the action has been executed. In other words, this representation must include the goal of the action, the means to reach it, and the consequences of achieving it on the environment and on the organism itself. How this mechanism can be conceived has been the subject of several influential hypotheses. The general idea is that neural signals are derived from the central commands for the action (the well-known corollary discharge or efference copy), with the function of influencing other levels of the nervous system. Because these signals are generated before the effectors are actuated (and often when no action is actually produced), their influence is exerted in anticipation of the action itself. As originally proposed by MacKay (1966), one of the main roles for such signals would be to provide cues for evaluating the effects of a movement. In a similar but more detailed hypothesis advanced by Wolpert and colleagues (1995), the brain builds an internal model of the action, which it uses to simulate the effects of the action. This simulation involves comparing the central command signals generated by the model with simulated reafferent signals that would result from potential execution. In other words, this hypothesis accounts for an entirely covert functioning of the action representation.

Most of the neural events leading to an overt action already seem to be present in the covert stages of that action. One might even contend that a covert action involves everything involved in an overt action except for the muscular contractions and the joint rotations. But such a contention would be factually incorrect: The musculo-articular events associated with an actual movement generate a flow of reafferent signals not present as such in a covert action. On the other hand, according to the simulation hypothesis of Wolpert and colleagues, the reafferent signals might also be simulated, just as the motor commands are. Their hypothesis, which is also the one advanced in this chapter, thus postulates that covert actions are actions in their own right, albeit not executed actions. Covert and overt stages represent a continuum, such that every overtly executed action implies the existence of a covert stage, whereas a covert action does not necessarily turn into an overt action. The hypothesis therefore predicts an identity, in neural terms, of the state where an action is simulated and the state immediately preceding execution of that action. The term *S-state* (where "S" stands for "simulation") will be used throughout this chapter to designate any mental state involving an action content, where brain activity can be shown to mimic or simulate what is overtly observed when that action is executed.

5.2   Covert Actions Are Simulated Actions

The idea that certain cognitive states correspond to simulated actions is by no means new. William James (1890, volume 2, p. 526) assessed that "every representation of a movement awakens in some degree the actual movement which is its object." Here we consider the term *representation* in a somewhat broader sense than James did so as to include the many situations that correspond to covert actions (see table 5.1). Some of these S-states are

Table 5.1
Taxonomy of behaviorally defined S-states

Type of S-state	Degree of awareness
Intended action	Conscious/nonconscious
Imagined action	Conscious
Prospective action judgments	Nonconscious
Perceptually based decisions	Nonconscious
Observation of graspable objects	Nonconscious
Observation of actions performed by others	Conscious/nonconscious
Action in dreams	Conscious

elicited from within (endogenously); some are elicited from outside. Some are accompanied by conscious experience; some are not. Despite their differences, all these states bear the same relationship to action, at both behavioral and neural levels. This section presents a behavioral description of the main aspects of covert actions.

Imagined Actions

Interest in mental imagery dates back to studies of hypnosis more than a century ago. To explain hypnotic phenomena, researchers (e.g., Binet, 1886) claimed that mental images of a sensation resulted from excitation of the same cerebral centers excited by the actual sensation. In the domain of motor images, they determined that the state of the motor centers influenced the possibility of generating a motor image showing, for example, that it was impossible to generate the image of pronouncing the letter *b* if one kept the mouth wide open: because the motor system could not engage in two contradictory actions at the same time (Stricker, as cited in Binet, 1886, p. 80).

Imagined actions or motor images have become a major tool for the study of representational aspects of action. Until quite recently, however, the field of motor imagery has developed far less than that of visual imagery, perhaps because, unlike visual images, motor images have no clear reference to which they can be compared: They are private events that can hardly be shared, if at all, by the experimenter. Among the most impressive behavioral findings of motor imagery studies is the fact that motor images and the executed actions to which they correspond share the same temporal characteristics. To cite two examples, it takes the same time mentally as it does actually to walk to a given place (Decety et al., 1989); mental and actual reciprocal tapping on targets of varying size observe the same temporal constraints (e.g., Fitts's law; Sirigu et al., 1996).

Likewise, subjects asked to make a perceptually based "motor" decision must covertly simulate the appropriate action in order to give the correct response. When they are asked, for example, to estimate the feasibility of grasping an object placed at different orientations, the time they take to respond is a function of the object's orientation, suggesting that they must first orient their arm mentally in an appropriate way. Indeed, the time to make this estimate closely corresponds to the time taken to actually reach to and grasp an object placed at the same orientation (Frak et al., 2001; for an extensive analysis of prospective judgments and their timing in a mental grasping task, see Johnson, 2000a). Similarly, Parsons (1994) found that, when subjects are presented with the picture of a hand at a given orientation, the time it takes them to determine its side is close to the time it takes them to actually achieve that orientation. This result suggests, first, that the perceptual decision requires a nonconscious process of mental simulation of hand position; and, second, that mental rotation of the hand is constrained by the biomechanics of the hand as a body part. (Not surprisingly, prospective judgments about geometrical objects have no such constraints; see Kosslyn et al., 1998.)

Another situation relevant to the concept of perceptually based "motor" decisions, viewing graspable objects and tools or even pictures of them (but not of other object types, such as a house or a car) elicits in the observer the covert action of using them. Here again, the timing of such covert action is subject to the biomechanical constraints of actually moving the object to achieve the depicted orientation (e.g., de Sperati and Stucchi, 1997). (Compulsive use of tools by certain pathological subjects suggests that the internal processing is directly transferred into execution, presenting strong homologies with compulsive imitation of actions, to which we will return.) Thus, motor imagery and its companion S-states, like perceptually based motor decisions are among the first situations for which it was specifically proposed that they should involve neural mechanisms in the motor brain similar to those operating during overt actions (see Jeannerod, 1994, 1997; Jeannerod and Frak, 1999).

Action Observation

Also relevant to the concept of S-states are covert actions elicited by observing the overt actions of others. To observe such actions with the purpose of understanding them or the intention behind them is by no means a passive process. However self-evident that statement may seem today, it was the subject of considerable analysis by philosophers and psychologists in the late nineteenth century. Among the several key concepts they elaborated is that of *empathy* (coined by Titchener as a translation of the German word *Einfühlung*). First used in the context of aesthetics, the concept of empathy was introduced in psychology by Theodor Lipps in an attempt to explain how we discover that other people have selves. He considered empathy to be the source of our knowledge about other individuals, just as sensory perception is the source of our knowledge about objects. According to Lipps (1903, p. 193; see also Pigman, 1995), we understand others' facial expressions, say, not because we compare them with our own, which we normally cannot see, but because seeing an expression on the face of someone else "awakens [in us] impulses to such movements that are suited to call just this expression into existence."

At present, empathy and its behavioral consequences are taken as roughly equivalent to *mind reading*, the ability of normal people to understand and predict the behavior of others. One of the recent explanations proposed for mind reading, quite reminiscent of Lipps's thinking, is that it represents an attempt to replicate and simulate the mental activity of the other agent. Thus the observed action activates the same mechanisms in the observer's brain that would be activated were the observer to intend or imagine that action. Or, as Gallese and Goldman (1998, p. 498) have put it, "when one is observing the action of another, one undergoes a neural event that is qualitatively the same as [the] event that triggers actual movement in the observed agent"; as a "mind reader," one "represents an actor's behavior by recreating in [oneself] the plans or movement intentions of the actor." The function of representing to oneself actions observed in others is primarily to process and exploit biological signals generated during interactions with them, signals critical for social communication.

Besides the social or intentional content of observing an action (What does it mean?), there is also its technical content (How is it done?). Think, for example, of the everyday experience of watching someone show another how to do something. Indeed, the simulation hypothesis predicts that, if the motor brain is rehearsed during action observation (as is indeed the case), the observed action should be facilitated when the observer attempts to replicate it, a straightforward basis for the form of learning called "observational learning." In the same vein, a second hypothesis, called the "motor theory of perception" (Liberman and Mattingly, 1985) and used as a framework for speech perception, postulates that we understand speech to the extent that we covertly simulate the corresponding speech movements.

Another concept, also developed during the nineteenth century, is that of *ideomotor action* (Lotze, 1852), which, at least in its narrow sense, accounts for the familiar observation that people tend to perform the movements they see, especially in situations where the observer feels strongly involved (a sports fan watching a game, for example). Thus empathy and ideomotor action seem to be complementary concepts. Empathy has us understand an observed action, not through perception, but through (normally covert) activation of the same mechanisms that would reproduce in us the action we are observing. By contrast, ideomotor action induces us (whether through perception or otherwise) to perform the action we are observing. Is ideomotor action based on the same mechanism as empathy, then (granted that action tends to become overt in the former, but not in the latter)? It is tempting to consider ideomotor action simply an exaggeration of empathy, whereby motor output, in principle blocked in S-states, becomes too strong to be controlled by the usual inhibitory mechanisms (see below). This possibility is potentially of great interest, accounting at once for empathy, ideomotor action, and imitation.

Or is ideomotor action instead a direct mapping of perceived movements onto the corresponding motor output? This possibility may sound familiar to adherents of "direct perception–action transformation" heralded by the Gibsonian school (see review in Jeannerod, 1993). It has been used, not only to explain interactions with the visual environment (such as steering locomotion, avoiding obstacles, or maintaining posture), but also to account for relationships between selves (Neisser, 1993). In this conception, ideomotor action represents a form of compulsive imitation where subjects cannot refrain from reproducing the perceived performance. Examples of this sort are contagious yawning or laughing, and perhaps also resonant behavior in animals, such as wing flapping in bird flocks. True imitation, by contrast, would not be temporally bound to the observed action, and could thus be delayed (see below). If ideomotor action were compulsive imitation, the ideomotor mechanism would depart from the general concept of S-states in at least two related respects: First, it would drive to "automatic" execution of the observed action, without the possibility of a covert stage; second, it would bypass the representational stages of S-states, which include levels of processing of the observed action not directly related to execution.

The two mechanisms may indeed coexist. Empathy, as a mechanism operating at the representational stages of action, including representation of other people's mental states, may be connected with the internal state of the observer, in continuity with other S-states, such as intentions or imagined actions. By contrast, ideomotor action, as a mechanism for immediate action, may bypass the representational stages under the direct influence of the environment, which would account for the inability of patients with frontal lesions to resist undertaking action induced by incoming events, even in neutral situations, hence their distractibility (see below).

5.3 Neurophysiological Validation of the Simulation Hypothesis

That S-states have many features in common with their overt counterparts does not in itself make them covert actions. Another important condition must be fulfilled, namely, the motor system must be activated during S-states. Researchers have found this to be the case. Early work by Ingvar and Philipsson (1977) measuring local cerebral blood flow with xenon-133 showed that "pure motor ideation" (e.g., thinking of rhythmic clenching movements) produced a marked frontal activation and a more limited activation in the Rolandic area. Roland and colleagues (1980) also found motor activation during imagined movements. This section will review the functional anatomy of S-states by mapping the anatomical locations found to be involved during those states from positron-emission tomography (PET) and functional magnetic resonance imaging (fMRI) data in human subjects. As can be seen in table 5.2 (for a more detailed overview of the same data, see Grèzes and Decety, 2001; see also Jeannerod, 1999), the activation network differs from one S-state to another, and from covert to overt actions, although networks corresponding to different conditions also overlap significantly. In other words, each S-state retains its own specific network, but there is a core network that pertains to all S-states.

Motor System

The most appropriate site of activity for testing the simulation hypothesis is of course the motor system itself. We will successively examine changes in primary motor cortex (M1) and the corticospinal tract, in subcortical motor structures (cerebellum and basal ganglia), and finally in premotor cortex and the supplementary motor area (SMA).

Table 5.2
Brain areas activated during S-states

Brain regions and Brodmann areas (BAs)	Conditions				
	Execute	Intend	Imagine	Observe actions	Observe objects
Precentral gyrus, BA 4	4,8,10,12,13		9,10,13	15	
Precentral gyrus dorsal BA 6	1,8,10,14		4,8,9,10,14	5,9	
Precentral gyrus ventral BA 6	1,14		4,14	2,5	3
Supplementary motor area rostral BA 6	6,10,13		8,9,10	5,9	
Cingular gyrus, BA 24	1,8,10,12,14	7	4,8,10,14		
Superior frontal gyrus, BA 10			4,8		
Middle frontal gyrus, BAs 9,46		7	4,8,9	5	
Inferior frontal gyrus, BAs 44,45			4,8,9	2,5,9,12	11
Inferior parietal lobule, BA 40	1,6,10,12,14		4,8,9,14	2,5,9	3

Note: Numbers in the table refer to the following studies documenting activation in a given area for a given condition: 1 = Binkofski et al., 1999; 2 = Buccino et al., 2001; 3 = Chao and Martin, 2000; 4 = Decety et al., 1994; 5 = Decety et al., 1997; 6 = Faillenot et al., 1997; 7 = Frith et al., 1991; 8 = Gerardin et al., 2000; 9 = Grafton et al., 1996; 10 = Lotze et al., 1999; 11 = Perani et al., 1995; 12 = Rizzolatti et al., 1996; 13 = Roth et al., 1996; 14 = Stephan et al., 1995; 15 = Hari et al., 1998.

Primary Motor Cortex As fMRI studies unambiguously demonstrate, areas activated during contraction of a group of muscles (the intrinsic hand muscles, for example) are also activated during imagery of a movement involving the same muscles (Roth et al., 1996). Porro and colleagues (1996) carefully demonstrated that fMRI signal intensity in primary motor cortex and in the posterior precentral gyrus was greater during two "motor" tasks, motor performance and motor imagery of repetitive finger opposition movements, than during a control task (visual imagery). They were also able to determine that areas activated during both motor performance and motor imagery represent a large fraction of all areas activated during motor performance (see also Lotze et al., 1999). Primary motor cortex activation during motor imagery is only 30% as strong as that during execution and may not be found in all subjects (indeed, it was found in only 4 of 8 subjects in Gérardin et al., 2000). Experiments using quantified electroencephalography and neuromagnetic techniques have confirmed these data (see Schnitzler et al., 1997). Similarly, during action observation, magnetoencephalography reveals a significant activation at the level of precentral motor cortex (Hari et al., 1998). That motor cortex activation during S-states might correspond to muscular contractions seems to be ruled out by the finding that activation was present during imaginary finger tapping movements in the left motor cortex in a man who had his right hand amputated (Ersland et al., 1996).

Corticospinal Pathway   A logical consequence of increased motor cortex excitability is that it should propagate down to the motoneuron level. This point was tested by directly measuring corticospinal excitability. Transcranial magnetic stimulation (TMS) of motor cortex was used to trigger motor evoked potentials (MEPs) in arm muscles during both observed and imagined arm movements (Fadiga et al., 1995 and 1999, respectively; see also Strafella and Paus, 2000). MEPs were found to be increased, but only in that or those muscles involved in the covert hand action. Accordingly, MEPs were selectively increased in a wrist flexor when the subject mentally activated wrist flexion, whereas MEPs in the antagonist extensor muscle remained unchanged. In addition, other types of imagery (e.g., visual) did not affect MEPs in any of the recorded muscles, although, as we will see, whether this increased excitability also affects the motoneuron level is still a controversial issue.

A closely related aspect of the motor system's generation of motor outflow is the concomitant activation of the vegetative system. Sympathetic outflow increases both during motor preparation (e.g., Krogh and Lindhard, 1913), and during motor exercise, an effect shown to be of a central origin (Vissing and Hjortso, 1996). Accordingly, an increase in heart rate during imagined movements has been observed by several authors (Decety et al., 1993; Oishi et al., 1994). Control of blood aeration and respiration rates also seems to be included among central commands generated by the motor system at the time of preparation to action. Indeed, volitional control of respiration activates areas involved in motor control, including primary motor cortex (Colebatch et al., 1991). Respiration rate is increased during imagination of exercise, and the increase is proportional to the imagined effort (Decety et al., 1993; Wuyam et al., 1995). A similar finding was made when subjects simply observed a runner on a treadmill: The respiration rate of the observers increased with the speed of the runner (Paccalin and Jeannerod, 2000). These findings stress a common property of covert actions and preparation of overt actions when metabolic changes due to muscular activity are anticipated.

Basal Ganglia   Decety and colleagues (1994) found that basal ganglia are activated during imagined actions. There are indications that execution and imagination engage different parts of the striatum (Gérardin et al., 2000). During execution, the putamen, which belongs to a sensorimotor cortico-cortical loop, is activated, whereas, during imagination, it is the head of the caudate, which belongs to a more cognitive loop.

Cerebellum   Activation of the cerebellum during covert actions is congruent with activation of the corticospinal system, if one considers the close functional linkage of the two systems during motor execution. Indeed, cerebellar activation was clearly found in imagined action (Ryding et al., 1993), in perceptually based motor decisions (Parsons et al., 1995), and during action observation (Grafton et al., 1996). The area involved, which includes both the medial and the lateral cerebellum, is more marked on the side ipsilateral to the limb involved in the covert action.

   A careful comparison of cerebellar activation during imagined and executed movements (Lotze et al., 1999) revealed that areas in the ipsilateral cerebellar hemisphere that are activated during execution (in the anterior lobe) are much less activated, if at all, during imagination. By contrast, imagined action (as well as observed action; Grafton et al., 1996) activates areas more posterior to these. This difference in activated areas might correspond to motor suppression during covert action (see below).

Premotor Cortex   Activation of premotor cortex is one of the most conspicuous findings across all S-states (see Table 5.2). Decety and colleagues (1994) found a large activation of the dorsal and ventral parts of lateral Brodmann area (BA) 6, and associated activation of neighboring BAs 44–45 during imagined hand movements. Their findings were subsequently replicated in studies dealing with imagined movements (Stephan et al., 1995; Grafton et al., 1996; Gérardin et al., 2000), with perceptually based motor decisions (Parsons et al., 1995; Kosslyn et al., 1998), and with visual presentation of graspable objects (Chao and Martin, 2000). During observation of hand movements, the same areas, principally in ventral area 6, were also found to be activated (Rizzolatti et al., 1996; Grafton et al., 1996; Decety et al., 1997; Iacoboni et al., 1999). More recently, Buccino and colleagues (2001) found that the anatomical location of this activation changed with the somatotopy of the observed movement: Activation was more ventral when observing mouth movements and more dorsal when observing hand and foot movements. Activation of lateral premotor cortex during covert actions was found to overlap extensively with activation of dorsal BA 6 during movement execution (Lotze et al., 1999; Gérardin et al., 2000; Rizzolatti et al., 1996). Moreover, the degree of activation (number of activated pixels) was found to be similar for covert and overt actions (Roth et al., 1996; Lotze et al., 1999). Activation of ventral BA 6 in the inferior frontal gyrus, however, so clearly found in covert action conditions, is less frequently mentioned during execution (e.g., by Binkofski et al., 1999, who observed activation of the ventral premotor area during a task of object manipulation).

The same degree of overlap between covert and overt action conditions exists for the SMA, whose activation has generally been found to be more rostral during imagined and observed movements than during executed movements (e.g., Stephan, 1995; Grafton, 1996; Lotze, 1999; Gérardin et al., 2000), although the active zones during S-states and action execution partially overlap. The function of the SMA, which acts as a parser for temporally segmenting the action and anticipating its successive steps, is thus retained during S-states.

Associative Cortical Areas

Parietal Cortex   Activation of areas caudal and ventral to the primary parietal cortex has been consistently observed during S-states. Areas in the inferior parietal lobule and in the intraparietal sulcus are activated during imagined grasping movements (Decety et al., 1994; Grafton et al., 1996), during perceptually based decisions (Parsons et al., 1995; Kosslyn et al., 1998), during action observation (Buccino et al., 2001; Grafton et al., 1996), and during visual presentation of graspable objects (Chao and Martin, 2000). It is worth mentioning that, in association with dorsal premotor cortex, this parietal area represents the cortical network for visuomotor transformation during the action of reaching toward objects (e.g., Faillenot et al., 1997). The results are less consistent for execution of grasping movements, where, according to monkey studies, one should expect a joint activation of posterior parietal cortex and ventral premotor cortex (see Jeannerod et al., 1995), but where, as mentioned previously, ventral BA 6 is activated only in some studies (e.g., Binkofski et al., 1999). Except for this latter point, the activation data in parietal cortex add to the evidence of an overlap between networks for covert and overt hand movements, which is indeed consistent with the finding that the networks overlap only partially (Gérardin et al., 2000).

Posterior parietal cortex (PPC) may be the site where action representations are stored, generated, or both. Because it integrates abundant visual and somatosensory information, PPC appears well suited for encoding the technical aspects of the action, such as transforming object spatial coordinates from a retinocentric framework into an egocentric framework or processing constraints related to the objects of the action. These aspects are present in many different S-states.

Prefrontal Cortex   Activation of prefrontal granular cortex occurs in most S-states, usually involving areas in the dorsolateral part (BAs 9 and 46), in the orbitofrontal zone (BAs 10 and 11), in the cingular gyrus, and in a ventral and caudal zone (BAs 44-45), which seem to be in continuity with the agranular zone of ventral BA 6 (Iacoboni et al., 1999). Dorsolateral prefrontal cortex is also typically activated during preparation states, when a decision has to be made about which finger to move (Frith et al., 1991) or when to start a movement. By contrast, prefrontal activation is far less marked during action execution. That activation of the prefrontal cortex seems to be limited to the covert stages of action suggests that this brain region may intervene in the simulation process itself, for example, by holding the goal of the action in a dedicated working memory.

The Problem of Execution Inhibition

The simulation hypothesis is faced with a difficult problem: How is it that covert actions, despite activation of the motor system, do not result in muscular activity? Although early studies (e.g., Jacobson, 1930) often reported electromyographic (EMG) activity during motor imagery, recent studies have observed no such activity in the relevant muscles during S-states.

There are two possible and perhaps complementary explanations for this absence of motor output. First, motor activation during S-states might be subliminal, thus insufficient to fire spinal motoneurons. Activation of primary motor cortex (M1) during an imagined movement, for example, is limited to about 30% of what is observed during effective muscular contraction for that same movement. Subjects engaged in covert actions might also voluntarily calibrate a level of pyramidal activity below the motoneuron recruitment threshold. And second, motor output might be blocked before it reaches the motoneuron level by an inhibitory mechanism generated in parallel to the motor activation. That motor cortex remains activated during S-states excludes an inhibitory role of corticocortical connections (e.g., at the premotor level); indeed, if this were the case, *no* activity would be found in primary motor cortex. To account for the data, the inhibitory mechanism must therefore operate downstream of motor cortex, for example, by blocking the descending corticospinal volleys at the level of the spinal cord or brain stem.

Data on spinal reflexes during S-states suggest just such a possibility. Bonnet and colleagues (1997) found increased spinal reflexes during mentally simulated isometric foot pressure, with T-reflexes increasing more markedly than H-reflexes. Oishi and colleagues (1994) found decreased H-reflexes in elite athletes, whereas Hashimoto and Rothwell (1999) found no significant increase in upper-limb H-reflexes during simulated wrist movements. In none of these studies was a significant increase in EMG activity observed in the muscles involved during covert action. Finally, studying H-reflexes in the upper limbs during action observation, Baldissera and colleagues (2001) found a subliminal activation of the motoneuron level during finger flexion or extension, although the pattern of activation appeared to be reversed with respect to that observed during imagined action: Flexor motoneurons were facilitated during extension and vice versa.

What emerges from these conflicting results is that motoneuron excitability is affected during action simulation. Different testing conditions (e.g., lower limbs versus upper limbs; trained athletes versus nonathletes) may account for the different amplitudes and directions of these changes. A tentative explanation for the observed patterns of motoneuron excitability could be that a dual mechanism operates at the spinal level: increased corticospinal tract activity governing a subthreshold preparation for overt movement and inhibitory influences governing a parallel suppression of overt movement. A similar explanation was put forward by Prut and Fetz (1999) to account for the early premovement activity in many motor structures of the monkey brain, including spinal interneurons, during an instructed delay period before a movement occurs.

5.4   Effects of Brain Lesions on S-States

Alteration of the simulation network by lesions may impair one or another aspect of motor cognition. Several conditions may be distinguished, whether the lesion affects the network at the output level (e.g., the motor system itself) or upstream of the motor system. The simulation hypothesis predicts that lesions affecting the motor system should impair the expression of all S-states, but should leave their content intact. By contrast, lesions affecting structures located upstream of the motor system should specifically affect the ability to produce a given S-state. Although data are still insufficient to confirm these predictions, as we will see, they tend to converge in the expected direction.

Lesions of the Motor System

Decety and Boisson (1990) and Sirigu and colleagues (1995) both reported that hemiplegic patients were still able to generate imagined movements with their affected limb. When tested with the mental reciprocal task described above, Sirigu and colleagues' patient showed the same regularities (e.g., Fitts's law) with both her normal and her affected hand. In these studies, the only difference between the mental performance of the two hands was that the affected hand was slower than the normal one. Such a difference was even not noticed in another series of hemiplegic patients tested in the perceptually induced motor decision paradigm (Johnson, 2000b).

A closely similar finding was reported from a study (Dominey et al., 1995) of patients suffering a dysfunction of the basal ganglia (Parkinson's disease), with akinesia more severe on one side. It was found that patients were still able to generate the motor image of a sequential finger task, although their performance was asymmetrical, with the worst affected hand slower than the other one. A PET study of motor imagery involving the akinetic hand in such patients showed a lack of activation of primary motor cortex and cerebellum, with normal activation of the parietal cortex and SMA (Thobois et al., 2000).

Lesions Upstream of the Motor System

Perhaps more interesting to consider are lesions located upstream of the motor system, which should disrupt S-states in different ways depending on the type or location of the lesions.

Posterior Parietal Cortex Lesions   Several studies have reported disruption of motor representations following lesions of posterior parietal cortex. A patient with a unilateral parietal lesion, although able to actually perform the reciprocal tapping task with her contralateral hand, was unable to imagine performing it with that hand (Sirigu et al., 1996). Another patient with a unilateral parietal lesion showed marked deficits in motor imagery tasks, but none in visual imagery tasks, whereas a patient with a bilateral inferotemporal lesion showed the opposite deficits (Sirigu and Duhamel, 2001).

Patients who exhibit left hemispatial neglect from right parietal lesions exhibit representational neglect as well: They fail to imagine the left side of the visual scenes they evoke mentally (Bisiach and Luzatti, 1978; Rode and Perenin, 1994). Although not directly related to disorders in motor cognition as reported here, this finding suggests that the concept of S-states should be generalized to other aspects of cognition as well.

Patients with posterior parietal lesions may also present difficulties in tasks that require representing an action: They may be unable to recognize pantomimed actions, to pantomime actions involving an object or a tool, or to distinguish their own actions from those performed by other people (Sirigu et al., 1999). These impairments, which are part of the apraxia syndrome, clearly correspond to a lack of action representation and recognition, which in turn can be attributed to defective simulation of the action shown or requested by the experimenter. As already stated, one possible conclusion to be drawn from these findings is that posterior parietal cortex, which is consistently activated during S-states, might be the site where action representations are stored, generated, or both. This conclusion is consistent with the central location of posterior parietal areas within the simulation network: They are directly connected with premotor cortex, they are reciprocally connected with prefrontal areas, and they receive abundant information about visual and somatosensory processing.

Prefrontal Cortex Lesions   Not surprisingly, lesions affecting the prefrontal cortex also alter the functioning of the simulation network. A critical example of this alteration can be observed in patients with orbitofrontal lesions (Lhermitte, 1983; Shallice et al., 1989): They tend to compulsively imitate gestures or even complex actions performed in front of them by another agent; when presented with common graspable objects, they cannot refrain from using them. This striking *imitation* or *utilization behavior* arises from impairment of the normal suppression, by the prefrontal areas, of inappropriate motor schemas. It would be interesting to know how such patients would behave during imagined actions: It is likely that they would be unable to generate motor imagery without immediately transferring it into motor output.

The opposite effect was described in a patient with hysterical paralysis of the left side of the body (Marshall et al., 1997), whose brain metabolism was mapped using PET scans. Normal activation of the left sensorimotor cortex was observed when the patient moved her right, "good" leg, whereas no such activation was observed in the right hemisphere when she attempted to move her left, "bad" leg. Instead, the right anterior cingulate and the right orbitofrontal cortex were significantly activated in this condition (and in this condition alone), suggesting that these prefrontal areas exerted a state-dependent inhibition on the motor system when the patient formed the intention to move her left leg. Whether, as predicted, this patient is unable to experience motor imagery with her affected leg, but not with her normal one, remains to be tested.

These findings suggest a twofold role for prefrontal cortex during S-states. First, the orbitofrontal and cingular areas might exert an inhibitory influence on other cortical areas involved in S-states. It is known that prefrontal cortex tends to become more active when inappropriate responses have to be suppressed (e.g., Paus et al., 1993). Because prefrontal cortex is interconnected with many of the areas involved in S-states (such as the inferior parietal lobule or premotor cortex), it might shape the appropriate network by either slowing down or releasing the activity of these areas depending on the S-state in which the subject is engaged. Findings from the pathological cases discussed above tend to support this view, although the proposed selective inhibition exerted by prefrontal cortex should not be confounded with the more global descending inhibition of motor commands already described at the spinal level. Second, dorsolateral prefrontal cortex, in conjunction with the basal ganglia, might be involved in short-term storage of information needed for anticipating the action goal and simulating the action to its completion.

Mindful of the proposed inhibitory role of prefrontal cortex, let us revisit ideomotor action. As suggested previously, the lack of inhibition in such action might well release activity in parts of the motor system specialized in visuomotor processing, thus bringing about a transfer of visual input into motor output, as illustrated above by the patients with prefrontal lesions. A similar explanation might also account for the behavior of psychotic patients (see below).

5.5   Conclusion: The Role of Simulation in Motor Cognition

The pattern of results on the mechanisms of covert action corresponds to the central stages of action organization, uncontaminated by the effects of execution. As such, it represents an interesting framework for the many S-states that compose motor cognition. Activation during S-states of brain areas involved in execution of actions, and particularly activation of motor cortex itself, provides a rationale for endogenous states arising as cognitive constructs largely independent of external events, thus also for the study of various aspects of action representation, such as intention, that are built from within using resources from semantic and episodic memory and cannot be accessed by following the usual stimulus-response track.

The common network associated with S-states as described here thus defines an *action brain*, which includes, besides motor areas, prefrontal cortex and posterior parietal areas. Assuming that prefrontal functions such as working memory and anticipation are involved in the S-states' remaining covert, the main activation network common to all S-states includes posterior parietal, premotor, and motor cortices. This network closely resembles one described in monkey and human studies for execution of visually goal-directed movements (e.g., Jeannerod et al., 1995), and referred to as the "dorsal visual pathway," specialized to process action toward objects. Although the proximity of covert goal-directed actions with overt ones fits the general framework of the simulation hypothesis, it clearly departs from the postulated function of the dorsal visual pathway: The dorsal pathway is supposed to rapidly process action-related visual features of objects, with the objective of immediate action. According to the proponents of the dorsal visual pathway hypothesis (e.g., Milner and Goodale, 1995), delaying execution of a movement toward its goal changes the modalities of control of this movement: Instead of being controlled by the dorsal pathway, it becomes controlled by a slower and less accurate route through the ventral pathway. Covert actions, which are in principle delayed actions, clearly do not fit this hypothesis: No sign of involvement of the ventral pathway has ever been reported in activation studies reported here.

The Role of Motor Cortex in Self-Generated Covert Actions

Activation of the motor cortex and the descending motor pathway seems to fulfill several critical functions. First, it puts the represented action in a *motor format,* whereby the represented action acquires the characteristics of a performed action and constraints for execution are encoded. These constraints become indeed apparent in the study of motor images and other S-states, as shown in this chapter. Thus, for example, judging the feasibility of the action of accurately grasping a glass full of water requires a simulation of the action that accounts for the initial position of the arm, its biomechanical limitations, the degree of force to apply to the grasp, and so on. To encode these constraints in S-states, the neural structures where the constraints are represented (cerebellum, spinal cord, basal ganglia) might send corollary signals to areas such as parietal and premotor cortex. This mechanism would be appropriate for updating the internal model, where the consequences of the potentially executed action are evaluated (Wolpert et al., 1995).

Logically, this mechanism, where all aspects of the motor system appear to be functionally involved, should facilitate the subsequent execution. In point of fact, various degrees of *mental training* have been found to occur during S-states: Mentally rehearsing an action (in the context of playing a sport, for example) produces a benefit in terms of speed of execution, degree of coordination, and force, when that action comes to execution. Thus Pascual-Leone and colleagues (1995) found that repetition of a mental task (imagining finger tapping) over several days produces an enlargement of the motor cortex area where a transcranial magnetic stimulation triggers motor potentials in the (mentally) trained finger muscles. This enlargement is in the same proportion as that produced by training with actual finger tapping.

Similarly, mental simulation while observing another perform an action, because it rehearses the same brain structures as a self-generated action, should produce the same effect as mental training: It should facilitate execution of that action by the observer. And, indeed, the well-known effect of observational learning is a commonly observed basis for the acquisition of motor skills.

The Role of Motor Cortex Activation in Social Interactions

Another function of motor cortex activation during S-states might be to provide one with information for consciously monitoring one's own S-states. The problem here is how, in the absence of overt behavior, to get enough information to disentangle whether one is the agent of a given covert action. The similarity of the cortical networks for different S-states, and particularly those related to imagined and observed action, stresses the need for specific cues for each category of S-states. First, when it is associated with perception of an action performed by an external agent, for example, motor cortex activation does not have the same significance as when it is associated with an imagined action: In the former case, the co-occurrence of third-person (e.g., visual) signals provides cues for attributing the action to the other agent. In addition, however similar, the networks activated in the respective brains of two socially interacting persons do not overlap entirely: The existence of nonoverlapping parts (see table 5.2) allows each agent to discriminate what belongs to whom, and thus to determine who is the author of an action (Georgieff and Jeannerod, 1998).

Imitation is a case where the simulation of an observed action and the simulation of one's own action interfere with each other. Meltzoff (1995) showed, in 18-month-old children, that they reenact, not what the observed agent actually did, but what he intended to do. If, for example, children are shown an adult who tried, but failed, to touch a certain target, they subsequently execute the complete movement, not the failed attempt. Children can thus infer the adult's intended act. As proposed in section 5.1, imitation may result from a process close to that of empathy, whereby an observed action is understood and encoded by matching the observed action onto an internal simulation of that action (see Iacoboni et al., 1999).

Psychotic States

The simulation hypothesis has been recently introduced as a possible framework for understanding psychotic symptoms (Georgieff and Jeannerod, 1998). Many of these symptoms bear on disorders of social behavior, that is, they relate to how people understand and predict each other's behavior. If, as above, we assume that mutual understanding of an action is based on simulation of the observed action or of the intention behind it, then we can hypothesize about the nature of the dysfunction responsible for misattribution of actions by schizophrenic patients. Changes in the pattern of cortical connectivity might alter the shape of the networks depending on different representations or on the relative intensity of activation in the areas composing these networks. In verbal hallucinations, for example, activity in primary temporal cortex is abnormally increased, which makes the patient feel that his voices originate from outside (Dierks et al., 2000). Similarly, in the delusion of influence, posterior parietal activation is abnormally high, hence the experience of alien control (Spence et al., 1997). As Frith and colleagues (1995) suggest, prefrontal cortex may well be a source of this perturbed activation in psychotic patients during S-states.

References

Baldissera, F., Cavallari, P., Craighero, L., and Fadiga, L. (2001). Modulation of spinal excitability during observation of hand action in humans. *Eur. J. Neurosci.* 13: 190–194.

Binet, A. (1886). *La psychologie du raisonnement: Recherches expérimentales par l'hypnotisme.* Paris: Alcan.

Binkofski, F., Buccino, G., Posse, S., Seitz, R.J., Rizzolatti, G., and Freund, H. J. (1999). A fronto-parietal circuit for object manipulation in man. *Eur. J. Neurosci.* 11: 3276–3286.

Bisiach, E., and Luzzatti, C. (1978). Unilateral neglect of representational space. *Cortex* 14: 129–133.

Bonnet, M., Decety, J., Requin, J., and Jeannerod, M. (1997). Mental simulation of an action modulates the excitability of spinal reflex pathways in man. *Cogn. Brain Res.* 5: 221–228.

Buccino, G., Binkofski, F., Fink, G. R., Fadiga, L., Fogassi, L., Gallese, V., Seitz, R. J., Zilles, K., Rizzolatti, G., and Freund, H. J. (2001). Action observation activates premotor and parietal areas in a somatotopic manner: An fMRI study. *Eur. J. Neurosci.* 13: 400–404.

Chao, L. L., and Martin, A. (2000). Representation of manipulable man-made objects in the dorsal stream. *NeuroImage* 12: 478–494.

Colebatch, J. G., Deiber, M.-P., Passingham, R. E., Friston, K. J., and Frackowiak, R. S. J. (1991). Regional cerebral blood flow during voluntary arm and hand movements in human subjects. *J. Neurophysiol.* 65: 1392–1401.

Decety, J., and Boisson, D. (1990). Effect of brain and spinal cord injuries on motor imagery. *Eur. Arch. Psychiatry Clin. Neurosci.* 240: 39–43.

Decety, J., Jeannerod, M., and Prablanc, C. (1989). The timing of mentally represented actions. *Behav. Brain Res.* 34: 35–42.

Decety, J., Jeannerod, M., Durozard, D., and Baverel, G. (1993). Central activation of autonomic effectors during mental simulation of motor actions. *J. Physiol.* 461: 549–563.

Decety, J., Perani, D., Jeannerod, M., Bettinardi, V., Tadary, B., Woods, R., Mazziotta, J. C., and Fazio, F. (1994). Mapping motor representations with PET. *Nature* 371: 600–602.

Decety, J., Grèzes, J., Costes, N., Perani, D., Jeannerod, M., Procyk, E., Grassi, F., and Fazio, F. (1997). Brain activity during observation of action: Influence of action content and subject's strategy. *Brain* 120: 1763–1777.

Dierks, T., Linden, D. E. J., Jandl, M., Formisano, E., Goebel, R., Lanferman, H., and Singer, W. (1999). Activation of the Heschl's gyrus during auditory hallucinations. *Neuron* 22: 615–621.

de Sperati, C., and Stucchi, N. (1997). Recognizing the motion of a graspable object is guided by handedness. *NeuroReport* 8: 2761–2765.

Dominey, P., Decety, J., Broussolle, E., Chazot, G., and Jeannerod, M. (1995). Motor imagery of a lateralized sequential task is asymmetrically slowed in hemi-Parkinson patients. *Neuropsychologia* 33: 727–741.

Ersland, L., Rosen, G., Lundervold, A., Smievoll, A. I., Tillung, T., Sundberg, H., and Hughdahl, K. (1996). Phantom limb imaginary fingertapping causes primary motor cortex activation: An fMRI study. *NeuroReport* 8: 207–210.

Fadiga, L., Fogassi, L., Pavesi, G., and Rizzolatti, G. (1995). Motor facilitation during action observation: A magnetic stimulation study. *J. Neurophysiol.* 73: 2608–2611.

Fadiga, L., Buccino, G., Craighero, L., Fogassi, L., Gallese, V., and Pavesi, G. (1999). Corticospinal excitability is specifically modulated by motor imagery: A magnetic stimulation study. *Neuropsychologia* 37: 147–158.

Faillenot, I., Toni, I., Decety, J., Gregoire, M. C., and Jeannerod, M. (1997). Visual pathways for object-oriented action and object recognition: Functional anatomy with PET. *Cereb. Cortex* 7: 77–85.

Frak, V. G., Paulignan, Y., and Jeannerod, M. (2001). Orientation of the opposition axis in mentally simulated grasping. *Exp. Brain Res.* 136: 120–127.

Frith, C. D., Friston, K., Liddle, P. F., and Frackowiak, R. S. J. (1991). Willed action and the prefrontal cortex in man: A study with PET. *Proc. R. Soc. Lond. B Biol. Sci.* 244: 241–246.

Frith, C. D., Friston, K., Herold, S., Silbersweig, P., Fletcher, P., Cahill, C., Frackowiak, R. S. J., and Liddle, P. F. (1995). Regional brain activity in chronic schizophrenic patients during the performance of a verbal fluency task. *Br. J. Psychiatry* 167: 343–349.

Gallese, V., and Goldman, A. (1998). Mirror neurons and the simulation theory of mind reading. *Trends Cogn. Sci.* 2: 493–501.

Georgieff, N., and Jeannerod, M. (1998). Beyond consciousness of external reality: A "who" system for consciousness of action and self-consciousness. *Conscious. Cognit.* 7: 465–472.

Gérardin, E., Sirigu, A., Lehéricy, S., Poline, J.-B., Gaymard, B., Marsault, C., Agid, Y., and Le Bihan, D. (2000). Partially overlapping neural networks for real and imagined hand movements. *Cereb. Cortex* 10: 1093–1104.

Grafton, S. T., Arbib, M. A., Fadiga, L., and Rizzolatti, G. (1996). Localization of grasp representations in humans by positron emission tomography: 2. Observation compared with imagination. *Exp. Brain Res.* 112: 103–111.

Grèzes, J., and Decety, J. (2001). Functional anatomy of execution, mental simulation, observation, and verb generation of actions: A meta-analysis. *Hum. Brain Mapp.* 12: 1–19.

Hari, R., Forss, N., Avikainen, S., Kirveskari, E., Salenius, S., and Rizzolatti, G. (1998). Activation of human primary motor cortex during action observation: A neuromagnetic study. *Proc. Natl. Acad. U. S. A.* 95: 15061–15065.

Hashimoto, R., and Rothwell, J. C. (1999). Dynamic changes in corticospinal excitability during motor imagery. *Exp. Brain Res.* 125: 75–81.

Iacoboni, M., Woods, R. P., Brass, M., Bekkering, H., Mazziotta, J. C., and Rizzolatti, G. (1999). Cortical mechanisms of human imitation. *Science* 286: 2526–2528.

Ingvar, D., and Philipsson, L. (1977). Distribution of the cerebral blood flow in the dominant hemisphere during motor ideation and motor performance. *Ann. Neurol.* 2: 230–237.

Jacobson, E. (1930). Electrical measurements of neuro-muscular states during mental activities: 3. Visual imagination and recollection. *Am. J. Physiol.* 95: 694–702.

James, W. (1890). *Principles of Psychology.* London: Macmillan.

Jeannerod, M. (1993). A theory of representation-driven actions. In *The Perceived Self: Ecological and Interpersonal Sources of Self-Knowledge*, U. Neisser (ed.). Cambridge: Cambridge University Press, pp. 89–101.

Jeannerod, M. (1994). The representing brain: Neural correlates of motor intention and imagery. *Behav. Brain Sci.* 17: 187–245.

Jeannerod, M. (1997). *The Cognitive Neuroscience of Action.* Oxford: Blackwell.

Jeannerod, M. (1999). To act or not to act: Perspectives on the representation of actions. *Q. J. Exp. Psychol.* 52A: 1–29.

Jeannerod, M. (2001). Neural simulation of action: A unifying mechanism for motor cognition. *NeuroImage* 14: S103–S109.

Jeannerod, M., and Frak, V. G. (1999). Mental simulation of action in human subjects. *Curr. Opin. Neurobiol.* 9: 735–739.

Jeannerod, M., Arbib, M. A., Rizzolatti, G., and Sakata, H. (1995). Grasping objects: The cortical mechanisms of visuomotor transformation. *Trends Neurosci.* 18: 314–320.

Johnson, S. H. (2000a). Thinking ahead: The case for motor imagery in prospective judgements of prehension. *Cognition* 74: 33–70.

Johnson, S. H. (2000b). Imagining the impossible: Intact motor imagery in hemiplegia. *NeuroReport* 11: 729–732.

Kosslyn, S. M., Digirolamo, G. J., Thompson, W. L., and Alpert, N. M. (1998). Mental rotation of objects versus hands: Neural mechanisms revealed by positron-emission tomography. *Psychophysiology* 35: 151–161.

Krogh, A., and Lindhard, J. (1913). The regulation of respiration and circulation during the initial stages of muscular work. *J. Physiol.* 47: 112–136.

Lhermitte, F. (1983). "Utilization behaviour" and its relation to lesions of the frontal lobe. *Brain* 106: 237–255.

Liberman, A. M., and Mattingly, I. G. (1985). The motor theory of perception of speech revisited. *Cognition* 21: 1–36.

Lipps, T. (1903). *Aesthetik: Psychologie des Schönen und der Kunst.* Hamburg: Voss.

Lotze, M., Montoya, P., Erb, M., Hülsmann, E., Flor, H., Klose, U., Birbaumer, N., and Grodd, W. (1999). Activation of cortical and cerebellar motor areas during executed and imagined hand movements: An fMRI study. *J. Cogn. Neurosci.* 11: 491–501.

Lotze, R. H. (1852). *Medizinische Psychologie oder Physiologie der Seele.* Leipzig: Weidmann.

MacKay, D. (1966). Cerebral organization and the conscious control of action. In *Brain and Conscious Experience*, J. C. Eccles (ed.). New York: Springer, pp. 422–445.

Marshall, J. C., Halligan, P. W., Fink, G. R., Wade, D. T., and Frackowiak, R. S. J. (1997). The functional anatomy of a hysterical paralysis. *Cognition* 64: B1–B8.

Meltzoff, A. N., (1995). Understanding the intentions of others: Re-enactment of intended acts by 18-month-old children. *Dev. Psychol.* 31: 838–850.

Milner, A. D., and Goodale, M. A. (1995). *The Visual Brain in Action.* Oxford: Oxford University Press.

Neisser, U. (1993). The self perceived. In *The Perceived Self: Ecological and Interpersonal Sources of Self-Knowledge*, U. Neisser (ed.). Cambridge: Cambridge University Press, pp. 3–21.

Oishi, K., Kimura, M., Yasukawa, M., Yoneda, T., and Maeshima, T. (1994). Amplitude reduction of H-reflex during mental movement simulation in elite athletes. *Behav. Brain Res.* 62: 55–61.

Paccalin, C., and Jeannerod, M. (2000). Changes in breathing during observation of effortful actions. *Brain Res.* 862: 194–200.

Parsons, L. M. (1994). Temporal and kinematic properties of motor behavior reflected in mentally simulated action. *J. Exp. Psychol. Human Percep. Perf.* 20: 709–730.

Parsons, L. M., Fox, P. T., Downs, J. H., Glass, T., Hirsch, T. B., Martin, C. C., Jerabek, P. A., and Lancaster, J. L. (1995). Use of implicit motor imagery for visual shape discrimination as revealed by PET. *Nature* 375: 54–58.

Pascual-Leone, A., Dang, N., Cohen, L. G., Brasil-Neto, J., Cammarota, A., and Hallett, M. (1995). Modulation of motor responses evoked by transcranial magnetic stimulation during the acquisition of new fine motor skills. *J. Neurophysiol.* 74: 1037–1045.

Paus, T., Petrides, M., Evans, A. C., and Meyer, E. (1993). Role of human anterior cingulate cortex in the control of oculomotor, manual and speech responses: A positron-emission tomography study. *J. Neurophysiol.* 70: 453–469.

Perani, D., Cappa, S. F., Bettinardi, V., Bressi, S., Gorno-Tempini, M., Matarrese, M., and Fazio, F. (1995). Different neural systems for the recognition of animals and man-made tools. *NeuroReport* 6: 1637–1641.

Pigman, G. W. (1995). Freud and the history of empathy. *Int. J. Psycho-Analysis* 76: 237–256.

Porro, C. A., Francescato, M. P., Cettolo, V., Diamond, M. E., Baraldi, P., Zuiani, C., Bazzochi, M., and di Prampero, P. E. (1996). Primary motor and sensory cortex activation during motor performance and motor imagery: A functional magnetic resonance study. *J. Neurosci.* 16: 7688–7698.

Prut, Y., and Fetz, E. E. (1999). Primate spinal interneurons show premovement instructed delay activity. *Nature* 401: 590–594.

Rizzolatti, G., Fadiga, L., Matelli, M., Bettinardi, V., Paulesu, E., Perani, D., and Fazio, F. (1996). Localization of grasp representations in humans by PET: 1. Observation versus execution. *Exp. Brain Res.* 111: 246–252.

Rode, G., and Perenin, M. T. (1994). Temporary remission of representational hemineglect following vestibular stimulation. *NeuroReport* 5: 869–872.

Roland, P. E., Skinhoj, E., Lassen, N. A., and Larsen, B. (1980). Different cortical areas in man in organization of voluntary movements in extrapersonal space. *J. Neurophysiol.* 43: 137–150.

Roth, M., Decety, J., Raybaudi, M., Massarelli, R., Delon-Martin, C., Segebarth, C., Morand, S., Gemignani, A., Décorps, M., and Jeannerod, M. (1996). Possible involvement of primary motor cortex in mentally simulated movement: A functional magnetic resonance imaging study. *NeuroReport* 7: 1280–1284.

Ryding, E., Decety, J., Sjolhom, H., Stenberg, G., and Ingvar, H. (1993). Motor imagery activates the cerebellum regionally: A SPECT rCBF study with ^{99m}Tc-HMPAO. *Cogn. Brain Res.* 1: 94–99.

Schnitzler, A., Salenius, S. Salmelin, R. Jousmäki, V., and Hari, R. (1997). Involvement of primary motor cortex in motor imagery: A neuromagnetic study. *NeuroImage* 6: 201–208.

Shallice, T., Burgess, P. W., Schon, F., and Baxter, D. M. (1989). The origins of utilization behavior. *Brain* 112: 1587–1592.

Sirigu, A., and Duhamel, J. R. (2001). Motor and visual imagery as two complementary but neurally dissociable mental processes. *J. Cogn. Neurosci.* 13: 910–919.

Sirigu, A., Cohen, L., Duhamel, J.-R., Pillon, B., Dubois, B., Agid, Y., and Pierrot-Deseiligny, C. (1995). Congruent unilateral impairments for real and imagined hand movements. *NeuroReport* 6: 997–1001.

Sirigu, A., Duhamel, J.-R., Cohen, L., Pillon, B., Dubois, B., and Agid, Y. (1996). The mental representation of hand movements after parietal cortex damage. *Science* 273: 1564–1568.

Sirigu, A., Daprati, E., Pradat-Diehl, P., Franck, N., and Jeannerod, M. (1999). Perception of self-generated movement following left parietal lesion. *Brain* 122: 1867–1874.

Spence, S. A., Brooks, D. J., Hirsch, S. R., Liddle, P. F., Meehan, J., and Grasby, P. M. (1997). A PET study of voluntary movements in schizophrenic patients experiencing passivity phenomena (delusions of alien control). *Brain* 120: 1997–2011.

Stephan, K. M., Fink, G. R., Passingham, R. E., Silbersweig, D., Ceballos-Baumann, A. O., Frith, C. D., and Frackowiak, R. S. J. (1995). Functional anatomy of the mental representation of upper extremity movements in healthy subjects. *J. Neurophysiol.* 73: 373–386.

Strafella, A. P., and Paus, T. (2000). Modulation of cortical excitability during action observation: A transcranial magnetic stimulation study. *NeuroReport* 11: 2289–2292.

Thobois, S., Dominey, P. F., Decety, J., Pollack, J., Grégoire, M. C., Le Bars, D., and Broussolle, E. (2000). Motor imagery in normal subjects and in asymmetrical Parkinson's disease: A PET study. *Neurology* 55: 996–1002.

Vissing, S. F., and Hjortso, E. (1996). Central motor command activates sympathetic outflow to the circulation in humans. *J. Physiol.* 492: 931–939.

Wolpert, D. M., Ghahramani, Z., and Jordan, M. I. (1995). An internal model for sensorimotor integration. *Science* 269: 1880–1882.

Wuyam, B., Moosavi, S. H., Decety, J., Adams, L., Lansing, R. W., and Guz, A. (1995). Imagination of dynamic exercise produced ventilatory responses which were more apparent in competitive sportsmen. *J. Physiol.* 482: 713–724.

III

Gesture and Tool Use

The ability to make and use tools is one of the defining characteristics of the human species. Drawing on studies of patients with manual apraxia, Sirigu and colleagues (chapter 6) review evidence indicating that human left parietal cortex is specialized for the representation of tool use actions. In their novel hypothesis, based on carefully delineated functional dissociations, hand action representations are organized modularly within left parietal cortex and play a critical role, not only in action production, but also in distinguishing one's actions from those of others.

Consistent with a specialized network in the left cerebral hemisphere for representing tool use actions, Johnson-Frey (chapter 7) argues for a specific "utilization system" that includes both the inferior parietal lobule and interconnected regions of frontal cortex. Under ordinary circumstances, the utilization system interacts with two other representational networks essential to skillful tool use: the "comprehension system," which constructs representations necessary for the identification and categorization of objects, including tools, and involves cortical areas within the ventral processing stream; and the "prehension system," which implements sensorimotor transformations necessary to manually engage objects on the basis of their perceptual attributes, and involves both parietal areas within the dorsal processing stream and the frontal areas with which they are interconnected. He presents neurophysiological, neuropsychological, and functional neuroimaging evidence indicating that these systems are functionally and anatomically dissociable.

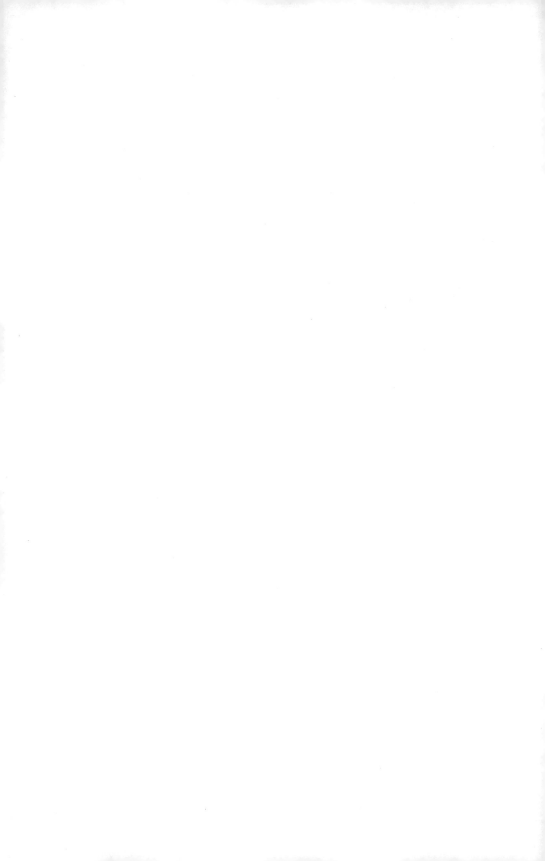

6

How the Human Brain Represents Manual Gestures: Effects of Brain Damage

Angela Sirigu, Elena Daprati, Laurel J. Buxbaum, Pascal Giraux, and Pascale Pradat-Diehl

One of the most felicitous definitions of the human hand comes from Aristotle, who described it as "the instrument of instruments." Indeed, the human hand serves a variety of goals, such as touching, feeling, holding, and manipulating objects. Hand gestures describe people's intentions and support social communication; more important for our purposes, however, they describe how people grasp objects and use tools.

In addressing where the brain represents manual gestures and how these representations are made available to generate meaningful actions, this chapter first describes the respective role of the arm and the hand in gesture organization and tool use, discussing the brain areas involved in gesture representation and focusing on the neuropsychological syndrome of apraxia to show that complex gestures, such as those involved in tool use, rely on specific motor representations within the left parietal cortex. Next, it proposes that a modular organization of hand actions exists in the brain; in support of this proposal, it then presents neuropsychological evidence from patients having lesions in the parietal cortex. And finally, in touching on the role of motor representations in programming and updating the course of an action, it suggests that such representations are crucial for recognizing self-generated actions.

6.1 Prehension and Tool Use

Phenomenologically, we can distinguish at least two components in the production of a gesture such as the use of an object. One relates to manual prehension, that is, to how the hand must be shaped; the second, to the movement pattern of the arm required to perform the intended function. This distinction is supported by psychophysical evidence that distinct visuo-motor mechanisms are involved in coding hand prehension and movement trajectory in reaching gestures. When we reach for an object, information about object features such as size and location are processed in parallel for efficient coordination of finger grasp and hand motion in space (Jeannerod, 1988). Furthermore, these two gestural parameters may change depending on whether we want simply to grasp the object or to use it. When grasping is part of a utilization behavior, grip selection depends not simply on the object's physical properties, but also on its functional properties. For instance, when subjects are asked to pick up a pair of scissors from a table, hand shaping depends chiefly on the orientation and size of the scissors, whereas when they are asked to cut a piece of paper with the scissors, hand shaping includes knowledge of how scissors are operated and of which fingers are involved in the act of cutting.

Although most of us execute the latter task with no particular effort, some patients suffering from a neuropsychological syndrome called "apraxia" find it impossible to access and use this "gestural repertoire." They are apparently unable to recall how to brush their teeth, how to use a knife and fork, how to tie their shoelaces, and so on, even if recognition of objects and of their functional properties and basic sensorimotor functions are well preserved (Liepmann, 1905; Heilman et al., 1982; De Renzi et al., 1982, 1988; Ochipa et al., 1989; Rothi et al., 1995b; Hermsdörfer et al., 1996). Although these patients can reach to and grasp objects, they have no knowledge of how to use them. The lesion responsible for this disturbance is most frequently located in the parietal region of the left hemisphere (Heilman et al., 1982; Poizner et al., 1990). This particular form of apraxia thus constitutes an interesting pathological model to investigate how complex movements are represented in the brain.

Since the work of Liepmann (1905), it has been recognized that skilled object use and pantomime requires integrity of stored gesture representations in the left parietal lobe. Liepmann characterized these representations as forming the "time-space-form" picture of the movement. Subsequently, Heilman and colleagues (e.g., 1982) suggested that there are at least two major subtypes of apraxia. In one subtype, where gesture representations are damaged, the ability to recognize gestures is impaired, suggesting that representations underlying gesture production are essential to gesture recognition; in the second subtype, where access of gesture representations to motor production systems is damaged, gesture recognition is intact.

Although important contributions on the representations underlying gesture, the studies discussed above specify neither how components of gestures (e.g., hand posture, arm trajectory) are integrated nor whether they may be dissociated. These theoretical gaps are filled in, at least in part, by the studies described below.

The Case of L.L.

A right-handed woman, L.L. sustained a severe hypotensive episode during an operation for uterine fibroma when she was 51 years old. Although her CAT scan was normal, a follow-up examination using single-photon emission computed tomography (SPECT) showed the existence of a bilateral occipitoparietal hypometabolism (Sirigu et al., 1995a). Although L.L. did not present any motor or sensory deficits, clinical evaluation showed a complex pattern of neuropsychological disturbance dominated by a severe apraxia.

Four years after onset, even though her sensory, motor, attentional, and linguistic functions were normal, the patient complained of difficulties doing simple everyday tasks such as cutting her nails, brushing her teeth, locking a door, and cutting meat with a knife and fork. Neuropsychological examination confirmed that gestural abilities were severely disturbed. Whether upon verbal command or on imitation of the examiner, L.L. was impaired in miming the use of objects, in making symbolic or meaningless gestures, and in using real objects, although her ability to recognize pantomimes was preserved.

L.L.'s gestures were investigated using several tasks involving a set of 20 familiar objects. In a first task, L.L. was asked to name each object, to take it in hand, and to show its use. The patient's performance was videotaped for later scoring. Four independent judges, naive about the purpose of the study, rated L.L.'s gestures on a two-point scale (0 = inadequate or incorrect; 1 = adequate or correct) during two separate sessions: paying attention to the global aspects of each gesture in the first; and rating separately hand prehension and movement trajectory in the second.

L.L. named all objects correctly, whereas almost all of the gestures she executed were rated as incorrect, regardless of the hand used to respond. More particularly, whereas L.L.'s arm trajectory was correctly goal-oriented, the judges rated her hand prehension as incorrect (figure 6.1). For example, when presented with a spoon and asked to use it ("eating soup with a spoon"), L.L. grabbed the spoon with her whole hand, and her prehension lacked a precise finger positioning on the object. It is noteworthy that during the transport movement toward the mouth, the patient rolled the

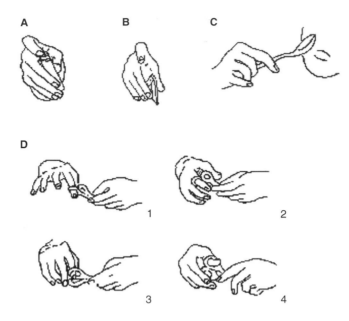

Figure 6.1
Spontaneous manual prehension by bilateral parietal patient L.L. during use of a (*A*) lighter, (*B*) nail clipper, (*C*) spoon. (*D*) L.L.'s four attempts (1 to 4) at inserting fingers in the loops of scissors. (Reprinted with permission from Sirigu et al. 1995a.)

spoon in her hand several times, as though searching for a better finger posture. Such corrective attempts were present on most trials.

This initial global evaluation identified L.L.'s impairment as the result of inadequate hand grasp when the object was manipulated with the intention to use it. To evaluate whether the deficit was specific to object use, in a separate task the patient was asked to reach for the object and hand it over to the examiner. Her videotaped performance was subjected to a frame-by-frame analysis of both the arm trajectory and the anticipatory finger grip formation. The maximum width of the index-thumb aperture at the finger tips (figure 6.2B) was measured for each trial. No qualitative or quantitative anomalies were observed in L.L.'s performance: The movements were smooth and correctly directed, the wrist's orientation matched the object's, and the size of the finger grip was highly correlated with the size of the grasped portion of the object (figure 6.2). As these last results indicate, L.L.'s incorrect hand posture seems to be specific to gestures involving the use of objects.

The dissociation between preserved hand shaping when *grasping to move* an object and incorrect hand shaping when *grasping to use* the same

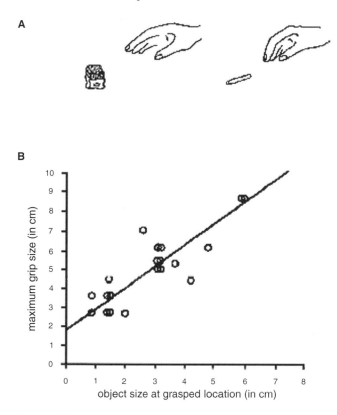

Figure 6.2
L.L.'s grip formation during combined reaching and grasping movements. (*A*) Examples of anticipatory finger positioning in relation to the object's size for a brush (*left*) and a cigarette (*right*). (*B*) Scatter plot and linear regression line for maximum grip size during the hand's transport phase as a function of the object size and grasped location. (Reprinted with permission from Sirigu et al., 1995a).

object raises the question of what distinguishes the processing involved in the control of finger movements during reaching and utilization behavior. Theories of limb motor coding postulate that grip formation in visually guided reaching gestures requires the transformation of retinal parameters into a series of body-centered (e.g., shoulder-, arm-, and hand-centered) reference frames, a process presumably applied in the same manner to any visual stimulus, regardless of its nature. In contrast, hand postures adopted during object utilization are determined by features unique to each object and must anticipate how the action is to be performed. Therefore, during utilization gestures, in addition to data about local object characteristics (e.g., orientation and size), the motor system for manual prehension needs to retrieve data from memory regarding functional properties of the object (e.g., the rings of the scissors must be grasped by the thumb and index finger to achieve the cutting movement).

To see whether knowledge of these complex manual configurations was impaired in L.L., we tested her capacity to recognize and to verbally evoke manual postures, using gesture discrimination and gesture description tasks. In the "gesture discrimination task," L.L. was asked to judge whether an object was held correctly by the examiner, and whether the correct movement of the limb was executed. For example, in one trial, the examiner grasped a hammer incorrectly (between the index and the middle finger), but moved it correctly. In a different trial, the examiner grasped the hammer correctly, but moved it incorrectly (with a twisting motion of the wrist and forearm). In the "gesture description task," the patient was told the names of the objects, and asked to verbally describe which fingers were involved in the prehension of each object during its use (for example, "Which fingers do you put in the rings of a pair of a scissors when you want to cut a piece of paper?").

Although L.L. correctly identified the incongruent movement patterns, she performed at chance level for hand postures, all of which she accepted as correct. Similarly, when asked about hand-object relations, she gave few correct answers. This behavior could not be attributed to impaired knowledge about finger names or objects: She could name and recognize all fingers, name all objects, and verbally define their function. Thus L.L. could neither visually discriminate nor verbally report how hand and finger postures related to objects and to specific functions, suggesting that her deficit was not merely one of translating a particular kind of representation or percept into action but rather in accessing and/or activating such a representation.

Neural Basis of Complex Hand Movements

The results obtained in patient L.L. suggest that distinct mechanisms underlie object prehension with respect to the action goal. Some clues as to whether there is an anatomical basis to this functional distinction for hand movement patterns can be found in the functional organization of the parietal lobe in nonhuman primates.

Here the intraparietal sulcus is the anatomical landmark separating the superior and inferior parietal lobule. Both are large regions containing multiple subdivisions, and in each lobule there are areas involved in hand prehension. Areas such as the medial intraparietal (MIP) and anterior intraparietal (AIP) areas all receive visual information via the dorsal cortical pathway, and they all separately project to premotor cortex (Colby and Duhamel, 1996; Matelli et al., 1998; Tanné et al., 1995). These output pathways remain to some extent segregated, inferior parietal areas projecting predominantly to the ventral premotor region and superior parietal areas projecting more predominantly to the dorsal premotor region. These pathways thus provide a route for carrying different types of information to the action systems in the frontal lobe, the ventral being more specialized for object grasping and manipulation (distal component), the dorsal being most involved in the transport phase of the movement (proximal component; Wise et al., 1997). Reciprocal connections in nonhuman primates also exist between the lateral intraparietal (LIP) area of the parietal lobe and the inferior temporal cortex (areas TE and TEO), known to be involved in object recognition in both humans and monkeys (Distler et al., 1993; Webster et al., 1994). Whether these anatomical connections also exist in humans remains to be established. We can speculate that the direct parietal-frontal route may subserve the "grasping to move" behavior, whereas the temporoparietal route may constitute an intermediate step necessary for the integration of objects' functional properties into complex movement patterns such as those required during "grasping to use" behavior. L.L.'s case suggests that these two systems can be dissociated.

6.2 Canonical Hand Postures

Having established that apraxic patients show deficits for a specific type of hand action, namely, skilled object manipulation, one still needs to characterize this behavior more precisely. The data presented thus far suggest that, in the case of complex movements, specialized mechanisms are required to encode functionally relevant manual postures. If hand postures have a distinct status, how are they represented in the brain?

Complex hand postures entail a large number of degrees of freedom. From a theoretical point of view, this suggests the need for the central nervous system to encode these movements as preassembled motor synergies (Napier, 1956; Arbib et al., 1985). Mackenzie and Iberall (1994) proposed that the variety of postures derived from hand-object interactions gives rise to the production of stabilizing forces, to engender movements and to collect sensory information. These three functions can be achieved by means of a restricted number of *canonical* prehension schemas defined by an opposition space centered on the hand. Within this coordinate system, two opposing vectorial forces produce a grip based on "virtual fingers." A virtual finger may be represented by one or several digits moving synergistically. When reaching for an object, the motor schemas for skilled hand movements, encoded as virtual grasp patterns in "hand space," are directly activated by the object's features (Iberall et al., 1986; Iberall and Arbib, 1990).

Is there a reality to the concept of canonical hand postures that would form distinct groups or clusters of postural types? Several lines of evidence support this hypothesis. Single-unit recording experiments made in the primate cortex have shown that individual neurons can be activated selectively by visual stimuli such as hands in various positions or performing certain actions (Taira, 1990). Although they pertain to relatively simple motor acts, these findings provide tentative support to the idea of a cerebral store of manual postures.

In humans, little is known about normal hand movements during complex actions. A novel virtual reality technology allows researchers to measure the displacement of each articulation of the five fingers and the palm of the hand by means of a large number of sensors inserted in the fabric of a glove. By recording hand movements during a variety of gestures, we can characterize them in terms of postural synergies and covariations between the different moving segments. Thus we can also identify strategies for grasping and object manipulation that reduce the number of degrees of freedom that need to be controlled in such a complex biomechanical system as the hand.

Results obtained in normal subjects instructed to pantomime the use of an object confirm that most hand postures can be represented by two basic statistical prototypes or principal components (Santello et al., 1998), derived from a characterization of the similarities and differences in a set of hand postures. By assuming a principal component captures the superordinate neural control that allows the different hand segments to move synergistically, Santello and colleagues showed that the distance between two postures can be defined as the measure of their degree of differentiation in a parametric space. Thus hand postures produced during the pantomime of the use of an object can be obtained by scaling the parametric value of each principal component appropriately.

Skilled Learned Hand Postures in Normal Subjects and in Brain-Damaged Patients

In a recent study, we tested the hypothesis that specialized mechanisms are required to encode functionally relevant manual postures. From the results of L.L.'s case, we expected that representation of hand postures involved in skilled gestures would be impaired after parietal lesions. To determine whether this was so, we measured hand movements in five apraxic patients with lesions in left parietal cortex and six normal controls during interactions with familiar objects under different instructions (Sirigu et al., 2002).

Subjects were required (1) to reach and grasp an object placed in front of them with their right hand; (2) to pantomime how they would handle the same object in order to use it; and (3) to actually reach for the object and to use it. Common objects such as a cigarette, lighter, or spoon were presented.

Angular variations of the different hand joints were recorded by means of an instrumented glove (CyberGlove; Virtual Technologies) that captured joint angles of 15 degrees of freedom of the right hand. Measured angles were at the metacarpal-phalangeal joints and at the proximal interphalangeal joints of the four fingers as well as at thumb joints (rotation, interphalangeal joint, and metacarpal-phalangeal joint). Abduction angles between adjacent fingers were also measured. A factorial analysis was performed on hand postures adopted by each subject at the end of each trial when grasping the object or pantomiming it. Each posture was characterized as a "waveform" (the value measured from the 15 sensors); the number of principal components that could account for the different hand postures was obtained for each subject.

In the normal control group, two principal components (PCs) accounted for more than 80% of the variance observed in all conditions and described the variety of hand postures subjects adopted in response to the sample of presented objects. Postures were distributed uniformly in the plane of the 2 PCs, forming a V shape similarly to that found in a pantomime task by Santello and colleagues (1998). No clusters were observed in any condition. Moreover, the profile of the first PC was found to be similar in all subjects and in each condition, suggesting that this factor may underlie a default posture corresponding to basic motor synergies such as an opening-closing movement pattern. In the case of object use, an additional PC was found that accounted for more than 80% of variance, and that was absent in the case of grasping and pantomime. We consider this factor to be the expression of finer motor adjustments necessary when actually using an object.

In the patient group, performance in the grasping condition was similar to that of the control group and showed the typical V-shaped distribution, whereas, in the pantomime condition, joint angles characterizing each hand posture clustered around one or both principal components and lacked the V-shaped distribution observed in the control group. These results show that patients adopted an undifferentiated posture across all objects shown.

These results confirm the behavioral dissociation described in L.L.'s case and suggest that apraxia specifically affects the production of learned hand postures during object use while preserving hand shaping involved in on-line "grasping to move" tasks.

Given that this study required gesture production, the question arises whether the apraxic deficit reflects damage to the representations underlying "grasping to use" or disconnection of intact representations from motor output. If the former, recognition of hand postures for "grasping to use" should be impaired; if the latter, it should be intact. In either case, production and recognition of hand postures for on-line "grasping to move" should be intact. To assess these hypotheses, we asked nine apraxic patients with left inferior parietal damage to produce and recognize hand postures most appropriate for contacting familiar and novel objects. We predicted that performance would be relatively intact with novel objects, indicating integrity of on-line procedures responsive to object structure. Performance of the apraxic patients was contrasted with ten healthy controls and six brain-lesioned nonapraxics (Buxbaum et al., in press).

Subjects were shown familiar objects and four pictures, each one depicting a different hand posture (clench, poke, palm, pinch). In a first condition, they were asked to point to the image that best described the hand posture adopted when manipulating the presented object. In a second condition, they were asked to pantomime how they would interact and manipulate the same object if holding it in their hand. The same task was repeated with a set of novel objects similar to those used by Klatzky and colleagues (1987).

Consistent with our predictions, the apraxics failed to recognize hand postures appropriate for familiar objects, but correctly recognized those appropriate for novel objects. Moreover, performance with objects calling for a prehensile response (pinch or clench) was superior to that with objects evoking a nonprehensile response (palm or poke). These data are consistent with the possibility, suggested earlier, that apraxic patients may produce relatively undifferentiated hand postures in response to objects; they suggest that the "default" postures may be generic representation of precision and power grip encoded by dorsal stream structures in the "grasp to move" system.

Taken together, the results of these two studies suggest that apraxia causes a degradation of hand posture representations associated with familiar objects. The lesion responsible for this disorder is located in the left inferior parietal cortex, indicating that this part of the brain may play a significant role in storing or accessing motor images associated with complex gestures.

6.3   Motor Imagery after Parietal Lesion

Having established that apraxics are unable to generate correct gestures because they cannot access stored motor images, we hypothesized the same deficit would be observed when motor images themselves are the object of investigation.

We tested this hypothesis by asking normal subjects, four patients suffering from parietal lesions and a patient with a right motor cortex lesion to mentally simulate hand movements (Sirigu et al., 1995b, 1996). In a first task, all subjects mentally simulated a continuous thumb-fingers opposition sequence with either the left or right hand in response to the sound of a metronome, whose beating speed was progressively augmented until subjects reported that the imagined hand could no longer keep up with the imposed speed. In a successive task, subjects actually executed the movement sequence, and the actual performance break point was recorded. Normal subjects showed excellent congruence between maximum imagined and executed movement speeds. This result is in agreement with several mental chronometry studies demonstrating that, in normal subjects, the time to mentally complete a particular movement is similar to the time needed to execute the corresponding motor act (Decety et al., 1989; Jeannerod, 1994; Jeannerod and Frak, 1999).

In contrast, patients with parietal cortex lesions systematically produced inaccurate estimates (too fast or too slow), which were inconsistent

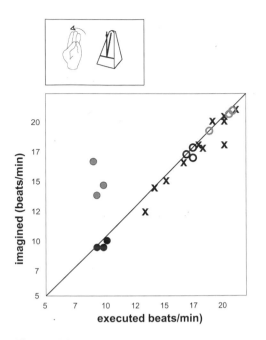

Figure 6.3
Correlation between imagined and executed movements in the thumb-fingers opposition task at the pace of a metronome for normal subject (Xs), right motor
patient (green circles), and right parietal patient (orange circles). Open circles =
ipsilateral movement; filled circles = contralateral. The data are represented as a
scatter plot of executed versus imagined movement speed. Points lying on the 45°
line represent a perfect match between the two movement conditions.

from one trial to the next. A different behavior was observed in the patient
with a right motor cortex lesion, whose simulated movement speed on the
metronome task mirrored exactly the asymmetrical motor performance of
the contra- and ipsilesional hands (figure 6.3).

   This result suggests that the ability to estimate manual motor performance through mental imagery is disturbed following parietal lobe damage.

   To address the effect of specific task factors, such as the complexity
of the motor program on motor imagery, we devised a second task, using
four sets of postures, empirically selected and rated on their degree of difficulty by a group of normal subjects. In this task, we also tested the apraxic
patient L.L. Both patients and controls were asked to mentally simulate the
production of each of the four postures. Movement duration was recorded
as the time elapsed between a go signal and the subject's report of having
completed five consecutive cycles of the same movement pattern. Once

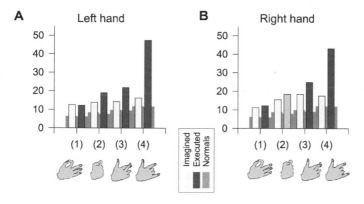

Figure 6.4
Bilateral parietal patient L.L.'s performance time for imagined and executed hand
movements of increasing complexity. 1 = easiest movement; 4 = most complex
movement; *y*-axis = movement time (s). Gray bars represent normal performance.

the imagery task was over, subjects executed each movement according to
the same procedure. In control subjects and in the motor cortex–lesioned
patient, imagined and executed movement times increased in parallel from
the simplest posture to the most complex one. In contrast, parietal patients
were unable to simulate the behavior of their contralesional hand, thus
indicating a reduced parallelism between the timing of motor performance
and imagery. L.L.'s performance was similar to that of the other parietal
patients; more particularly, the decoupling between actual and mentally
simulated movements increased with motor complexity (figure 6.4).

At the beginning of this chapter, we presented data showing that
apraxic patients with parietal damage cannot access motor representations
linked to object use. This is consistent with the classical view of apraxia as
first described by Liepmann (1905). We also presented evidence that apraxia
affects hand motor synergies *only* during object utilization but *not* during
simple grasping. The last piece of data we presented further suggests that
complex movements after parietal lesions are impaired even in the context
of mental rehearsal and independently of the interaction with objects. If
imagining a complex movement is difficult for these patients, then not only
should the access of a gesture engram be deficient (as suggested by Liepmann), but also the ability to manipulate and update such motor representations. This deficit likely implies a failure to generate or monitor an internal
model of one's own movement, or both. If this hypothesis is correct, apraxia
should also affect the perception of self-generated actions.

6.4   Recognition of Self-Generated Actions

Wolpert and colleagues (1995) have suggested that one of the main stages in motor control is the comparison between an internal model and the expected and actual sensory consequences of the movement. If such an internal model is faulty or unavailable in apraxic subjects, then the capacity to compare or match predicted and actual sensory feedback is likely to be impaired as well.

We tested this hypothesis by investigating the behavior of three apraxic patients with left parietal damage (Sirigu et al., 1999). Patients were asked to execute simple (single-finger extension) and complex (multifinger extension) gestures with their unseen hand, and to observe the motor output on a TV screen. A special device (Daprati et al., 1997) allowed real-time presentation of the patient's or examiner's hand. In the latter case, the examiner could either perform the same movement as the patient or a different movement. Subjects were asked to decide whether the hand moving on the screen was their own or not. We compared patients' responses to those produced by normal controls and nonapraxic brain-lesioned patients. All subjects accurately recognized their own hand when it appeared on the screen. Similarly, they correctly identified the viewed hand as the examiner's when it performed a movement that departed from the one they were performing, but when it performed a movement that matched the one they were performing, apraxic patients incorrectly identified the examiner's hand as their own significantly more often than did controls.

This deficit was especially evident in the case of complex gestures, which, as used in our paradigm, required precise multifinger patterns and fine synchrony between the moving digits. Not surprisingly, apraxic patients often made those gestures rather clumsily: When we showed them the examiner's hand correctly executing the same movement, instead of attributing the movement to its proper source, apraxic patients modified the perception of their own movement, and identified the examiner's movement as their own, though improved, performance.

The patients' impairment was unique, and cannot be accounted for by a general consequence of brain damage or by the presence of a general motor disturbance. In fact, control patients suffering from a motor-premotor lesion and from inferotemporal damage, respectively, performed at the same level as normal controls. More noteworthy, none of them showed a dissociation between simple and complex gestures.

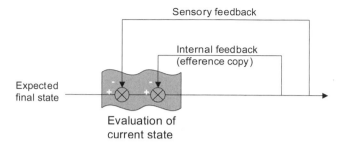

Figure 6.5
Hypothetical processing model for imagining, executing, and recognizing self-produced movements. The orange area shows the putative level of dysfunction in apraxic patients.

Requiring subjects to judge the origin of an action likely activates an internal representation of the expected visual and kinesthetic feedback generated by the movement. To decide whether the movement displayed on the screen is congruent with what the subject's hand is actually doing, this representation has to be compared with the actual visual and kinesthetic feedback (figure 6.5). When the movement on the screen matches that of the subject, but is executed by someone else, the role of visual cues is minimized and subjects must use the subtle position and timing differences between kinesthetic and visual feedback to distinguish their own hand from the viewed alien hand. This discrimination, though difficult even for normal subjects, is disproportionately hard for apraxic patients. These results are consistent with the existence of a selective impairment in the ability to form or monitor internal models for complex movements, or both. Such a deficit is likely to play an important role in the difficulties experienced by apraxic patients in disambiguating the visual stimulus in the congruent movement condition. As shown in figure 6.5, our data indicate that either the suggested predictive model is defective or that it cannot be adequately updated on-line during movement execution.

To conclude, the data presented in this chapter support the view that the parietal cortex plays key role in generating and storing models of complex hand postures. The selective impairment for one class of movements suggest that a modular organization is likely to exist within the parietal lobe for human hand gestures. This modular representation is perhaps necessary to account for the variety of goals the "instrument of instruments" may attain.

References

Arbib, M. A., Iberall, T., and Lyons, D. (1985). Coordinated control programs for movements of the hand. In *Hand Function and the Neocortex*, A. W. Goodman and I. Darian-Smith (eds.). Berlin: Springer, pp. 135–170.

Buxbaum, L., Sirigu, A., Schwartz, M., and Klatzky, R. (in press). Cognitive representations of hand posture in ideomotor apraxia. *Neuropsychologia*.

Colby, C. L., and Duhamel, J.-R. (1996). Spatial representations for actions in parietal cortex. *Cog. Brain Res.* 5: 105–115.

Daprati, E., Franck, N., Georgieff, N., Proust, J., Pacherie, E., Dalery, J., and Jeannerod, M. (1997). Looking for the agent: An investigation into consciousness of action and self-consciousness in schizophrenic patients. *Cognition* 65: 71–86.

Decety, J., Jeannerod, M., and Prablanc, C. (1989). The timing of mentally represented actions. *Behav. Brain Res.* 34: 35–42.

Decety, J., and Michel, F. (1989). Comparative analysis of actual and mental movement times in two graphic tasks. *Brain Cogn.* 11: 87–97.

De Renzi, E., and Luchelli, F. (1988). Ideational apraxia. *Brain* 111: 1173–1185.

De Renzi, E., Faglioni, P., and Sorgato, P. (1982). Modality-specific and supramodal mechanisms of apraxia. *Brain* 105: 301–312.

Distler, C., Boussaud, D., Desimone, R., and Ungerleider, L. G. (1993). Cortical connections of inferior temporal area TEO in macaque monkeys. *J. Comp. Neurol.* 334: 125–150.

Heilman, K. M., Rothi, L. J., and Valenstein, E. (1982). Two forms of ideo-motor apraxia. *Neurology* 32: 342–346.

Hermsdörfer, J., Mai, N., Spatt, J., Marquardt, C., Veltkamp, R., and Goldenberg, G. (1996). Kinematic analysis of movement imitation in apraxia. *Brain* 119: 1575–1586.

Iberall, T., and Arbib, M. A. (1990). Schemas for the control of hand movements: An essay on cortical localization. In *Vision and Action: The Control of Grasping*, M. A. Goodale (ed.). Norwood, N.J.: Ablex, pp. 204–242.

Iberall, T., Bingham, G., and Arbib, M. A. (1986). Opposition space as a structuring concept for the analysis of skilled hand movements. *Exp. Brain Res. Ser.* 15: 158–173.

Jeannerod, M. (1988). *The Neural and Behavioural Organization of Goal-Directed Movements*. Oxford: Clarendon Press.

Jeannerod, M. (1994). The representing brain: Neural correlates of motor intention and imagery. *Behav. Brain Sci.* 17: 187–245.

Jeannerod, M., and Frak, V. (1999). Mental imaging of motor activity in humans. *Curr. Opin. Neurobiol.* 9: 735–739.

Klatzky, R. L. McCloskey, B., Doherty, S., and Pellegrino, J. (1987). Knowledge about hand shaping and knowledge about objects. *J. Mot. Behav.* 19: 187–213.

Liepmann, H. (1905). Die linke Hemisphäre und das Handeln. *Münch. Med. Wochenschr.* 49: 2322–2326.

Mackenzie, C., and Iberall, T. eds. (1994). *The Grasping Hand*. Amsterdam: North-Holland.

Matelli, M., Govoni, P., Galletti, C., Kutz, D. F., and Luppino, G. (1998). Superior area 6 afferents from the superior parietal lobule in the macaque monkey. *J. Comp. Neurol.* 402: 327–352.

Napier, J. R. (1956). The prehensile movements of the human hand. *J. Bone Jt. Surg.* 38B: 902–913.

Ochipa, C., Rothi, L. J. G., and Heilman, K. M. (1989). Ideational apraxia: A deficit in tool selection and use. *Ann. Neurol.* 25: 190–193.

Poizner, H., Mack, L., Verfaellie, M., Rothi, L. J. G., and Heilman, K. M. (1990). Three-dimensional computergraphic analysis of apraxia. *Brain* 113: 85–101.

Rothi, L. J. G., Heilman, K. M., and Watson, R. T. (1985b). Pantomime comprehension and ideomotor apraxia. *J. Neurol. Neurosurg. Psychiatry* 48: 207–210.

Santello, M., Flanders, M., and Soechting, J. F. (1998). Postural hand synergies for tool use. *J. Neurosci.* 18: 10105–10115.

Sirigu, A., Cohen, L., Duhamel, J. R., Pillon, B., Dubois, B., and Agid, Y. (1995a). A selective impairment of hand posture for object utilization in apraxia. *Cortex* 31: 41–56.

Sirigu, A., Cohen, L., Duhamel, J. R., Pillon, B., Dubois, B., Agid, Y., and Pierrot-Deseilligny, C. (1995b). Congruent unilateral impairments for real and imagined hand movements. *NeuroReport* 6: 997–1001.

Sirigu, A., Duhamel, J. R., Cohen, L., Pillon, B., Dubois, B., and Agid, Y. (1996). The mental representation of hand movements after parietal cortex damage. *Science* 273: 1564–1568.

Sirigu, A., Daprati, E., Pradat-Diehl, P., Frank, N., and Jeannerod, M. (1999). Perception of self-generated movement following left parietal lesion. *Brain* 122: 1867–1874.

Sirigu, A., Didi, N., Baron, S., and Pradat-Diehl, P. (Forthcoming). Control of distal movements in apraxia.

Taira, M., Mine, S., Georgopoulos, A. P., Murata, A., and Sakata, H. (1990). Parietal cortex neurons of the monkey related to the visual guidance of hand movement. *Exp. Brain Res.* 83: 29–36.

Tanné, J., Boussaoud, D., Boyer-Zeller, N., Rouiller, E. M. (1995). Direct visual pathways for reaching movements in the macaque monkey. *NeuroReport* 7: 267–272.

Webster, M. J., Bachevalier, J., and Ungerleider, L. G. (1994). Connections of inferior temporal areas TEO and TE with parietal and frontal cortex in macaque monkeys. *Cereb. Cortex* 4: 470–483.

Wise, S. P., Boussaoud, D., Johnson, P. B., and Caminiti, R. (1997). Premotor and parietal cortex: Corticocortical connectivity and combinatorial computations. *Annu. Rev. Neurosci.* 20: 25–42.

Wolpert, D. M., Ghahramani, Z., and Jordan, M. (1995). An internal model for sensorimotor integration. *Science* 269: 1880–1882.

7

Cortical Representations of Human Tool Use

Scott H. Johnson-Frey

7.1   Introduction

The ability to rapidly transform sensory representations of one's external environment into object-oriented actions is common throughout the animal kingdom. Primates and nonprimates alike pursue and engage mates, food items, and other desired objects with remarkable dexterity. Although many animals are known to use external objects to effect changes in their surroundings (see review in Bradshaw, 1997), only in humans has the capacity for tool use become a defining characteristic, arguably on a par with language.

This chapter has assembled and organized heretofore disparate observations concerning the neural substrates of primate tool use with an eye toward understanding the mechanisms that support our vastly expanded repertoire. It begins with the largely self-evident observation that skillful tool use demands something more than simply the capacity for dexterous sensorimotor control. To illustrate, consider the problem of reaching to grasp a familiar tool such as a hammer or pliers. Figure 7.1A illustrates two stable grips that will enable an actor to move the tool from one location to another. Although both grips represent successful transformations of sensory information into motor programs, neither is suitable for using these tools to perform their common functions. As shown in figure 7.1B, functional grips often differ substantially from those chosen solely on the basis of perceptual information: The skillful tool-user must also possess representations of functional actions that have come to be associated with objects through past interactions. I contend that the ability to represent functional actions involving one's body and external objects is the key to understanding the human proclivity for tool use.

A. GRASPING TO MOVE   B. GRASPING TO USE

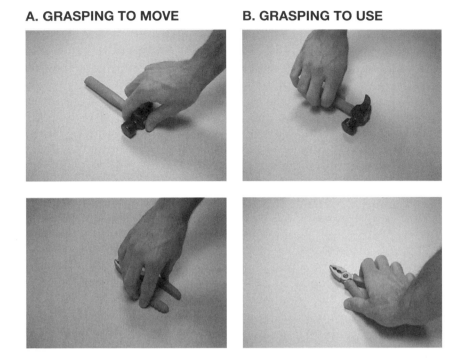

Figure 7.1
Interactions with objects guided by their perceptual properties alone (*A*) or by their perceptual properties and knowledge of their functions (*B*). Achieving a stable grip for object prehension requires transforming sensory information into motor plans for prehension. These grips often differ from those adopted based on knowledge of how objects are used.

As I will argue below, there are reasons to believe that humans have evolved a specialized network in the left cerebral hemisphere for this purpose. This network, which I will refer to as the "utilization system," includes much of the inferior parietal lobule (IPL), ventral regions of the superior parietal lobule (SPL), and interconnected regions of frontal cortex. Under ordinary circumstances, the utilization system interacts with two other representational networks on which skillful tool use depends: (1) the *comprehension system,* which constructs representations necessary for the identification and categorization of objects, including tools, and involves temporal areas of the ventral processing stream; and (2) the *prehension system,* which implements sensorimotor transformations necessary to manually engage objects on the basis of their perceptual attributes. Although the utilization system involves SPL and IPL areas associated with the dorsal processing stream, and frontal areas with which they are reciprocally interconnected, under experimental conditions, it becomes apparent that the utilization system is dissociable from both comprehension and prehension systems. Drawing on evidence from a variety of different areas including neurophysiology, neurology, and functional neuroimaging, I will make a case for distinguishing between the parietofrontal anatomy of the utilization system and that of the prehension system (for a similar distinction, see Buxbaum, 2001).

7.2 The Prehension System

Most of what is currently known about the substrates of prehension comes from electrophysiological investigations of monkeys. Although the debate continues over their roles in specific behaviors, it is generally acknowledged that posterior parietal areas within the dorsal visual stream of humans and monkeys are involved in constructing representations of objects' spatial properties (Milner and Goodale, 1995; Ungerleider and Haxby, 1994). These representations are integrated with somatosensory information regarding the positions of actors' effectors and transformed into action plans within reciprocally interconnected regions of premotor cortex (Hoshi and Tanji, 2000). Electrophysiological studies of monkeys have revealed the existence of parallel parietofrontal circuits functionally specialized for actions involving different effectors (Jeannerod et al., 1995). This chapter will confine itself to circuits directly implicated in the dexterous control of manual prehension and tool use, first reviewing some of the key anatomy before focusing on physiological data. (For comprehensive summaries of parietofrontal, parietoparietal, and frontofrontal circuitry, see Andersen et al., 1997; Battaglia-Mayer et al., 2001; Cavada and Goldman-Rakic, 1989a, 1989b; Kurata, 1991; Marconi et al., 2001; Rizzolatti and Luppino, 2001; Wise et al., 1997.)

Parietofrontal Anatomy

The many conventions used for parceling parietal and frontal areas in the monkey are continuously reevaluated and revised as new data become available. In this section, I will adopt the conventions of Pandya and Seltzer (1982; see also Petrides and Pandya, 1984), as used in Rizzolatti and Luppino, 2001. Although, as we will see, there are important differences between human and monkey cortical anatomy, particularly with respect to the inferior parietal lobule (IPL), the monkey brain nevertheless provides a useful blueprint for understanding the functional architecture of prehension.

As shown in figure 7.2 and plate 4, posterior parietal cortex (PPC) of primates can be grossly partitioned into superior and inferior parietal lobules (SPL and IPL), separated by the intraparietal sulcus (IPs). In the monkey, SPL consists of several areas that have been defined based on their anatomical or functional characteristics or both, including areas PE, PEa, PEc, PEci, the medial intraparietal (MIP) area, and a portion of the ventral intraparietal (VIP) area located on the rostral bank of the IPs. The IPL includes areas PF, PFG, PG, the anterior and lateral intraparietal (AIP and LIP) areas, and a portion of the ventral intraparietal (VIP) area located on the caudal bank of the IPs.

Areas within the superior and inferior parietal lobules are directly interconnected with premotor cortex, and also provide indirect input to premotor areas via distinct sectors of prefrontal cortex (figure 7.2). Premotor (PM) cortex can be grossly divided into dorsal and ventral (PMd and PMv) regions, which appear not to be densely interconnected (Kurata, 1991). Further, PMd is subdivided into rostral (area F7) and caudal (area F2) regions, whereas PMv consists of areas F4 and F5. Area F2 is interconnected with primary motor area F1, and is also known to project directly to the spinal cord (He et al., 1993; Wise et al., 1997).

Most of the direct visual input to area PMd in the monkey originates in the superior parietal lobule (Caminiti et al., 1996), although area V6a (the pars opercalis or area PO) also provides direct visual input to area F7. Area PO is the only known visual area that lacks foveal magnification, and its response properties suggest that it may be important for detecting and localizing objects in ambient vision (Battaglia-Mayer et al., 2001; Wise et al., 1997), an important characteristic of many manual actions. Area MIP also receives visual input from area V6a and projects to areas F2 and F7. As discussed below, this circuit appears to be specialized for visuomotor transformations necessary for the control of reaching. Somatosensory information concerning limb position is provided to PMd via a circuit interconnecting areas PEc-PEip and F2 (Matelli et al., 1998). Recent data suggest that cells in PEc are involved in the integration of eye-hand information for coordinated movements (Ferraina et al., 2001). The portion of area VIP within the SPL also projects to area F2.

It is important to recognize that many areas within the inferior parietal lobule are also connected directly to dorsal premotor cortex (Tanné et al.,

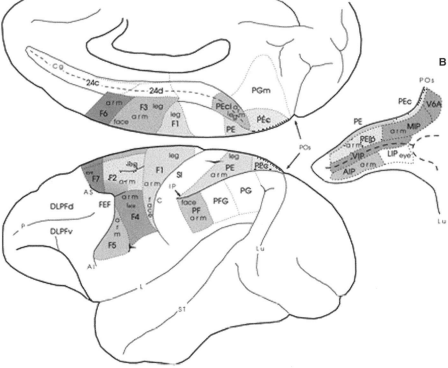

Figure 7.2
Cortical areas involved in sensorimotor behavior. Interconnected regions of parietal and frontal areas are shown in the same colors; areas receiving prefrontal input are shown in blue. (A) Mesial and lateral views of the monkey brain showing the parcellation of the motor, posterior parietal, and cingulate cortices. (B) Unfolded view of areas within the intraparietal sulcus. AI, inferior arcuate sulcus; AIP, anterior intraparietal area; AS, superior arcuate sulcus; C, central sulcus; Cg, cingulate sulcus; DLPFd, dorsolateral prefrontal cortex, dorsal; DLPFv, dorsolateral prefrontal cortex, ventral; FEF, frontal eye field; L, lateral fissure; LIP, lateral intraparietal area; Lu, lunate sulcus; MIP, medial intraparietal area; P, principal sulcus; POs, parieto-occipital sulcus; ST, superior temporal sulcus; VIP, ventral intraparietal area. (Adapted with permission from Rizzolatti and Luppino, 2001.) See plate 4 for color version.

1995), albeit less densely (Marconi et al., 2001). These areas include caudal VIP, LIP, PF, PFG, and PG (Wise et al., 1997). Although not considered part of premotor cortex, it is also worth noting that the frontal eye fields (FEFs) receive input from area LIP, which itself houses neurons that represent eye position relative to the head and body (Andersen et al., 1997).

The rostral portion of the inferior parietal lobule is a major source of afferent projections to ventral premotor cortex (Godschalk et al., 1984; Kurata, 1991; Luppino et al., 1999). The PMv area contains two functional subdivisions, areas F4 and F5, whose inputs arise from segregated regions of parietal cortex (Luppino et al., 1999). Area F5 receives input from prefrontal cortex and the anterior intraparietal area and appears to be concerned with visuomotor transformations involved in grasping. Area F4 is directly interconnected with ventral and medial intraparietal areas and with area V6a; this circuit may play a role in constructing representations of peripersonal space (Graziano and Gross, 1998).

There is also evidence that input from the inferior and superior parietal lobules may reach premotor cortex indirectly via prefrontal areas. Regions within the IPL project to distinct subdivisions of dorsolateral prefrontal cortex (Cavada and Goldman-Rakic, 1989b). Area PFG projects to dorsolateral prefrontal cortex, ventral (DLPFv), as well as to the FEFs. Area PG is connected with dorsolateral prefrontal cortex, dorsal (DLPFd), DLPFv, FEFs, and F7 (Petrides and Pandya, 1984). By contrast, areas within the superior parietal lobule project to dorsomedial prefrontal cortex (Petrides and Pandya, 1984). In turn, dorsolateral and dorsomedial prefrontal regions provide input to dorsal premotor areas (F2 and F7) and medial premotor areas (F3), respectively (Barbas, 1988). Prefrontal inputs to PMd are more concentrated in F2, and may provide an indirect route for sensory information from both IPL and SPL (Wise et al., 1997).

Finally, it is important to note that dorsal and ventral premotor cortex are not densely interconnected (Kurata, 1991), although the caudal aspect of dorsal premotor cortex (PMdc) is interconnected with F1 and also projects directly to the spinal cord.

An important principle that has emerged from electrophysiological investigations of these areas is that parietofrontal circuits are specialized for computing different sensorimotor transformations. Recent functional neuroimaging studies suggest a homologous organization in humans.

Functionally Specialized Parietofrontal Circuits

Constructing representations of actions involves integrating sensory information on target objects' intrinsic and extrinsic spatial properties with information on the spatial properties of the effector system and surrounding space. Over the past decade, an understanding of the roles played by functionally specialized parietofrontal circuits in these sensorimotor transformations has emerged. This section reviews several of the circuits most pertinent to the planning and control of prehensile actions, specifically, those involved in reaching, grasping, and the representation of peripersonal space.

Sensorimotor Transformations for Reaching

Psychophysical observations by Jeannerod and colleagues first suggested that sensorimotor transformations underlying reaching versus grasping actions involve dissociable mechanisms (Jeannerod, 1981), a finding supported by subsequent physiological data (Jeannerod et al., 1995). Reaching toward a target involves transforming a representation of objects' extrinsic spatial properties (i.e., location, orientation) and knowledge of the limb's position into a motor plan. These transformations are accomplished within a circuit interconnecting the medial intraparietal area of the superior parietal lobule and dorsal premotor cortex (Johnson et al., 1993; Johnson and Ferraina, 1996). Cells within the MIP area appear to represent the intention to move an arm along a specific trajectory in space; moreover, PMd is well situated for computing premovement plans for reaching, receiving direct visual (Caminiti et al., 1996) and higher-level proprioceptive (Lacquaniti et al., 1995) input from the SPL. Likewise, somatosensory information concerning limb position is provided to PMd via a circuit interconnecting PEc-PEip-F2 (Matelli et al., 1998). Neurons in PMd represent both the location of visual targets and the direction of intended forelimb movements needed to acquire them, even under conditions of nonstandard mappings (Shen and Alexander, 1997). Indeed, it appears that single PMd neurons represent specific reaching actions: A subpopulation of PMd neurons selectively responds to specific combinations of sensory cues specifying target location and the limb to use during manual pointing (Hoshi and Tanji, 2000). Work in my laboratory suggests that a homologue of the medial intraparietal area–dorsal premotor cortex (MIP-PMd) circuit may be involved in reach planning in humans.

Reach Circuit Homologue in Humans

Results of several PET studies (Colebatch et al., 1991; Deiber et al., 1991; Grafton et al., 1992) suggest the existence of a human homologue of the MIP-PMd circuit. Because of both spatial constraints and movement-related artifacts, however, it has proven challenging to investigate reaching with the higher-resolution technique of functional magnetic resonance imaging (fMRI). Recently, my colleagues and I (Johnson et al., 2002) developed an event-related fMRI paradigm that enabled us to circumvent these obstacles by having subjects plan object-oriented reaching movements without overt execution. In this implicit motor imagery paradigm, subjects were required to select whether an under- or overhand posture would be the most comfortable way to grip a handle appearing in a variety of different three-dimensional orientations. For these choices to be consistent with grip preferences displayed on a comparable task that involved actually grasping handles, subjects had to accurately represent both the stimulus orientation and the biomechanical constraints on pronation and supination of the hand (Johnson, 2000b). Grip selection judgments were made in the absence of overt hand movements and, as a consequence, without associated sensory feedback. We reasoned that selecting a grip in this task requires computing plans for both reaching toward and orienting the hand to engage the handle correctly, without changing the configuration of the hand. Therefore, to the extent that mechanisms involved in reach planning are organized similarly in the human and the monkey, this task should involve a homologue of the MIP-PMd pathway.

As expected on the basis of earlier psychophysical studies (Johnson, 2000a, b, Johnson et al., 2001; Johnson, Sprehn, and Saykin, 2002), subjects performed these tasks in a manner highly consistent with the biomechanical constraints of the two arms. As illustrated in figure 7.3, these biomechanically constrained judgments induced bilateral activation on the dorsal aspect of the precentral gyrus (putative PMd) regardless of whether they were based on the left or right hand. This observation is consistent with earlier observations suggesting that that caudal PMd is involved in preparation and selection of conditional motor behavior (Grafton et al., 1998; Passingham, 1993).

In contrast to the bilateral effects observed in dorsal premotor cortex, activations within posterior parietal cortex were dependent, in part, on the hand on which grip decisions were based. Left and right hand grip selection judgments each activated regions located within the medial extent of the intraparietal sulcus in the hemisphere contralateral to the involved hand.

A. Left Hand Reach Planning

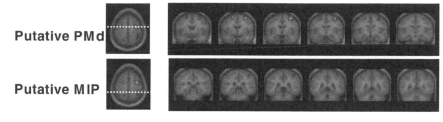

B. Right Hand Reach Planning

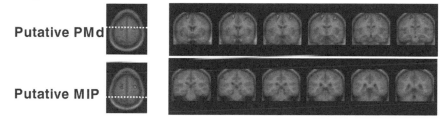

Figure 7.3
Putative homologue of the monkey parietofrontal reach circuit. Implicit motor imagery involving either the left or right hands is associated with bilateral activation of Brodmann area 6 (putative dorsal premotor cortex) and medial intraparietal sulcus (putative medial intraparietal area) contralateral to the hand on which grip selection decisions are based.

On the basis of both their locations and their functional involvement in reach planning, we believe that these sites represent homologues of the medial intraparietal area in the monkey. Consistent with this interpretation, responses of cells within the MIP area are known to be most pronounced when actions involve the contralateral hand (Colby and Duhamel, 1991). Together, these findings suggest that the MIP area in humans and monkeys may compute spatial representations according to a frame of reference centered on the involved limb.

Finally, grip decisions involving either hand also activated a common region of the right superior parietal lobule. As noted earlier, it is well known that the SPL is the major source of parietal visual input to dorsal premotor cortex in monkeys and is also involved in higher-level proprioception. In humans, the SPL participates in the representation of finger, hand, and arm movements (Deiber et al., 1991; Grafton et al., 1992; Roland et al., 1980), as well as high-level spatial cognitive processes like mental rotation (Haxby et al., 1991, 1994), and imitation of hand movements (Iacoboni et al.,

1999). Involvement of the SPL is therefore consistent with our behavioral investigations in suggesting that this grip selection task involves implicitly transforming representations of the cued arm in order to evaluate the awkwardness of over- versus underhand responses.

In sum, results from functional neuroimaging are consistent with electrophysiological studies in monkeys in showing that dorsal premotor cortex integrates visual information from the medial intraparietal area on a target object's spatial disposition with proprioceptive information from the superior parietal lobule on the involved limb into a premovement plan for reaching.

Sensorimotor Transformations for Grasping

In contrast to reaching, grasping involves integrating representations of objects' intrinsic spatial properties (e.g., shape, size, texture) with properties of the hand and fingers. In the monkey, this is accomplished in a more ventral parietofrontal circuit connecting the anterior intraparietal area of the inferior parietal lobule with area F5 of ventral premotor cortex (figure 7.2). The AIP area contains several subpopulations of "manipulation" cells that represent specific types of hand postures necessary for grasping objects of differing shapes (Sakata et al., 1995; Taira et al., 1990). Motor dominant neurons require no visual input and therefore discharge in either the light or dark during grasping. Visuomotor neurons respond more strongly in light, but also in dark when neither the hand nor target are visible. Finally, visual neurons only respond in the light, and some appear to selectively represent the three-dimensional shapes of "graspable" objects even in the absence of hand movements (Murata et al., 1996).

Area F5 contains interleaved representations of the fingers, hands, and mouth. Cells within F5 appear to be involved in the preparation and execution of visually guided grasping actions (Rizzolatti et al., 1988). This area is subdivided into F5ab, in the posterior bank of the inferior arcuate sulcus, and area F5c, in the dorsal convexity (Rizzolatti and Luppino, 2001). Both subdivisions receive major inputs from secondary somatosensory cortex (SII), and from the inferior parietal lobule (Godschalk et al., 1984), which also contains a representation of the face and arm. Area F5ab also receives a major projection from the AIP area. Like visual neurons in AIP, some F5ab units respond selectively to three-dimensional shapes even when no hand movements are involved. Effective stimuli are typically of a shape that is compatible with the particular cells' preferred hand configuration

(Rizzolatti et al., 1996a). It is believed that these visual units code objects' 3-D features and are involved in the selection of appropriate grasping and manipulation movements (Luppino et al., 1999, p. 181).

Similar to cells in the anterior superior temporal sulcus (STS; Jellema et al., 2000), many F5c units represent specific hand configurations, such as power or precision gripping. However, unlike STS neurons, F5c cells do not appear to code arbitrary postures or movements. Instead, they seem to represent the goal of, rather than the specific movements involved in, manual actions, such as holding, grasping, or tearing an object. In this sense, F5c units' responses are context dependent (Rizzolatti and Luppino, 2001). If the same hand movements are made in the context of a different action (e.g., grooming instead of feeding), F5c responses will be weak or absent. This has led to the hypothesis that area F5c contains a "vocabulary" of hand *actions* (Rizzolatti et al., 1988). Furthermore, F5c units appear to differentially code the temporal properties of hand movements, with some units responding selectively during early, intermediate, or later phases of an action (Rizzolatti and Luppino, 2001). Although not discussed here, it is noteworthy that a subset of these units, known as "mirror cells," responds when the monkey either performs or observes an experimenter performing a goal-oriented movement (e.g., manipulating an object, or grasping a piece of food; see Iacoboni, chapter 4, this volume).

Grasp Circuit Homologue in Humans

Identification of a parietofrontal circuit specifically associated with grasping in humans has proven challenging. Several early positron-emission tomography (PET) studies observed that grasping was associated with a site in the superior frontal gyrus (GFs) or Brodmann area (BA) 6 that would be a more likely homologue of dorsal than ventral premotor cortex (Grafton et al., 1996; Rizzolatti et al., 1996b). Grafton and colleagues (1996) suggested that difficulties identifying a more ventral anterior intraparietal area–ventral premotor cortex (AIP-PMv) homologue may be related to methodological limitations including use of relatively undemanding tasks and reliance on the limited spatiotemporal resolution of (PET) imaging. They also raised another admittedly more speculative possibility, that the functional architecture of human prehension may differ considerably from that of other primate prehension. More recent work using higher-resolution fMRI appears to support the former hypothesis. Binkofsky and colleagues (1998) first reported significant activation within the anterior intraparietal sulcus (putative AIP) when subjects grasped versus pointed at rectangular visual objects; moreover they reported that lesions in this region produced deficits in configuring the hand to engage objects effectively. Putative AIP also seems to be active when subjects grasp objects without vision, as haptic manipulation of complex versus simple spherical shapes induced significant activations in putative AIP as well as BA 44 (putative F5; Binkofski et al., 1999). This later observation is consistent with the existence of motor dominant AIP neurons that respond even when objects are grasped in the dark.

My colleagues and I recently undertook an fMRI study of visually guided grasping using a more varied set of stimuli that have geometrically irregular bounding contours. In earlier psychophysical experiments (Johnson, 2001), I found evidence that the human visual system is especially sensitive to objects' two-dimensional bounding contours or silhouettes, and that this may reflect the importance of this information in grasping. Earlier work by Goodale and colleagues (1994) had demonstrated that the shape of the bounding contour is used to achieve stable precision grips where opposing forces of the thumb and forefinger pass directly through objects' centers of mass. As illustrated in figure 7.4A (and plate 5), subjects in our imaging study also showed this pattern when they were required to grasp visually presented, complex, three-dimensional shapes with their dominant right hands. Figure 7.4B shows that in 90% of our subjects grasping was associated with a consistent activation in putative AIP as well as the secondary somatosensory region (SII). As noted above, in monkeys both areas provide major sensory projections to F5. Conspicuously absent, however, are activations in frontal cortex (BA 44) that might be homologous with F5. The reasons for this are unknown, and additional work on mechanisms of grasping in humans is clearly needed. Nevertheless, these results do indicate that, as in monkeys, a highly localized region of the anterior intraparietal sulcus contralateral to the effector participates in the transformation of objects' intrinsic spatial properties into hand configurations for grasping.

In addition to representations of objects' extrinsic and intrinsic spatial properties, accurate representations of one's limbs and their relationships to target objects and to the surrounding environment are necessary to manipulate objects effectively. Indeed, we know that such representations are requisite for dexterous tool use. Although less is presently known about substrates involved in representing peripersonal space, recent evidence sug-

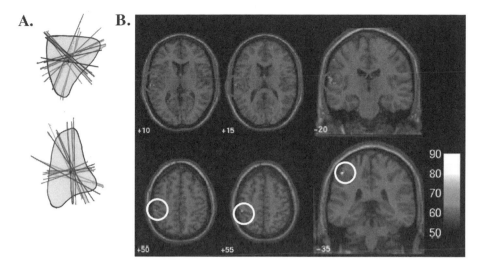

Figure 7.4
Putative homologue of the anterior intraparietal area of the monkey parietofrontal grasp circuit. (*A*) Two of the shapes used in the grasping experiment. Each line represents the opposing force vectors from two points on the objects' surfaces contacted by the thumb and forefinger on a given trial. Across four different orientations, subjects consistently chose grips that caused these opposing forces to cancel through objects' centers of mass. (*B*) Approximately 90% of participants showed activation in the anterior intraparietal sulcus (yellow circles; putative anterior intraparietal area) and secondary somatosensory cortex (SII; blue circles) during visually guided precision gripping as contrasted with pointing. See plate 5 for color version.

gests that they may include a specialized parietofrontal circuit interconnecting the subregions of the inferior parietal lobule and ventral premotor cortex.

Visuotactile-Motor Transformations for Object Manipulation

Electrophysiological investigations suggest that visuotactile representations of peripersonal space are constructed in a circuit connecting the ventral intraparietal area of the inferior parietal lobule with area F4 in ventral premotor cortex (Fogassi et al., 1992, 1996). Area F4, which contains a representation of the face, neck, trunk, and limbs, lies caudal to grasp-related area F5 (figure 7.2). Most units in area F4 are bimodal, having tactile receptive fields (RFs) that are in register with three-dimension visual RFs of space immediately adjacent to the animal. However, these representations are not affected by variations in gaze direction. Similar RF properties can be found in the VIP area (Colby et al., 1993; Duhamel et al., 1998), which provides direct afferent input to F4 (Luppino et al., 1999). These observations have prompted the hypothesis that the VIP-F4 circuit represents peripersonal space in a frame of reference centered on the body part involved in a given visually guided action such as object manipulation (Fogassi et al., 1996; Graziano et al., 1994).

It is also worth noting that recent work in electrophysiology has also identified cells distributed throughout the intraparietal sulcus that appear to have visuotactile properties similar to those observed in area F4 (Iriki et al., 2001; Obayashi et al., 2000). Interestingly, the visual receptive fields of these units appear to *increase* when monkeys use tools to retrieve other objects (e.g., food pellets; Iriki et al., 1996). Visual RFs normally in register with tactile RFs of the hand expand to encompass peripersonal space occupied by the tool. Such expansion was not observed when tools were merely held, only when they were actively used to accomplish an intentional action (e.g., food retrieval). Similarly, a recent PET study of monkeys showed increased activation that included VIP and F4, as well as basal ganglia, pre–supplementary motor area (pre-SMA), and cerebellum when monkeys used a tool to retrieve food (Obayashi et al., 2001).

Recent studies of humans with parietal lesions have revealed behavioral effects that nicely complement these observations in monkeys (Farne and Ladavas, 2000; Maravita et al., 2001). For instance, right parietal patient P.P. evidenced unilateral left neglect when performing a line bisection task positioned within reach and when bisecting lines at a distance with a handheld stick, but no such neglect when bisecting distant lines with a laser pointer (Berti and Frassinetti, 2000). It was suggested that, as with changes in the receptive field properties of intraparietal sulcus neurons in monkeys, the use of a stick caused distant space to be remapped as "within reach," leading to neglect-related bias in performance.

In a recent pilot study, my colleagues and I used fMRI to compare areas activated when performing a repetitive object transfer task using either the right hand or a handheld set of tongs. Using tongs to transfer a set of rings from one peg to another resulted in increased activation within the contralateral inferior frontal gyrus (GFi, putative PMv), which may reflect an expansion in the representation of the hand to encompass peripersonal space covered by the tool.

Together, these findings are consistent with the existence of parieto-frontal mechanisms specialized to maintain and update representations of peripersonal space during object manipulation in both monkeys and humans. These mechanisms represent an important bridge between circuits underlying prehension and those involved in more sophisticated tool utilization behaviors elaborated below.

To summarize, evidence from studies of nonhuman primates and humans suggests that functionally specialized parietofrontal circuits are involved in the sensorimotor transformations necessary for manual prehension of objects. These circuits involve parietal regions within both inferior and superior parietal lobules and the segregated regions of frontal cortex to which they project. Together, these circuits constitute a prehension system that is well suited to control reaching, grasping, and manipulating objects on the basis of the perceptual information. As noted at the outset, however, complex tool utilization demands more than sensorimotor transformations. Actors must also have the ability to acquire and access representations of the tools' functional properties and the actions with which they are associated. Nevertheless, the possibility of a separate system dedicated to controlling skilled actions involving other objects has been largely overlooked (see Buxbaum, 2001). Drawing on evidence from neurology and neuroimaging, section 7.3 makes a case for a utilization system that is functionally and anatomically dissociable from the prehension and comprehension systems.

7.3   The Utilization System

Although the skillful use of tools demands seamless cooperation between prehension and tool use systems, on closer examination, it becomes clear that representations involved in tool use are dissociable from the sensorimotor transformations underlying prehension.

Dissociating Utilization from Prehension

As more than a century of neurological research suggests, tool use behaviors involve a system that is functionally and anatomically dissociable from the system that controls dexterous prehension. On the one hand, patients with optic ataxia (OA) have difficulties using visual information to control manual actions, regardless of their familiarity with the task—reflecting impairment of the sensorimotor transformations of the prehension system. On the other hand, patients with ideomotor apraxia (IM) can use objects' perceptual properties to control manual actions relatively normally, but have selective difficulties at manual tasks that require accessing representations of skilled actions, most notably tool use. These deficits reflect impairment, not of the prehension system per se, but rather of a separate utilization system.

Optic Ataxia   In 1909, Balint (see Balint, 1995) coined the term *optic ataxia* to describe the deficit of a patient with bilateral parietal damage who misreached for objects when using the right hand. This deficit could not be accounted for in purely perceptual or motor terms. The patient remained capable of reaching accurately for objects with the left hand, and retained the ability to access representations within the comprehension system (ventral processing stream) necessary to recognize, and perform perceptual judgments about, objects that could not be successfully engaged.

Consistent with observations in monkeys that reaching and grasping are controlled by separate parietofrontal circuits, some OA patients display deficits in visually guided reaching, while still retaining the ability to correctly preshape the hand when grasping (Tzavaras and Masure, 1976, cited in Milner and Goodale, 1995). Conversely, grasping can also be affected while reaching remains intact (Jakobson et al., 1991).

Traditionally, optic ataxia has been associated with lesions to the superior parietal lobule (Perenin and Vighetto, 1988). Given the substantial spatial variation in brain injuries among these patients, however, it is quite likely that this disorder also reflects damage to regions within the inferior parietal lobule (e.g., Guard et al., 1984). Indeed, on the basis of functional imaging results discussed above, one would expect lesions to the anterior intraparietal area of the IPL to be an important factor in cases of OA where grasp is affected (e.g., Goodale et al., 1994; Jeannerod, 1986). Indeed, Binkofski and colleagues (1998) have shown that damage to putative AIP results in impairments of visually guided grasping.

Recent work in monkey electrophysiology has suggested a more detailed hypothesis concerning the sensorimotor impairment in optic ataxia that emphasizes the interdependence of parietal and frontal areas. Specifically, misreaching may reflect a failure of systems involved in the "early and context-dependent combination of eye and hand signals within the global tuning fields of parietal neurons" (Battaglia-Mayer et al., 2001, p. 543). Normally, this combined information would be available to premotor areas involved in action planning. However, as a result of their injury, OA patients fail when the tasks demand combining eye and hand position information to contact a visual target. As a consequence, it is hypothesized that patients may realize that movements have occurred, but are unaware of their direction. OA lesions may therefore impair not just parietal functions, but also the interplay between parietal and premotor areas that occurs within the prehension system during manual actions.

One of the more astounding observations in the optic ataxia literature is that, despite substantial difficulties with on-line prehension, at least some patients may still accurately acquire familiar objects. This suggests that the prehension system can be damaged without disrupting the execution of learned skills. Jeannerod and colleagues (1994) reported an intriguing case of patient A.T., who suffered bilateral parietal lesions, but whose ability to reach for unfamiliar objects (cylinders of different sizes) remained largely intact. However, the hand configurations she adopted when attempting to grasp these items were grossly impaired; she failed to appropriately scale her grip aperture to the objects' sizes and to correctly time the closing of her grasp with both her left and right hands, although the deficit was more pronounced for her right. Strikingly, when A.T. was instead required to grasp familiar, meaningful objects, her performance improved dramatically; indeed, her maximum grip apertures correlated with objects' sizes at a level comparable to that of normal controls. This finding was interpreted as evidence that dorsal (prehension) and ventral (comprehension) systems are interactive, that stored semantic representations of familiar objects' physical properties can be used as cues for prehension (Jeannerod, pp. 66–67). On the other hand, it might as easily be interpreted as evidence for the existence of two dissociable systems for the control of manual actions: a prehension system that relies exclusively on the physical properties of the objects and is damaged in optic ataxia, and a utilization system that represents movements associated with objects' functional properties and remains intact. This alternative interpretation is consistent with evidence for the opposite dissociation manifest in patients with ideomotor apraxia (IM).

Ideomotor Apraxia   Leipmann (1900) coined the term *ideomotor apraxia* to describe loss of skilled movements that could not be attributed to elementary motor or perceptual deficits. IM patients have difficulties in performing one or more of the following actions: pantomiming tool use, gesturing to command, imitating movements, and, in some instances, actually using tools or objects (for a comprehensive review, see Heilman and Rothi, 1997). Leipmann's original patient (M.T.) exhibited a loss of skilled movement involving the right arm following diffuse brain damage associated with syphilis. Subsequently, Leipmann showed that right hemisphere damage did not appear to result in apraxia: Many left hemisphere patients were apraxic even when performing movements with the non-hemiplegic, left hand. However controversial Leipmann's interpretation of these impairments may be, numerous subsequent investigations have supported his primary contention—that the posterior left cerebral hemisphere of humans plays a dominant role in representing skilled action (Geschwind, 1965; Leiguarda and Marsden, 2000). In contrast to optic ataxia, ideomotor apraxia is associated with damage to areas within and adjacent to the left intraparietal sulcus, including BA 7, the angular gyrus (BA 39), and the supramarginal gyrus (BA 40), as well as the middle frontal gyrus (GFm; Haaland et al., 2000; these areas will be treated in greater detail in section 7.4).

Although the standard test for ideomotor apraxia includes having subjects pantomime tool use, at least some patients display impairments that are consistent with the model of separate prehension and utilization systems when attempting to actually use tools. For instance, Sirigu and colleagues (1995; see also Sirigu et al., chapter 6 this volume) reported that left parietal patient L.L. committed errors when grasping common objects in order to use them, whereas she was able to grasp the same objects in appropriately stable grips when she was simply asked to pick them up. In other words, L.L. was capable of performing the sensorimotor transformations necessary for accurate prehension, but could not access information required for utilization.

In short, contrasting deficits displayed by optic ataxia versus ideomotor apraxia patients suggest the existence of two functionally independent systems for controlling object-oriented, manual actions (Buxbaum, 2001). The prehension system relies on sensorimotor transformations to perform actions based on objects' perceptual properties, whereas the utilization system guides skilled actions based on representations of previously acquired skills. Despite considerable intersubject variation, analyses of lesion locations in these populations raise the possibility that different parietal or frontal areas, or both, may be contributing to these functions. More precise details of the functional architecture of the utilization systems has emerged from a recent series of fMRI experiments in my laboratory.

7.4   Mapping the Utilization System

As noted earlier, over a century of research on ideomotor apraxia patients
has consistently shown that the left posterior parietal lobe plays a critical
role in representing the skilled actions of right-handers. Although the traditional view is that ideomotor apraxia results from damage to regions of the
left parietal lobe resulting in a loss of movement formulas or engrams, some
IM patients have damage exclusive to, or encompassing, the left frontal
lobe, which suggests that, like prehension, representations of skilled action
involve interconnected parietal and frontal mechanisms.

Lesion Localization

Analysis of lesion locations in a population of 41 ideomotor apraxia patients
by Haaland and colleagues (2000) provides a more refined portrait of the
regions, whether frontal, parietal, or both, involved in skilled praxis. Lesion
locations in these patients were compared with those in a group of nonapraxic controls who also had left hemisphere damage. IM patients were
divided into three categories based on whether their lesions included parietal, frontal, or parietal and frontal cortex. As illustrated in figure 7.5 and
plate 6, results for the parietal group indicate 68–84% lesion overlap in
regions within and adjacent to the intraparietal sulcus, in both the ventral
extent of the superior parietal lobule and, more extensively, into the inferior
parietal lobule. Key sites included Brodmann area (BA)7, the angular gyrus
(BA 39), and the supramarginal gyrus (BA 40). Results for the frontal group
showed 100% lesion overlap within the middle frontal gyrus, particularly
BAs 46 and 9. As would be expected, the group with both parietal and
frontal lesions showed maximum lesion overlap in BAs 9, 46, 7, 39, and
40. Further, nonapraxic controls tended not to have lesions in these regions.

These areas do overlap somewhat with regions associated with the
prehension system. That damage associated with ideomotor apraxia often
includes regions within the intraparietal sulcus and ventral superior parietal
lobule may explain why some patients exhibit kinematic abnormalities
when interacting with perceptually available objects (Haaland et al., 1999;
Poizner et al., 1995; Rapcsak et al., 1995). This would be expected if damage included circuits within the prehension system that are functionally
specialized for specific sensorimotor transformations (e.g., putative AIP for
grasping or MIP for reaching, or both). On the other hand, the core deficit
that distinguishes ideomotor apraxia from optic ataxia—loss of access to

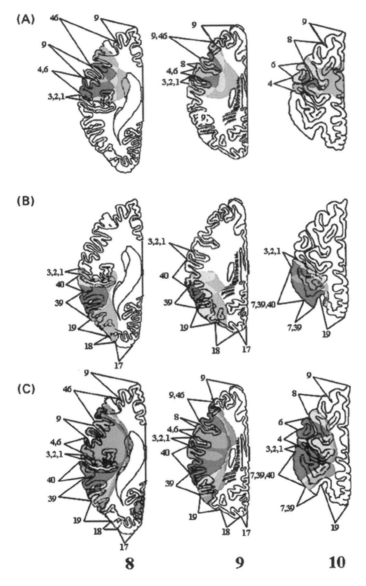

Figure 7.5

Overlap of lesions in patients who are limb-apraxic (*A*, *B*, and *C*) and patients who are not (*D*, *E*, and *F*). Patients with damage anterior (*A* and *D*), posterior (*B* and *E*), or both anterior and posterior (*C* and *F*) to the central sulcus are shown separately. Overlapping the lesions in the anterior apraxic group (*A*) produced 100% overlap (yellow) in the middle frontal gyrus including Brodmann areas (BAs) 46, 9, 8, 6, and 4 on sections 8 and 9. Lesion overlap of the same areas in the nonapraxics (*B*) was much less, especially for BAs 46 and 9 on section 8. Overlapping the lesions in the posterior apraxic group (*B*) produced an area of maximum overlap (pink)

(D)

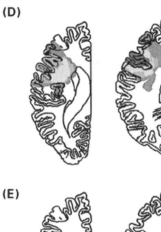

Percent of overlap

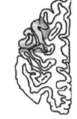

(E)

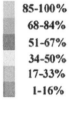

	85-100%
	68-84%
	51-67%
	34-50%
	17-33%
	1-16%

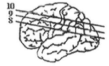

(F)

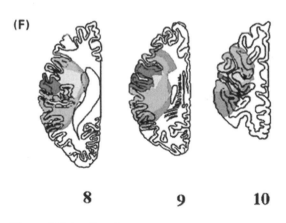

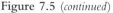

8　　　**9**　　　**10**

Figure 7.5 (*continued*)
in BAs 7, 39, and 40 on section 10. Comparison with the nonapraxics with posterior lesions (*E*) showed much less overlap (dark blue) in that area. Overlapping the lesions in the apraxic patients with anterior and posterior damage (*C*) produced 100% overlap (yellow) in BAs 9 and 46 on section 8 with much less overlap (green) in the nonapraxics (*F*); BAs 7, 39, and 40 on section 10 showed an area of maximum overlap (red) relative to the minimal overlap (blue) in the nonapraxics; the area of maximum parietal overlap was in area 40 on section 9 (pink), with less overlap (red and green) in the nonapraxics. (Reprinted with permission from Haaland et al., 2000, p. 2310.) See plate 6 for color version.

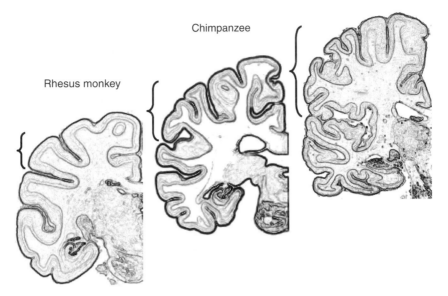

Figure 7.6
Comparisons between the relative size of the inferior parietal lobule (IPL) in rhesus monkey, chimpanzee, and human. As illustrated in these coronal brain slices of the left hemisphere, there has been a substantial expansion in the relative size of the human parietal cortex, particularly within the IPL (bracketed). Note that slices have been rescaled to achieve similar overall dimensions to aid in direct comparison.

representations needed for skilled actions—cannot be explained solely by disruption of these sensorimotor transformations.

The implication of BAs 39–40 in the representation of tool use is intriguing from an evolutionary perspective. As illustrated in figure 7.6, when overall brain volume is controlled, human inferior parietal lobule is considerably larger than rhesus monkey or even chimpanzee IPL (Eidelberg and Galaburda, 1984). It has long been known that the IPL underwent significant expansion during human evolution. In particular, Brodmann himself only identified the angular gyrus (BA 39) and the supramarginal gyrus (BA 40) in the human neocortex, leading to protracted debate over whether homologous regions exist in monkeys (Kolb, 1996, p. 266). It is therefore tempting to speculate that the greatly expanded repertoire of tool use behaviors in humans may indeed be related to these anatomical differences.

Another interesting finding that emerged from Haaland et al., 2000, is the implication of the left middle frontal gyrus in skilled action representations. As with prehension, this finding emphasizes the role of parietal and interconnected frontal sites in the representation of skilled action.

In sum, results of lesion analysis suggest that the utilization system may reside within a parietofrontal circuit in the human left cerebral hemisphere. A recent series of fMRI studies in my laboratory were undertaken in an attempt to more precisely identify areas involved in representing tool use.

Functional Neuroimaging

The most common bedside screening for ideamotor apraxia involves having patients attempt to pantomime familiar actions, including use of familiar tools (e.g., a comb to comb their hair or a hammer to drive a nail). Success on this task requires that they perform three related subtasks. First, they must engage in linguistic processing in order to identify the stimulus object and retrieve the function associated with the tool. According to the present model, these processes should take place within the comprehension system. Second, they must access representations of specific movements, or motor engrams, that constitute the appropriate tool use actions. This process should take place within the left, parietofrontal utilization system. Finally, they must execute tool use actions in peripersonal space. Control of these movements should involve parietofrontal circuits of the prehension system.

Using fMRI, my colleagues and I attempted to replicate this screening test with the goal of isolating the areas within the healthy brain that are involved in the processes of these subtasks. Each trial in this randomized, event-related design consisted of three components: (1) an instructional cue (IC); (2) a delay period of either 3s or 5s; and (3) a movement cue (MC). On 50% of trials, ICs named familiar tools that were commonly manipulated in a characteristic way with the dominant hand (e.g., knife, hammer, or pencil). When hearing one of these object ICs, subjects used the delay interval to prepare to pantomime the associated action. If the subsequent MC was a go signal, they executed the pantomime. If the MC was a no-go signal, they merely relaxed until the next IC occurred. An equal number of randomly intermixed trials began with the IC "Move." During the delay interval on these control trials, subjects simply prepared to move their hand in a random fashion. If the MC was a go signal, they would then execute the random movements. If it was a no-go signal, they would do nothing. All cues were auditory, and subjects' eyes remained closed throughout the task.

In our initial experiment, subjects used their dominant, right hand to produce all pantomimes and movements. Of primary interest were those areas activated during the delay interval when subjects were retrieving a tool–associated action as contrasted with preparing a random, nonmeaningful, hand movement. We reasoned that this comparison should isolate areas involved in representing actions associated with tool use, namely, those of the hypothesized utilization system. As shown in figure 7.7A (and plate 7), data were highly consistent with the lesion localization results discussed above. Gesture preparation was associated with a significant activation in the left inferior parietal lobule extending into the intraparietal sulcus and the ventral superior parietal lobule. This pattern is also highly consistent with Leipmann's century-old hypothesis that the left parietal lobule plays a key role in storage of motor programs for skilled actions, and Haaland and colleagues' (2000) lesion analysis (figure 7.5). Further, these results are consistent with the position that both parietal and frontal mechanisms are equally important in representing praxis (Heilman et al., 1982). As predicted on the basis of Haaland et al. (2000), the middle frontal gyrus was significantly activated during gesture retrieval. In contrast to the patient literature, however, we observed bilateral GFm involvement. One possibility is that the action representations are stored within the left parietal cortex but accessed via computations performed in bilaterally in GFm. According to this hypothesis, these processes would be interdependent rather than redundant, thus explaining why left unilateral frontal lesions can induce ideomotor apraxia. Another is that lesions of the middle frontal gyrus result in a disconnection between parietal action representations and primary motor cortex (Heilman et al., 1982).

Left posterior activations were also apparent in temporal cortex. These areas are likely involved in the linguistic processing necessary to identify stimuli and retrieve their associated functions (e.g., hammer → pounding). Consistent with this possibility, previous work (Fiez et al., 1996; Martin et al., 1995; Warburton et al., 1996) has shown a similar pattern during generation of action verbs.

A potential limitation of this experiment is that subjects always prepared and produced gestures with their dominant, right hand. Consequently, the left asymmetry in parietal and middle frontal gyrus activation is open to two interpretations. On the one hand, it may indeed reflect a left-hemisphere specialization for the representation of tool use actions, as expected on the basis of brain lesions in ideomotor apraxia, namely, that tool use actions are acquired and performed with the dominant, right hand, which is in turn controlled by the left hemisphere, or it might be

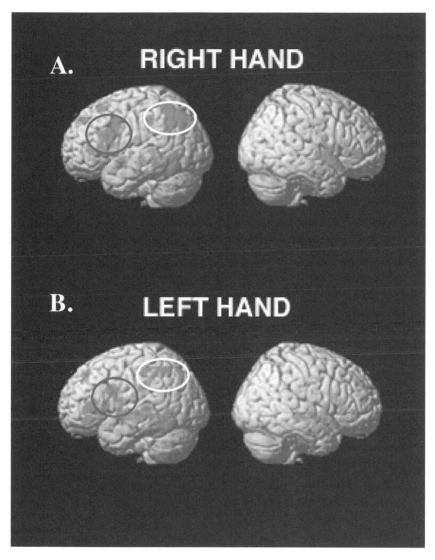

Figure 7.7
(*A*) Areas involved in preparing tool use gestures for the right hand. Preparing tool use actions is associated with activations in the left inferior parietal lobule (yellow circle) and middle frontal gyrus (blue circle). (*B*) This left lateralized parietofrontal network is also activated when gestures are prepared with the left hand. See plate 7 for color version.

the left hemisphere's overall specialization for constructing symbolic representations, most notably, language. Although not truly arbitrary, gestures certainly bear an abstract relationship to the tools with which they are associated. On the other hand, it could indicate a bilateral organization of the utilization system, with each hemisphere representing tool use actions involving the contralateral limb. Given the contralateral organization inherent in lower-level functions, this would allow quicker access to sensorimotor processes when planning and implementing actions with either limb, as the need for interhemispheric transfer would be eliminated. If the utilization system is specific to the left hemisphere, then requiring subjects to prepare gestures for the left hand should have no effect on the observed asymmetry. If, however, the utilization system is bilaterally organized, then preparing gestures for the left hand should induce a shift of these activations to homotopic areas of the right hemisphere.

A second experiment, undertaken in an attempt to distinguish between these alternative interpretations, consisted of a direct replication of the initial study with one exception: Subjects were now required to prepare and—depending on the identity of the movement cue, produce gestures with their nondominant, left hands. As shown in figure 7.7B, the results were highly consistent with a left-hemisphere specialization for representing tool use. As in the initial study, both the left inferior parietal lobule and the left middle frontal gyrus were activated during gesture preparation on the basis of the left hand.

7.5   Conclusions

Tool use in humans encompasses a remarkably diverse set of behaviors, from the fine skills of performing microsurgery or playing a violin to the mundane skills of drinking a glass of wine or shaving one's face. Underlying these behaviors is a parietofrontal system within the left cerebral hemisphere of humans that acquires and represents movements necessary for skilled tool use. An important component of this utilization system is the inferior parietal lobule, which has undergone significant expansion during evolution of the human brain. Although the IPL is interconnected with both ventral (comprehension system) and dorsal (prehension system) processing streams, it can be argued that it belongs to neither (see Milner and Goodale, 1995, p. 110). A similar argument has been made for the monkey anterior superior temporal polysensory (STP) area (Boussaoud et al., 1990), which some have suggested may be a homologue of BAs 39 and 40 (Milner, 1995; Morel and Bullier, 1990). Just as the STP area appears to integrate form processing associated with the ventral stream and motion processing associated with the dorsal stream (Oram and Perrett, 1996), so the utilization system conspires with the comprehension and prehension systems to enable skillful tool use in the everyday world.

References

Andersen, R. A., Snyder, L. H., Bradley, D. C., and Xing, J. (1997). Multimodal representation of space in the posterior parietal cortex and its use in planning movements. *Annu. Rev. Neurosci.* 20: 303–330.

Balint, R. (1995). Psychic paralysis of gaze, optic ataxia, and spatial disorder of attention, M. Harvey (trans.). *Cogn. Neuropsychol.* 12: 261–282.

Barbas, H. (1988). Anatomic organization of basoventral and mediodorsal visual recipient prefrontal regions in the rhesus monkey. *J. Comp. Neurol.* 276: 313–342.

Battaglia-Mayer, A., Ferraina, S., Genovesio, A., Marconi, B., Squatrito, S., Molinari, M., Lacquaniti, F., and Caminiti, R. (2001). Eye-hand coordination during reaching: 2. An analysis of the relationships between visuomanual signals in parietal cortex and parieto-frontal association projections. *Cereb. Cortex*, 11: 528–544.

Berti, A., and Frassinetti, F. (2000). When far becomes near: Remapping of space by tool use. *J. Cogn. Neurosci.* 12: 415–420.

Binkofski, F., Dohle, C., Posse, S., Stephan, K. M., Hefter, H., Seitz, R. J., and Freund, H. J. (1998). Human anterior intraparietal area subserves prehension: A combined lesion and functional MRI activation study. *Neurology* 50: 1253–1259.

Binkofski, F., Buccino, G., Posse, S., Seitz, R. J., Rizzolatti, G., and Freund, H. (1999). A fronto-parietal circuit for object manipulation in man: Evidence from an fMRI-study. *Eur. J. Neurosci.* 11: 3276–3286.

Boussaoud, D., Ungerleider, L. G., and Desimone, R. (1990). Pathways for motion analysis: Cortical connections of the medial superior temporal and fundus of the superior temporal visual areas in the macaque. *J. Comp. Neurol.* 296: 462–495.

Bradshaw, J. L. (1997). *Human Evolution: A Neuropsychological Perspective.* East Sussex, UK: Psychology Press.

Buxbaum, L. (2001). Ideomotor apraxia: A call to action. *Neurocase* 7: 445–458.

Caminiti, R., Ferraina, S., and Johnson, P. B. (1996). The sources of visual information to the primate frontal lobe: a novel role for the superior parietal lobule. *Cereb. Cortex* 6: 319–328.

Cavada, C., and Goldman-Rakic, P. S. (1989a). Posterior parietal cortex in rhesus monkey: 1. Parcellation of areas based on distinctive limbic and sensory corticocortical connections. *J. Comp. Neurol.* 287: 393–421.

Cavada, C., and Goldman-Rakic, P. S. (1989b). Posterior parietal cortex in rhesus monkey: 2. Evidence for segregated corticocortical networks linking sensory and limbic areas with the frontal lobe. *J. Comp. Neurol.* 287: 422–445.

Colby, C. L., and Duhamel, J. R. (1991). Heterogeneity of extrastriate visual areas and multiple parietal areas in the macaque monkey. *Neuropsychologia* 29: 517–537.

Colby, C. L., Duhamel, J. R., and Goldberg, M. E. (1993). Ventral intraparietal area of the macaque: Anatomic location and visual response properties. *J. Neurophysiol.* 69: 902–914.

Colebatch, J. G., Deiber, M. P., Passingham, R. E., Friston, K. J., and Frackowiak, R. S. (1991). Regional cerebral blood flow during voluntary arm and hand movements in human subjects. *J Neurophysiol.* 65: 1392–1401.

Deiber, M. P., Passingham, R. E., Colebatch, J. G., Friston, K. J., Nixon, P. D., and Frackowiak, R. S. (1991). Cortical areas and the selection of movement: A study with positron-emission tomography. *Exp. Brain Res.* 84: 393–402.

Duhamel, J. R., Colby, C. L., and Goldberg, M. E. (1998). Ventral intraparietal area of the macaque: Congruent visual and somatic response properties. *J. Neurophysiol.* 79: 126–136.

Eidelberg, D., and Galaburda, A. M. (1984). Inferior parietal lobule: Divergent architectonic asymmetries in the human brain. *Arch. Neurol.* 41: 843–852.

Farne, A., and Ladavas, E. (2000). Dynamic size-change of hand peripersonal space following tool use. *NeuroReport* 11: 1645–1649.

Ferraina, S., Battaglia-Mayer, A., Genovesio, A., Marconi, B., Onorati, P., and Caminiti, R. (2001). Early coding of visuomanual coordination during reaching in parietal area PEc. *J. Neurophysiol.* 85: 462–467.

Fiez, J. A., Raichle, M. E., Balota, D. A., Tallal, P., and Petersen, S. E. (1996). PET activation of posterior temporal regions during auditory word presentation and verb generation. *Cereb. Cortex* 6: 1–10.

Fogassi, L., Gallese, V., di Pellegrino, G., Fadiga, L., Gentilucci, M., Luppino, G., Matelli, M., Pedotti, A., and Rizzolatti, G. (1992). Space coding by premotor cortex. *Exp. Brain Res.* 89: 686–690.

Fogassi, L., Gallese, V., Fadiga, L., Luppino, G., Matelli, M., and Rizzolatti, G. (1996). Coding of peripersonal space in inferior premotor cortex (area F4). *J. Neurophysiol.* 76: 141–157.

Geschwind, N. (1965). Disconnexion syndromes in animals and man. Part 2. *Brain* 88: 585–644.

Godschalk, M., Lemon, R. N., Kuypers, H. G., and Ronday, H. K. (1984). Cortical afferents and efferents of monkey postarcuate area: An anatomical and electrophysiological study. *Exp. Brain Res.* 56: 410–424.

Goodale, M. A., Meenan, J. P., Bulthoff, H. H., Nicolle, D. A., Murphy, K. J., and Racicot, C. I. (1994). Separate neural pathways for the visual analysis of object shape in perception and prehension. *Curr. Biol.* 4: 604–610.

Grafton, S. T., Mazziotta, J. C., Woods, R. P., and Phelps, M. E. (1992). Human functional anatomy of visually guided finger movements. *Brain* 115: 565–587.

Grafton, S. T., Arbib, M. A., Fadiga, L., and Rizzolatti, G. (1996). Localization of grasp representations in humans by positron-emission tomography: 2. Observation compared with imagination. *Exp. Brain Res.* 112: 103–111.

Grafton, S. T., Fagg, A. H., & Arbib, M. A. (1998). Dorsal premotor cortex and conditional movement selection: A PET functional mapping study. *J. Neurophysiol.* 79: 1092–1097.

Graziano, M. S., and Gross, C. G. (1998). Spatial maps for the control of movement. *Curr. Opin. Neurobiol.* 8: 195-201.

Graziano, M. S., Yap, G. S., and Gross, C. G. (1994). Coding of visual space by premotor neurons. *Science* 266: 1054–1057.

Guard, O., Perenin, M. T., Vighetto, A., Giroud, M., Tommasi, M., and Dumas, R. (1984). Bilateral parietal syndrome approximating a Balint syndrome. *Rev. Neurol.* 140: 358–367.

Haaland, K. Y., Harrington, D. L., and Knight, R. T. (1999). Spatial deficits in ideomotor limb apraxia: A kinematic analysis of aiming movements. *Brain* 122: 1169–1182.

Haaland, K. Y., Harrington, D. L., and Knight, R. T. (2000). Neural representations of skilled movement. *Brain* 123: 2306–2313.

Haxby, J. V., Grady, C. L., Horwitz, B., Ungerleider, L. G., Mishkin, M., Carson, R. E., Herscovitch, P., Schapiro, M. B., and Rapoport, S. I. (1991). Dissociation of object and spatial visual processing pathways in human extrastriate cortex. *Proc. Natl. Acad. Sci. U. S. A.* 88: 1621–1625.

Haxby, J. V., Horwitz, B., Ungerleider, L. G., Maisog, J. M., Pietrini, P., and Grady, C. L. (1994). The functional organization of human extrastriate cortex: A PET-rCBF study of selective attention to faces and locations. *J. Neurosci.* 14: 6336–6353.

He, S. Q., Dum, R. P., and Strick, P. L. (1993). Topographic organization of corticospinal projections from the frontal lobe: Motor areas on the lateral surface of the hemisphere. *J. Neurosci.* 13: 952–980.

Heilman, K. M., and Rothi, L. J. G. (1997). Limb apraxia: A look back. In *Apraxia: The Neuropsychology of Action*, L. J. G. Rothi and K. M. Heilman (Eds.). Sussex: Psychology Press, pp. 7–28.

Heilman, K. M., Rothi, L. J., and Valenstein, E. (1982). Two forms of ideomotor apraxia. *Neurology* 32: 342–346.

Hoshi, E., and Tanji, J. (2000). Integration of target and body-part information in the premotor cortex when planning action. *Nature* 408: 466–470.

Iacoboni, M., Woods, R. P., Brass, M., Bekkering, H., Mazziotta, J. C., and Rizzolatti, G. (1999). Cortical mechanisms of human imitation. *Science* 286: 2526–2528.

Iriki, A., Tanaka, M., and Iwamura, Y. (1996). Coding of modified body schema during tool use by macaque postcentral neurones. *NeuroReport* 7: 2325–2330.

Iriki, A., Tanaka, M., Obayashi, S., and Iwamura, Y. (2001). Self-images in the video monitor coded by monkey intraparietal neurons. *Neurosci. Res.* 40: 163–173.

Jakobson, L. S., Archibald, Y. M., Carey, D. P., and Goodale, M. A. (1991). A kinematic analysis of reaching and grasping movements in a patient recovering from optic ataxia. *Neuropsychologia* 29: 803–809.

Jeannerod, M. (1981). *The Neural and Behavioral Organization of Goal-Directed Movements.* Vol. 10. New York: Oxford Science.

Jeannerod, M. (1986). The formation of finger grip during prehension: A cortically mediated visuomotor pattern. *Behav. Brain Res.* 19: 99–116.

Jeannerod, M., Decety, J., and Michel, F. (1994). Impairment of grasping movements following a bilateral posterior parietal lesion. *Neuropsychologia* 32: 369–380.

Jeannerod, M., Arbib, M. A., Rizzolatti, G., and Sakata, H. (1995). Grasping objects: The cortical mechanisms of visuomotor transformation. *Trends Neurosci.* 18: 314–320.

Jeannerod, M. (1996). The cognitive neuroscience of action. Blackwell.

Jellema, T., Baker, C. I., Wicker, B., and Perrett, D. I. (2000). Neural representation for the perception of the intentionality of actions. *Brain Cogn.* 44: 280–302.

Johnson, P. B., and Ferraina, S. (1996). Cortical networks for visual reaching: Intrinsic frontal lobe connectivity. *Eur. J. Neurosci.* 8: 1358–1362.

Johnson, P. B., Ferraina, S., and Caminiti, R. (1993). Cortical networks for visual reaching. *Exp. Brain Res.* 97: 361–365.

Johnson, S. H. (2000a). Imagining the impossible: Intact motor representations in hemiplegics. *NeuroReport* 11: 729–732.

Johnson, S. H. (2000b). Thinking ahead: The case for motor imagery in prospective judgments of prehension. *Cognition* 74: 33–70.

Johnson, S. H. (2001). Seeing two sides at once: Effects of viewpoint and object structure on recognizing three-dimensional objects. *J. Exp. Psychol. Hum. Percept. Perform.* 27: 1468–1484.

Johnson, S. H., Corballis, P. M., and Gazzaniga, M. S. (2001). Within grasp but out of reach: Evidence for a double dissociation between imagined hand and arm movements in the left cerebral hemisphere. *Neuropsychologia* 39: 36–50.

Johnson, S. H., Rotte, M., Grafton, S. T., Kanowski, M., Gazzaniga, M. S., and Heinze, J. (2002). Action-specific representation in implicitly imagined reaching. *NeuroImage* 17: 1693–1704.

Johnson, S. H., Sprehn, G., and Saykin, A. J. (2002). Intact motor imagery in chronic upper limb hemiplegics: Evidence for activity-independent action representations. *J. Cogn. Neurosci.* 14: 841–852.

Kolb, B. W., and Whishaw, I. Q. (1996). *Fundamentals of Human Neuropsychology.* 4th ed. New York: Freeman.

Kurata, K. (1991). Corticocortical inputs to the dorsal and ventral aspects of the premotor cortex of macaque monkeys. *Neurosci. Res.* 12: 263–280.

Lacquaniti, F., Guigon, E., Bianchi, L., Ferraina, S., and Caminiti, R. (1995). Representing spatial information for limb movement: Role of area 5 in the monkey. *Cereb. Cortex* 5: 391–409.

Leiguarda, R. C., and Marsden, C. D. (2000). Limb apraxias: Higher-order disorders of sensorimotor integration. *Brain* 123: 860–879.

Leipmann, H. (1900). Das Krankheitshild der Apraxie (motorischen Asymbolie). *Monatschr. Psychiatrie Neurol.* 8: 15–44, 102–132, 182–197.

Luppino, G., Murata, A., Govoni, P., and Matelli, M. (1999). Largely segregated parieto-frontal connections linking rostral intraparietal cortex (areas AIP and VIP) and the ventral premotor cortex (areas F5 and F4). *Exp. Brain Res.* 128: 181–187.

Maravita, A., Husain, M., Clarke, K., and Driver, J. (2001). Reaching with a tool extends visual-tactile interactions into far space: Evidence from cross-modal extinction. *Neuropsychologia* 39: 580–585.

Marconi, B., Genovesio, A., Battaglia-Mayer, A., Ferraina, S., Squatrito, S., Molinari, M., Lacquaniti, F., and Caminiti, R. (2001). Eye-hand coordination during reaching: 1. Anatomical relationships between parietal and frontal cortex. *Cereb. Cortex* 11: 513–527.

Martin, A., Haxby, J. V., Lalonde, F. M., Wiggs, C. L., and Ungerleider, L. G. (1995). Discrete cortical regions associated with knowledge of color and knowledge of action. *Science* 270: 102–105

Matelli, M., Govoni, P., Galletti, C., Kutz, D. F., and Luppino, G. (1998). Superior area 6 afferents from the superior parietal lobule in the macaque monkey. *J. Comp. Neurol.* 402: 327–352.

Milner, A. D. (1995). Cerebral correlates of visual awareness. *Neuropsychologia* 33: 1117–1130.

Milner, A. D., and Goodale, M. A. (1995). *The Visual Brain in Action.* Vol. 27. New York: Oxford University Press.

Mishkin, M., Ungerleider, L. G., and Macko, K. A. (1983). Object vision and spatial vision: Two cortical pathways. *Trends Neurosci.* 6: 414–417.

Morel, A., and Bullier, J. (1990). Anatomical segregation of two cortical visual pathways in the macaque monkey. *Vis. Neurosci.* 4: 555–578.

Murata, A., Gallese, V., Kaseda, M., and Sakata, H. (1996). Parietal neurons related to memory-guided hand manipulation. *J. Neurophysiol.* 75: 2180–2186.

Obayashi, S., Tanaka, M., and Iriki, A. (2000). Subjective image of invisible hand coded by monkey intraparietal neurons. *NeuroReport* 11: 3499–3505.

Obayashi, S., Suhara, T., Kawabe, K., Okauchi, T., Maeda, J., Akine, Y., Onoe, H., and Iriki, A. (2001). Functional brain mapping of monkey tool use. *NeuroImage* 14: 853–861.

Oram, M. W., and Perrett, D. I. (1996). Integration of form and motion in the anterior superior temporal polysensory area (STPa) of the macaque monkey. *J. Neurophysiol.* 76: 109–129.

Pandya, D. N., and Seltzer, B. (1982). Intrinsic connections and architectonics of posterior parietal cortex in the rhesus monkey. *J. Comp. Neurol.* 204: 196–210.

Passingham, R. E. (1993). *The Frontal Lobes and Voluntary Action.* Oxford: Oxford University Press.

Perenin, M. T., and Vighetto, A. (1988). Optic ataxia: A specific disruption in visuomotor mechanisms: 1. Different aspects of the deficit in reaching for objects. *Brain* 111: 643–674.

Petrides, M., and Pandya, D. N. (1984). Projections to the frontal cortex from the posterior parietal region in the rhesus monkey. *J. Comp. Neurol.* 228: 105–116.

Poizner, H., Clark, M. A., Merians, A. S., Macauley, B., Gonzalez Rothi, L. J., and Heilman, K. M. (1995). Joint coordination deficits in limb apraxia. *Brain* 118: 227–242.

Rapcsak, S. Z., Ochipa, C., Anderson, K. C., and Poizner, H. (1995). Progressive ideomotor apraxia: Evidence for a selective impairment of the action production system. *Brain Cogn.* 27: 213–236.

Rizzolatti, G., and Luppino, G. (2001). The cortical motor system. *Neuron* 31: 889–901.

Rizzolatti, G., Camarda, R., Fogassi, L., Gentilucci, M., Luppino, G., and Matelli, M. (1988). Functional organization of inferior area 6 in the macaque monkey: 2. Area F5 and the control of distal movements. *Exp. Brain Res.* 71: 491–507.

Rizzolatti, G., Fadiga, L., Gallese, V., and Fogassi, L. (1996a). Premotor cortex and the recognition of motor actions. *Brain Res. Cogn. Brain Res.* 3: 131–141.

Rizzolatti, G., Fadiga, L., Matelli, M., Bettinardi, V., Paulesu, E., Perani, D., and Fazio, F. (1996b). Localization of grasp representations in humans by PET: 1. Observation versus execution. *Exp. Brain Res.* 111: 246–252.

Roland, P. E., Skinhoj, E., Lassen, N. A., and Larsen, B. (1980). Different cortical areas in man in organization of voluntary movements in extrapersonal space. *J. Neurophysiol.* 43: 137–150.

Sakata, H., Taira, M., Murata, A., and Mine, S. (1995). Neural mechanisms of visual guidance of hand action in the parietal cortex of the monkey. *Cereb. Cortex* 5: 429–438.

Shen, L., and Alexander, G. E. (1997). Preferential representation of instructed target location versus limb trajectory in dorsal premotor area. *J. Neurophysiol.* 77: 1195–1212.

Sirigu, A., Cohen, L., Duhamel, J. R., Pillon, B., Dubois, B., and Agid, Y. (1995). A selective impairment of hand posture for object utilization in apraxia. *Cortex* 31: 41–55.

Taira, M., Mine, S., Georgopoulos, A. P., Murata, A., and Sakata, H. (1990). Parietal cortex neurons of the monkey related to the visual guidance of hand movement. *Exp. Brain Res.* 83: 29–36.

Tanné, J., Boussaoud, D., Boyer-Zeller, N., and Rouiller, E. M. (1995). Direct visual pathways for reaching movements in the macaque monkey. *NeuroReport* 7: 267–272.

Tzavaras, A., and Masure, M. C. (1976). Aspects différents de l'ataie optique selon la latéralisation hémisphérique de la lésion. *Lyon Médicale* 236: 673–683.

Ungerleider, L. G. (1996). What and where in the human brain? Evidence from functional brain imaging studies. In *Vision and Movement Mechanisms in the Cerebral Cortex*, K.-P. H. R. Caminiti, F. Lacquaniti, and J. Altman (eds.). Strasbourg: Human Frontiers in Science Program, pp. 23–30.

Ungerleider, L. G., and Haxby, J. V. (1994). "What" and "where" in the human brain. *Curr. Opin. Neurobiol.* 4: 157–165.

Ungerleider, L. G., and Mishkin, M. (1982). Two cortical visual systems. In *Analysis of Visual Behavior*, D. J. Ingle, M. A. Goodale, and R. J. W. Mansfield (eds.). Cambridge, Mass.: MIT Press, pp. 549–586.

Warburton, E., Wise, R. J., Price, C. J., Weiller, C., Hadar, U., Ramsay, S., and Frackowiak, R. S. (1996). Noun and verb retrieval by normal subjects: Studies with PET. *Brain* 119: 159–179.

Wise, S. P., Boussaoud, D., Johnson, P. B., and Caminiti, R. (1997). Premotor and parietal cortex: Corticocortical connectivity and combinatorial computations. *Annu. Rev. Neurosci.* 20: 25–42.

IV

Sequencing, Coordination, and Control

Complex actions, from suckling to computer programming, can be understood to consist of simpler units that must be assembled in the proper sequence to successfully achieve the intended behavior. How this sequencing is accomplished in the brain is a fundamental yet unresolved issue. Ivry and Helmuth (chapter 8) take on this significant challenge by focusing on how brain lesions disrupt the ability to sequence actions properly. Brain-lesioned patients provide insights into mechanisms responsible for sequential actions and reveal important commonalities with other sequential activities like thought.

In addition to proper sequencing, complex actions often depend on the ability to effectively coordinate the two hands in both time and space. Franz (chapter 9) argues that, to understand bimanual coordination, we must span traditionally discrete areas of inquiry. Toward this end, she integrates a wide range of findings, from those on split-brain patients to those on amputees with phantom limb syndrome, into a coherent picture of how bimanual actions are represented in the brain.

Even for the simplest of actions, one can ask whether movements are planned entirely in advance of their execution (feedforward) or are undertaken in a manner that depends entirely on incoming sensory information (feedback). Desmurget and Grafton (chapter 10) argue convincingly that, as with most dichotomies, the truth resides somewhere in the middle: Rough action plans are computed in advance of movement generation, whereas internal forward models are used to predict the current and upcoming states of the motor system on the basis of both efferent and afferent signals. They present evidence that this hybrid system is instantiated in a distributed network of interconnected cerebellar and parietal structures.

Representations and Neural Mechanisms of Sequential Movements

Richard B. Ivry and Laura L. Helmuth

8.1 Introduction

Over a half century ago, Karl Lashley (1951), called serial order in behavior the "most important and most neglected problem of cerebral physiology." Despite significant advances since then, it remains a difficult problem. Neuropsychological and neurophysiological studies are currently adapting the analytic tools of cognitive psychology to develop a finer understanding of the contributions of different neural regions to sequencing. Earlier efforts in this direction sought to develop taxonomies for the types of tasks associated with different brain regions as guides to identifying the particular computations these regions are performing.

To appreciate the cognitive neuroscience of sequencing, we need to explore this topic at many different levels of analysis. How are seemingly innate behavioral sequences, some appearing in the first days of life, "hardwired" in the brain? How are acquired sequences learned, represented, and produced? Are there fundamental similarities between the sequencing of movements and thoughts? Do these two domains share common neural mechanisms? These questions can be answered in part by examining how different neurological disorders disrupt sequential behavior.

8.2 The Ethological Perspective

The systematic study of sequential behavior took hold with the emergence of ethology in the first half of this century. Partly in reaction to the behaviorists' single-minded focus on the association of discrete stimuli and responses, ethologists pursued a "more appropriate" level of analysis, based on complex behaviors. Arguing that careful study of animal behavior revealed innate fixed action patterns that were species specific, Lorenz (1950) suggested that a "comparative anatomy of behavior" could be constructed, using similarities and differences in behavior patterns to deduce taxonomic relationships.

Whereas Lorenz described the innate sequential behaviors of his animals as "fixed action patterns," implying an invariance across individuals and through time, Barlow (1977) suggested a less restrictive designation for such behaviors, "modal action patterns." These spatiotemporal patterns of movement were characteristic of particular species; they could be recognized and quantified by skilled observers. But, rather than being fixed, they interacted in interesting and complex ways with the environment: Motivational states, the strength of a triggering stimulus, experience, or feedback from the environment could alter the expression of a particular sequence in subtle ways.

The level of analysis at which we choose to study a behavioral system, indeed, how we define a sequence of behavior, will determine what we can learn. Suggesting that we adopt frameworks, in particular ontogeny, that provide complementary insights into behavior, Fentress (1973, p. 1544) pointed to the swimming abilities in rodents, where "actions are assembled, refined, disassembled, and reassembled during ontogeny in ways simply too rich to be squeezed into simple categories such as local to global or global to local." Thus, rather than pose binary questions such as whether a sequence of movements is triggered by central or peripheral mechanisms, or by internal or external cues, we need to pose more refined questions, ones that consider the relative contributions of different processes and that explore how these contributions change over time.

Grooming Behavior in the Rat

Golani (1992) has applied a rich system of movement description to characterize and reveal patterns of behavior in vertebrates. By viewing the postures and movements of an animal in terms of the animal's gravitational support and range of possible movements, he has found properties to describe movements that apply throughout the animal kingdom. He has found that the *mobility gradient*, which he defines as the range of possible motions, given an animal's position, changes through ontogeny and in the course of a movement. It is also a factor in dominance encounters. The dominant animal adopts a position affording the greatest mobility gradient, whereas submissive animals adopt positions that limit their mobility gradient.

Of particular relevance to the current chapter, Golani (1992) suggests that the basal ganglia may modulate the expression of mobility gradient variables by regulating the activity levels of different parts of the body. Furthermore, the degree to which an animal is stimulus-bound may depend critically on dopamine projections from the basal ganglia. The generality of the mobility gradient suggests that it may be hardwired into the vertebrate brain, and the basal ganglia are the prime candidates for controlling this complex phenomenon.

Rodent grooming patterns constitute an excellent model system for studying natural sequential patterns of behavior. Although rodents often groom in a random manner or in response to a peripheral cue, there are also well-defined, relatively invariant grooming syntaxes that are phylogenetically ancient and seen throughout the rodent order (Fentress, 1973). Several interesting properties suggest that these sequences are innate, centrally programmed, and species specific. For one, a particular sequence can be seen very early in ontogeny—before the movements are actually effective: The young mouse will move its paws in the stereotypical manner without actually coming into contact with the face, which implies that the sequence is not dependent on peripheral feedback, or at least not on feedback from a tactile sensory system. For another, the sequence can be seen even in rodents who have had limbs amputated or deafferented

Grooming is composed of four basic behavioral elements: body licking, small elliptical strokes that extend to the vibrissae, small unilateral strokes that extend to the eyes, and large bilateral strokes extending past the ears. These four elements are organized into specific sequences that are characteristic of a species. The serial order of different elements and the rate and number of times a given element is performed, are highly stereotyped. Thus there are both a semantics and a syntax in this behavior. The individual elements can be considered the fundamental semantic units, whereas the particular ordering constitutes the syntax (figure 8.1).

The neurobiology of rodent grooming behaviors has been explored in lesion and electrophysiological studies. Berridge and Whishaw (1992) compared the effects of striatal, cortical, and cerebellar lesions on grooming behavior. Little effect on the grooming sequence was found following cortical lesions, whether in motor cortex or the entire neocortex, or following cerebellar lesions; the impairments proved transient. In contrast, the striatal lesions produced a severe and permanent disruption of the syntactic chain.

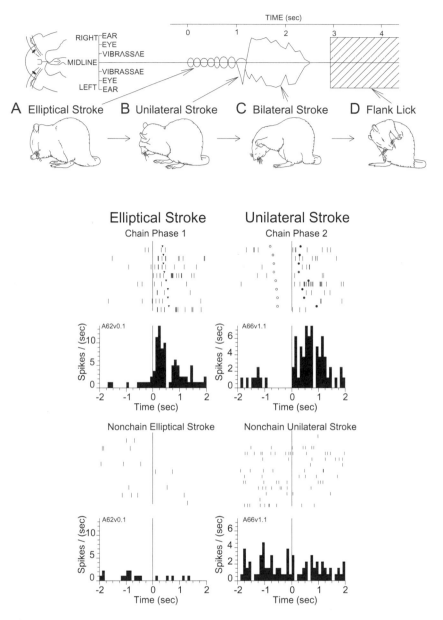

Figure 8.1

(*Top*) Grooming sequence in the rat consists of four components, produced in a fixed order extending over approximately 4 s. The choreography diagram shows the excursion of the forepaw in the medial-lateral direction. (*Bottom*) Activity in two dorsolateral striatal neurons during component movements. The neuron on the left responds vigorously following the onset of the elliptical stroke when performed within the grooming sequence (chain), but not when the same movement was performed outside the grooming chain (nonchain). The neuron on the right shows a similar sequence-specific response correlated with the unilateral stroke component. (Adapted with permission from Aldridge and Berridge, 1998.)

Even after full recovery, these animals performed only about 50% of the sequences to completion. They would frequently complete the early elements of the sequence, but then fail to terminate with the correct body lick. Instead, their sequences would end with a dysfunctional paw lick. Subsequent studies involving local injections of neurotoxic agents have identified a region within anterior dorsolateral striatum as critical for the production of grooming sequences. Lesions as small as 1 mm in diameter and as large as near-complete striatal ablation can produce similar effects (Cromwell and Berridge, 1996).

At least two interpretations of the role of the striatum in rodent grooming patterns should be considered. The striatum could be the site of some element of the engram for the grooming syntax: The representation of the sequence could require an intact striatum in order to be accessed. That the rodent grooming syntax may have evolved more than 60 million years ago and that the striatum is involved in various other naturalistic sequential actions such as birdsong (Brainard and Doupe, 2000) would be consistent with this hypothesis. Similarly, imaging and patient studies of "habit" formation in humans across a range of tasks have generally been interpreted as reflecting a shift in the locus of sequence representation from cortex to basal ganglia over the course of learning.

Alternatively, the striatal contribution could take the form of a progression mechanism. Accurate completion of a grooming sequence may require the striatum to pass through the representation correctly. The physiological evidence favors the hypothesis that the anterior dorsolateral striatum is related to sequence implementation rather than sequence encoding or generation. Cells in this region exhibit sequence specificity. For example, a vigorous response might be found in a cell when the unilateral stroke element is performed within the sequence, but not when the same gesture is performed outside a grooming chain (Aldridge and Berridge, 1998), although the increased firing almost always occurs after the onset of the specified element. The activation of the successive elements may come from other brain structures, perhaps in a distributed manner, with the basal ganglia providing a mechanism to link these actions together. The failure of animals with striatal lesions to complete a sequence is consistent with this view.

Innate Behavioral Sequences in Humans

In studying our behavior patterns, ethologists rely on at least three different types of evidence to determine whether a pattern of movements is innate.

First, if the identical stereotyped movement sequence is found in many different and isolated cultures, it can be concluded that cultural transmission has little impact on the behavior's development. Second, if the behavior appears very early in ontogeny, there is less opportunity for learning to play a part. This is particularly relevant if the behavior emerges under special circumstances that minimize physical limitations. Third, if the behavior develops reliably in people who have been deprived of sensory stimuli (blind or deaf people), it is likely that the behavior reflects a centrally generated pattern of movement.

Several interesting examples of innate behavior patterns have been described in humans. These sequences of movements almost invariably constitute a behavior that has probable adaptive advantage, either now or in our evolutionary history. For example, human infants rub their eyes in a stereotyped fashion: They close their eyes and rub one eye with the back of the first two fingers of the hand. This behavior minimizes the risk of harming the eye (Eibl-Eibesfeldt, 1989). Expressive behaviors also appear to be highly determined. Facial expressions of basic emotions are quite similar across cultures (Ekman, 1973). Eyebrow flashes, indicating interest or welcoming, also occur in all cultures studied and in the blind (Eibl-Eibesfeldt, 1989).

One of the more dramatic displays of innate sequenced movement in humans occurs in newborn infants, who, if held so that the muscles in their legs do not have to support their weight, will walk along with their carriers. Thus, even though maturation of the skeletomuscular system is necessary before the behavior can be independently performed, the neural circuitry for locomotion is present at birth (Thelen, 1984).

Pathology of an Innate Behavioral Sequence: Obsessive-Compulsive Disorder

A complex syndrome that has provided insights into habitual behaviors in humans, obsessive-compulsive disorder (OCD) is characterized by intrusive, uncontrollable thoughts (obsessions) and irresistible urges to perform specific behaviors repetitively (compulsions). The incidence rate has been estimated to be as high as 2% of the population (Rapoport, 1989).

Ethologists have focused on the most frequent sorts of compulsive behaviors: grooming behaviors and safety behaviors. For example, many OCD patients repetitively wash their hands or become preoccupied with germs and dirt. Others cannot resist the urge to repetitively check potentially dangerous situations. They may lock and relock the door many times a night or return repetitively to the kitchen to make sure that the stove has been turned off. Rapoport (1989) has suggested that these behaviors are important from an evolutionary standpoint, and that OCD may represent a pathological repetition of a behavioral system that is innate and usually adaptive. She compares the repetitive performance of grooming behaviors to the modal action patterns described in animals. One particularly striking property of the compulsions is that they must be carried out in full once the behavior has begun, much as the greylag goose continues to move as if rolling an egg into the nest even when the egg has been removed.

Neuroimaging studies indicate that obsessive-compulsive disorder is associated with abnormal activity in orbitofrontal cortex, the caudate nucleus of the basal ganglia, and, less consistently, the anterior cingulate (reviewed in Baxter, 1999). OCD patients exhibit hypermetabolism in these areas when at rest and enhanced activation when compulsive behaviors are provoked more often than do control participants, with activation levels returning to the normal range in OCD patients responding to treatment, whether pharmacological or behavioral. Furthermore, the co-occurrence of Tourette's syndrome and other disorders of the basal ganglia with OCD is high.

An interesting aspect of obsessive-compulsive disorder is that the affected patterns of behavior may be either movements or thoughts. In both cases, a sequential behavior is repetitive, irresistible, and unbidden. The expression of OCD in the motor and cognitive domains may arise from a common basal ganglia pathology. As reviewed above, the basal ganglia are associated with a range of tasks involving sequential activity. Although the sequencing properties of the striatum may have evolved for purely motoric sequencing, this operation may now be invoked across a variety of task domains (Hayes et al., 1998). The class of elements that the striatum acts on may have changed during the course of evolutionary history, but the computation performed by the striatum may have been conserved. Namely, the striatum may "modulate the serial activation of brain circuits that represent discrete functions" (Berridge and Whishaw, 1992, p. 288).

8.3 Representational Issues in Sequence Learning

Animals are clearly capable of learning complex, arbitrary sequences of action. A horse can be trained to traverse an equestrian course. We learn to tie our shoes or to drive a car with a manual transmission. A central concern for cognitive psychology has been to explore how these complex behaviors are represented. What constraints limit our ability to learn sequential actions, and how are learned actions structured in memory?

Introduced by Nissen and Bullemer (1987), the serial reaction time (SRT) task has emerged as a model task for studying sequence acquisition in humans over the past decade. Participants are told to tap a key when a stimulus appears on the computer screen. In the spatial version of this task there are four keys, one for each finger, and four stimulus locations that correspond to the four fingers. The mapping of stimulus to response is direct: The rightmost light indicates that the participant should tap with the rightmost finger. Participants are told that this is a reaction time task, and that they should press the appropriate key as soon as possible after the stimulus appears.

The critical manipulation in this experiment is whether the positions of the stimuli occur in a fixed or a random sequence. In their original study, Nissen and Bullemer presented participants with blocks of sequenced key presses in which the stimuli followed a ten-element pattern, such as 4231324321. This pattern would repeat within a block of trials so that the tenth element was always followed by the first element. In other blocks, the stimulus positions were randomly chosen with the constraint that a position (and therefore response) could not occur on two successive trials. In a typical experiment, testing begins with random blocks, switches to sequence blocks, and then returns to random blocks. This procedure provides two measures of learning. First, if participants are learning the sequence, then reaction times should decrease over the blocks with the sequenced pattern. Second, and more important, when the random patterns are reintroduced, participants should show a large cost in performance: Reaction times and perhaps error rates should increase. To account for possible order effects, some studies include control groups who are tested only on random blocks.

This paradigm and several variations of the basic task have been used extensively to answer questions about declarative versus procedural knowledge, the necessity of attention for different kinds of learning, the nature of the learned representation, and the role of different neural structures in sequence learning.

Procedural versus Declarative Knowledge
Damage to the hippocampus and syndromes such as Korsakoff's disease, which destroys mammilary bodies, lead to severe memory deficits. Such

patients suffer from anterograde amnesia: They are unable to form new memories of events, although they are able to learn new skills without remembering having performed the action (e.g., Corkin, 1968). A fundamental distinction in the memory literature has been made between declarative knowledge (the ability to explicitly recollect an event) and procedural knowledge (the ability to perform a new skill). Many of the tasks that amnesiac patients are able to learn to perform involve motor skills. Writing mirror-reversed words or performing a rotor pursuit task are two examples. Because the patients show improved performance on successive trials without any memory for the task, their learning must not rely on structures shown to be involved in explicit, episodic memory.

Nissen and Bullemer (1987) tested Korsakoff's patients on the serial reaction time task. When the stimuli followed a fixed sequence, reaction times improved for patients and control participants alike, even though the amnesiac patients expressed neither awareness nor recognition of the sequence. Similar effects were found when healthy college-age students were given scopolamine, a drug that produces a transient amnesiac disorder: They also were found to have learned the sequence as measured by the difference between sequenced and random blocks, but showed no awareness of the sequence (Nissen et al., 1987). From these results, the serial reaction time task can clearly be added to the list of tasks that reflect procedural learning.

Declarative knowledge may also influence performance of the serial reaction time task. The magnitude of learning can be correlated with the level of awareness and, as would be expected, informing the participants of the sequence can facilitate performance (Curran and Keele, 1993). Learning to perform the SRT task does not require declarative knowledge, but declarative knowledge, whether developed by the participant independently or explicitly imparted by the researcher, can augment performance.

Attentional versus Nonattentional Forms of Sequence Learning

Nissen and Bullemer (1987) also tested a condition in which participants performed the serial reaction time task under dual-task conditions: As they tapped keys in response to the spatial locations of visual stimuli, tones sounded between each response and the following stimulus. The tones were either high or low in pitch; participants were instructed to count the number of high-pitched tones. Under these conditions, the participants showed no evidence of sequence learning: Their performance was no different from that of participants responding to a random sequence of lights. The authors concluded that whereas awareness was not required for sequence learning, attention was.

The nature of the sequence to be learned, however, modulates the effect of the distracter task on learning (Cohen et al., 1990). As noted above, the original SRT task involved ten-element sequences (Nissen and Bullemer, 1987). Cohen and colleagues (1990) tested participants on simpler sequences of six elements under similar dual-task conditions. They contrasted two types of sequences. In one type, each of three positions occurred twice (e.g., 132123). In the other type, there were four possible positions with two positions occurring once and two positions occurring twice (e.g., 132423). Participants in the first condition showed no evidence of learning, whereas those in the second showed evidence of implicit sequence learning: When they were transferred to a random sequence, there was a large increase in their mean reaction time. Furthermore, when the tone counting task was made more difficult, the overall reaction times increased, although the difference between random and sequenced conditions remained the same.

What is the difference between the two types of sequences such that one cannot be learned under conditions of attentional distraction, whereas the other can? Cohen and colleagues (1990) proposed that the key difference was whether the sequences contained unique pairwise elements. In a sequence such as 132423, position 1 is always followed by position 3, and position 4 is always followed by position 2. For sequences such as 132123, however, there are no unique pairwise associations. Each position is followed by the other two possible positions at different points in the sequence. Cohen and colleagues argued that sequences with unique pairwise associations could be learned by a simple associative mechanism. When these unique associations were not available, a hierarchic representation had to be formed for learning to occur. Hierarchic representations are assumed to require attentional resources. Indeed, hierarchic representation may be a prominent feature of declarative forms of learning.

Cohen et al., 1990, does not make clear the relationship between the cognitive processes required for hierarchic and nonhierarchic sequence learning. One possibility is that hierarchic representations are formed by extracting chunks from an associative learning mechanism. Alternatively, attentional and nonattentional sequence learning may operate independently. Curran and Keele (1993) provide evidence in favor of the latter hypothesis. In a series of transfer experiments where participants were transferred between distraction, full attention, and dual-task conditions, their performance under one condition did not predict performance under different task conditions. For example, when participants tested without distraction were informed of the sequence in advance, they showed greater sequence learning than naive participants, whereas when the two groups were transferred to the dual-task situation, their performance was comparable (but see Frensch et al., 1998). Other permutations showed that learning under dual-task conditions was lost when participants were transferred to a distraction-free condition.

Other studies have explored why distraction disrupts sequence learning. The influence of the distracter task may not be strictly related to attentional capacity. For example, observing that participants were able to learn sequences that lacked unique pairwise associations when a distracter task did not disrupt the temporal structure of the sequential events, Stadler (1995) proposed that the timing of the distracter task may interfere with the formation of sequential associations.

Schmidtke and Heuer (1997) provided an important extension to this idea. Their dual-task condition involved the pairing of the spatial SRT task with a distracter tone discrimination task modified in two important ways: First, responses were required following each target tone (go-no-go condition); second, the tones could also occur in a fixed sequence. The tone sequence was either matched in length to the spatial sequence (i.e., both sequences were six elements long) or mismatched (i.e., spatial sequence of six elements and tone sequence of five elements). The matched-length condition produced a consistent cross-modal sequence, 12 elements in

Table 8.1a
Matched and mismatched sequences in dual-task conditions

Matched length										
Visual sequence	1	2	4	2	3	4	1	2		4. . .
Auditory sequence		A	B	B	A	B	A	A	B. . .	
Mismatched length										
Visual sequence	1	2	4	2	3	4	1	2		4. . .
Auditory sequence		A	B	B	A	B	A	B	B. . .	

Source: Schmidtke and Heuer, 1997.
Note: Numbers refer to one of four visual locations; letters refer to high- or low-pitched tones. Both visual and auditory sequences are six elements long for the matched-length condition. The auditory sequence is only five elements long in the mismatched-length condition.

Table 8.1b
Increases in reaction time (ms) associated with probe type

	Probe type			
	Random sequences		Phase-shift sequences	
	Visual	Auditory	Visual	Auditory
Matched length	153	135	109	63
Mismatched length	85	83	—	—

Note: Phase shift applies only in the matched-length condition; in the mismatched-length condition, visual and auditory sequences are uncorrelated.

length, whereas, in the mismatched-length condition, the two sequences were uncorrelated.

As evidenced by the increases in reaction time when either the spatial or tone sequences were randomized, learning of the sequential associations within each dimension was observed for the matched-length and mismatched-length groups (table 8.1b). The increases were greater for the matched-length condition. Moreover, increase in reaction time was also found in this condition following the phase-shift probe in which the events for one dimension were shifted in phase by one position. These results indicate that learning is not limited to the formation of within-dimension associations, but rather can also involve interdimensional associations. Accordingly, rather than the distracter task taking up resources that could be allocated to sequence learning, it may be that distracter events such as random tones interfere with the formation of cross-dimensional associations (by definition, there are no cross-dimensional regularities when the events on one dimension are randomized).

Keele and colleagues (forthcoming) propose that the ability to form multidimensional associations is fundamental to many complex skills such as speech comprehension (e.g., integration of auditory and visual cues; Massaro, 1998). They distinguish between two types of computational processes, an intradimensional process and a general-access associative process. The former consists of modules, each tuned to extract regularities occurring along a single dimension and insulated from information along other channels. The latter has access to all task-relevant information and will thus exhibit learning when there are regularities across dimensions.

Their proposal provides a computational account of the distinction between procedural and declarative memory. Keele and colleagues postulate that only representations within the general-access associative process can be accessible to awareness. Thus learning will be outside awareness when the distracter events are random because associations will only develop in an intradimensional module. One prediction of this proposal is that amnesiacs should also show deficits in cross-dimensional learning, even if these associations occur outside awareness. It is the inability to integrate information across dimensions that is central to their impairment rather than a deficit in awareness per se. Consistent with this prediction, recent studies (e.g., Chun and Phelps, 1999) have shown context-learning deficits associated with medial temporal lobe amnesia, even when such learning occurs outside awareness in healthy controls.

What Is Learned in Sequence Learning?

Although the serial reaction time task can be used to show that something is learned and under what conditions learning takes place, the question of exactly what is learned is somewhat unclear. In the original Nissen and Bullemer (1987) experiment involving four spatial stimuli and four fingers, there are several different regularities that participants could take advantage of in order to improve performance. Participants could be learning to attend to a sequence of positions in space. That is, they could be learning to direct attention to one of the four stimulus locations in anticipation of the stimulus. A second possibility is that they could be learning a motor response sequence. The learning could reside in the order in which the fingers should be tapped. A third possibility is that participants could be learning an abstract representation of the sequence that is tied neither to the spatial location of the stimulus nor to the motor response.

Willingham and his colleagues (1989, 2000; Willingham, 1999) have conducted a series of studies to explore these issues. For example, Willingham et al., 1989, tested whether purely motor procedural learning could be observed in a serial reaction time task. Participants first learned the sequence by responding to a set of four spatial stimuli. The four spatial positions were then replaced by four color patches. For some participants, the color patches followed the same movement pattern as the spatial locations, whereas, for others, the color patches followed a random pattern. Little evidence of transfer was found, indicating that learning was not purely motor.

Further evidence that learning does not occur at the level of specific movement patterns is provided by studies showing substantial transfer between different response formats. For example, participants who are initially trained to respond by making finger movements exhibit near-perfect transfer when switched to a response format that requires arm movements (Cohen et al., 1990; Grafton et al., 1998). However, when key press responses were replaced with vocal responses, transfer was incomplete, suggesting that some of the sequence learning is effector system dependent (Keele et al., 1995).

Effector specificity is likely related to skill level (Rand et al., 1998, 2000). It is unlikely that expert violinists could switch to bowing with the left hand and fingering with the right hand without cost. Similarly, right-handers have difficulty learning to throw a ball with the left hand; the cost is primarily associated with the fine timing required for coordinating the opening of the hand to release the ball with the rotation of the arm (Hore et al., 1996). Although it is possible that effector specificity is primarily limited to multijoint movements, intermanual transfer is also limited for serial key-pressing tasks with highly practiced participants (Karni et al., 1995). The evidence in favor of effector independence has typically been obtained in studies involving only limited amounts of practice.

Neural Correlates of Learning in the Serial Reaction Time Task

Neuropsychological research and neuroimaging studies using the serial reaction time task have further confirmed two basic ideas emerging from the behavioral studies: (1) Sequence learning requires the contribution of a number of different brain regions; and (2) procedural and declarative forms of sequence learning involve separable neural mechanisms.

Numerous studies have examined the performance of neurological patients on the serial reaction time task. The results for patients with basal ganglia damage, from either Huntington's or Parkinson's disease, are mixed (Ferraro et al., 1993; Helmuth et al., 2000; Jackson et al., 1995; Pascual-Leone et al., 1993; Willingham and Koroshetz, 1993). In some studies, the patients show no evidence of learning; in others, the magnitude of learning is reduced or even reaches normal levels. A more consistent picture has emerged from studies involving patients with cerebellar damage. These patients fail to exhibit learning in the SRT task (e.g., Pascual-Leone et al., 1993). Interestingly, the learning deficit is limited to the ipsilesional side in patients with unilateral lesions (Gómez-Beldarrain et al., 1998; Molinari et al., 1997). Thus, even though the transfer studies suggest that a learned representation may be accessible to different effector systems, learning appears to require an intact ipsilateral cerebellum. Although the SRT task has not been extensively employed with patients with cortical lesions, the few studies conducted indicate that deficits can be found following lesions in right prefrontal cortex (Grafman, personal communication).

Imaging studies have further demonstrated that sequence learning involves functional changes in a number of brain structures. Pascual-Leone and colleagues (1994) creatively applied transcranial magnetic stimulation (TMS) to study changes in primary motor cortex as participants performed the serial reaction time task. Before training, the motor fields of the fingers were mapped by stimulating the primary motor strip of the left hemisphere. Participants then performed the SRT task, using a 12-element sequence with no unique pairwise elements. After every block of ten sequence repetitions, the participants were indirectly queried to determine if they were aware of the sequential nature of the stimuli. In addition, the magnetic stimulation procedure was repeated to assess changes in the motor fields. Two primary results were obtained in this study. First, as sequence learning progressed, the motor fields expanded. Second, when participants became aware of the sequence, these motor fields shrank, quickly returning to their initial size. These findings led Pascual-Leone and colleagues to propose that procedural sequence learning involves rapid plasticity in the primary motor cortex. Moreover, the acquisition of declarative knowledge abolishes this transient reorganization. It is as if other neural systems have assumed control, and the motor cortex is free to reshape itself for new learning.

Converging evidence for multiple pathways for sequence learning comes from a series of PET studies involving the SRT task. Grafton and colleagues (1995) measured changes in cerebral blood flow that were correlated with two types of sequence learning. In both conditions, a six-element sequence was used in which two spatial positions occurred only once in the sequence (i.e., the sequence type that can be learned with attentional distraction). The dual-task procedure was used in the first condition with the spatial events interleaved with random tones and the participants required to keep a running count of the number of low-pitched tones. All participants showed learning, in that mean reaction times increased when the stimuli were presented at random locations, although none of the participants reported any awareness of the sequence. As in Pascual-Leone et al., 1994, metabolic correlates of sequence learning were found over the contralateral primary motor cortex. Blood flow increased in this region over the three PET scans obtained during blocks containing sequenced stimuli.

Increased blood flow was also found in the parietal cortex (Brodmann area 40), supplementary motor cortex, and putamen (figure 8.2).

In the second condition, participants were tested on a new sequence, but the secondary task was eliminated. The amount of learning was greater, primarily because most of the participants became aware of the sequential nature of the stimuli. In fact, many of the reaction times were less than 100 ms for these participants. In this condition, the metabolic correlates of sequence learning shifted. No changes in blood flow were observed over the contralateral primary motor cortex. Rather, prominent changes were found in the ipsilateral right frontal cortex, including dorsolateral and premotor cortex, as well as in right temporal and right parieto-occipital cortex.

Hazeltine and colleagues (1997) repeated these two conditions but used color instead of spatial location to cue the responses. Despite this change in stimulus dimension, the overall pattern of results was similar to that reported by Grafton and colleagues (1995). Dual-task learning was associated with changes in motor areas of the left hemisphere, whereas neural correlates of single-task learning were primarily in the right hemisphere. The effect of stimulus dimension in both single- and dual-task conditions consisted of a shift toward more ventral regions in posterior cortex and, in the single-task condition, prefrontal cortex.

The neuroimaging studies indicate that distinct neural systems are engaged during sequence learning both with and without attentional distraction. Dual-task learning was correlated with changes in motor cortex, the supplementary motor area (SMA), and parietal cortex. It is likely that these associations reflect, not successive stimulus events, but rather the development of a series of stimulus-response associations, defined as a series of "stimulus-triggered spatially directed responses" (Willingham et al., 2000). This hypothesis is supported by the results of an imaging study (Grafton et al., 1998) that used a transfer paradigm. Behaviorally, positive transfer was found to arm movements after training with finger movements. Activation during sequential blocks remained high in the SMA and in parietal cortex, whereas the center of activation within motor cortex shifted to a more dorsal location, consistent with the motor homunculus. Interestingly, an increase in cingulate activity was found at transfer. One interpretation of these results is that the parietal activation reflects the abstract representation of a sequence of spatial goals or relative locations. Activation in the SMA and in motor cortex reflects the translation of these goals into a particular movement sequence, with cingulate cortex involved in selecting

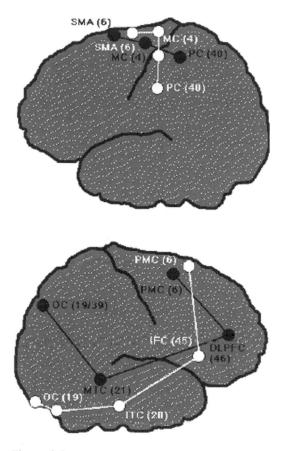

Figure 8.2
Primary cortical regions identified in positron–emission tomography (PET) studies with sequence learning. (*Top*) Areas in which neural activity was positively correlated with learning under conditions of attentional distraction. (*Bottom*) Corresponding areas under conditions without distraction. Black lines connect areas identified during learning of spatial sequences (adapted with permission from Grafton et al., 1995); white lines connect areas identified during learning of color sequences (adapted with permission from Hazeltine et al., 1997). DLPFC, dorsolateral prefrontal cortex; IFC, inferior frontal cortex; ITC, inferotemporal cortex; MC, motor cortex; MTC, middle temporal cortex; OC, occipital cortex; PC, parietal cortex; PMC, primary motor cortex; SMA, supplementary motor area. Numbers in parentheses signify Brodmann areas.

which effector system will be used to accomplish the goal (Botvinick et al., 1999).

Surprisingly, with the exception of premotor cortex, the neural correlates of learning under single-task conditions are not part of what are traditionally considered motor areas. Without the distracter tone-counting task, changes were seen in prefrontal cortex, temporal lobe, and inferior regions of parietal and occipitoparietal cortex. In posterior cortex, these loci are clearly more ventral than those associated with dual-task learning. This division corresponds to the what-where, or more appropriately, the what-how distinction that has been proposed to account for a major functional division in the visual pathways (Milner and Goodale, 1995). Sequence learning with distraction might be thought of as the development of predictions about where the next response will be directed, a type of association that would be well suited for the dorsal stream. Without distraction, these predictions might be more stimulus centered, associations of what the next event will be in the sequence. Such associations appear to be formed along the ventral stream.

We have yet to address two important issues that emerge from the imaging studies of sequence learning. First, there is a striking laterality effect. With distraction, changes are almost exclusively in the left hemisphere. In contrast, the loci were in the right hemisphere when the distracter task was eliminated, a result that is especially surprising given that only right-hand finger movements were produced. The shift to the right hemisphere is intriguing. It is consistent with the hypothesis that sequence learning here was more stimulus based and less movement oriented. It may also suggest that learning here involved active memory retrieval (as opposed to priming), given the association of the right hemisphere in such processes (Tulving et al., 1994). About half of the participants in the single-task condition became aware of the sequence (see also Honda et al., 1998).

Second, the imaging work suggests that the two associative systems operate in an exclusive manner. There were no areas that showed similar learning-related changes under both single- and dual-task conditions, although behavioral studies indicate that learning within each system will occur in parallel (Curran and Keele, 1993; Schmidtke and Heuer, 1997; Willingham and Goedert-Eschmann, 1999). Perhaps the lack of overlap in the imaging studies reflects a limitation when measuring a relatively fixed resource such as blood flow.

8.4 Neurological Disorders Affecting Sequential Behavior

That sequence learning is associated with a widespread change in brain metabolism can be attributed to the inherent complexity of sequential behavior. Not only do motor demands require the coordinated activity of a number of different effectors, but these actions must be integrated with perceptual information. The perceptual input consists of the afferent inflow from the moving limbs, exteroreceptive information concerning the general layout of external space, and task-specific information about stimuli to be responded to or objects to be manipulated. Moreover, sequential behavior is goal directed: The actions are designed to accomplish a specific goal that satisfies internal needs and motivations.

Given this degree of complexity, it is not surprising that many neural regions have been linked to the production of sequential behavior. This section provides a brief overview of this literature, focusing on neurological disorders that affect sequencing. In considering these and neuroimaging studies, it points to some constraints on the cognitive architecture underlying sequencing.

Parkinson's Disease as a Model of Basal Ganglia Pathology

As described in section 8.2, researchers working with a number of different species have hypothesized that the basal ganglia play a central role in the production of learned, sequential movements. Much of the work with neurological patients has centered on Parkinson's disease, with an eye to determining whether the impairment of these patients on sequencing tasks goes beyond a more basic impairment in motor control.

One approach has been to focus on cognitive manipulations in which the motor demands are roughly constant across conditions. For example, are Parkinson's patients able to use precued information to plan a series of sequential responses? Stelmach and colleagues (1987) observed that reaction times of Parkinson's patients versus control participants increased disproportionately as sequence complexity increased. Harrington and Haaland (1991) have reported similar programming deficits as well as a problem in switching between hand gestures within a heterogeneous sequence (see also Agostino et al., 1992; Roy et al., 1993).

A problem with varying the actions within a response sequence is especially marked when the movements must be based on internal referents, rather than on external cues (e.g., Henderson and Goodrich, 1993).

Georgiou and colleagues (1994) had participants produce a sequence of ten successive responses, each of which required a binary decision. In one condition, external cues for each of the ten response decisions were always provided; in the others, these cues were reduced. As the participants made one response, either the next cue (moderate reduction) or next two cues (high reduction) were removed. This manipulation forced the participants to rely on memory in selecting the sequential responses. Although the Parkinson's patients were slower to move than control participants in all conditions, this difference became accentuated when the external cues were reduced. Thus, like the SMA, the basal ganglia may be especially important in the generation of internally guided movements.

Such results have been interpreted in a different manner in Robertson and Flowers, 1990, where Parkinson's participants were taught two different sequences of button presses, both of which they learned to perform accurately. When required to switch back and forth between the two sequences within one trial, however, Parkinson's participants were impaired relative to control participants. The errors the patients made were not random: They were likely to press a key that would have been a correct next response if the other sequence were being performed. To rule out working memory as a simple explanation for the effect, Robertson and Flowers demonstrated that patients could perform a sequence that required a complex mental transformation. When lights were used to indicate which sequence was required, the Parkinson's patients performed as well as controls, even if the sequences were alternating within a trial. Because their deficit emerged only when they were required to switch between the sequences without external cues, Robertson and Flowers concluded that the Parkinson's patients' primary deficit was an inability to select and maintain one plan of action in the face of competition from other plans of action.

Hayes and colleagues (1998) provided a strong, explicit test of this hypothesis. In a training phase, Parkinson and control participants learned to produce two sequences. For example, sequence A might require successive presses of buttons 1, 2, then 3, and sequence B might require the order 1, 3, then 2. In the test phase, one of four letter pairs was presented for each trial (AA, AB, BB, BA). The participants were required to produce a series of six responses, the first three according to the letter on the left and the second three dictated by the letter on the right. The participants were instructed to begin responding as soon as possible and to make all of the responses as rapidly as possible. The primary measure was the intertap interval separating the two sequences. Note that for all four conditions, the key press that begins the second sequence (which is the fourth key press) is always identical: In this example, the response would be to press button 1. However, for stimuli AB and BA, this response is part of a new sequence, whereas for stimuli AA and BB, this response initiates a second repetition of a single sequence.

The results of Hayes et al., 1998, show that, in both conditions, the interval preceding the fourth response was inflated, a pattern quite similar to that observed in Povel and Collard, 1982, which demonstrated the presence of a hierarchic representation of extended response strings. More important, this increase was largest for the Parkinson's patients when they were required to shift to a new sequence.

The preceding work provides some of the strongest evidence in support of the hypothesis that the basal ganglia play a critical role in set shifting, a hypothesis that may prove parsimonious in linking together several functions associated with the basal ganglia. First, according to the set-shifting hypothesis, the inability of Parkinson's patients to initiate movement may be seen as an extreme manifestation of an inability to change motor set. Bradykinesia may reflect this same deficit, but an ongoing movement may impose a weaker inertial force. Second, the set-shifting hypothesis is also consistent with the observed effects on rat grooming behavior following lesions to the striatum (Berridge and Whishaw, 1992). As noted above, rats in this study would frequently initiate a grooming sequence in the appropriate manner, but would fail to switch between the successive elements in order to complete the sequence. Third, and perhaps most provocative, the set-shifting hypothesis may offer new insight into the cognitive problems associated with pathologies of the basal ganglia. Perhaps the domain of the set-shifting operation extends beyond motor control to more covert realms of cognition (Hayes et al., 1998; Owen et al., 1993).

Cerebellum

The cerebellum is essential for the production of skilled, sequential movements; indeed, the cardinal symptoms associated with cerebellar pathology are seen in the production of sequential acts. For example, patients with cerebellar damage are severely limited in their ability to produce rapid, alternating movements about a single joint (Holmes, 1939). As with apraxic patients, their behavior on sequential tasks has the appearance of a series of discrete movements (Beppu et al., 1984). Cerebellar patients tend to slow down the speed of their movements, thus reducing the likelihood that the gestures will produce neuromuscular interactions. Relatively little work has directly examined the consequences that such a strategy might have in terms of movement preparation. Inhoff and colleagues (1989) found that reaction time did not tend to increase as a function of sequence length in cerebellar patients, a result consistent with the idea that the patients are not planning the entire sequence in advance.

One explanation of this behavior is that cerebellar damage disrupts the precise timing required to coordinate a sequence of muscular events (Timmann et al., 1999). Indeed, a general computational account of cerebellar function has centered on the idea that the cerebellum is specialized to represent the temporal relationship between events (Ivry, 1997). The timing hypothesis is supported by the well-established involvement of the cerebellum in Pavlovian eye blink conditioning. Successful conditioning requires that the animal not only learn that a neutral stimulus such as a tone predicts the unconditioned, aversive air puff, but also the precise timing between these events. It is this timing that makes the response adaptive, occurring just prior to the air puff. Trained rabbits with focal lesions of the cerebellar cortex continue to produce the conditioned response, but the adaptive timing is abolished (Perrett et al., 1993).

As noted above, patients with cerebellar atrophy fail to show any learning on the serial reaction time task (Pascual-Leone et al., 1993) and unilateral cerebellar lesions produce similarly dramatic deficits when patients perform the task with the ipsilesional hand (Molinari et al., 1997). It is not obvious how a timing hypothesis could account for this consistent pattern. If learning consists of forming associations between successive stimulus-response associations or a series of spatial goals, why would precise timing be required? One possibility is that associative mechanisms require a consistent temporal relationship between successive events, even if this timing is incidental to the task (but see Willingham et al., 1997). With cerebellar damage, the representation of the timing of successive events may be noisy, reducing the likelihood that associations will be formed.

Alternatively, timing may be one form of a more general function associated with the formation of predictions (Bower, 1997; Courchesne and Allen, 1997; Ivry, 2000). That is, the cerebellum may be essential for developing an internal representation of future events, a prerequisite for a sequential associative process. This idea has been developed computationally as a process of forward modeling. Just as the cerebellum has been central to models of efference copy in the production of movements (Gellman et al., 1985), so it may also generate forward models for learning in a general manner (Imamizu et al., 2000). For example, predictions could be shaped within the cerebellum through the use of salient error signals.

Apraxia

The study of ideomotor apraxia, a disorder of the execution of skilled movement that cannot be attributed to motor problems of weakness, ataxia, sensory loss, or failures of comprehension (Heilman et al., 1981), has furthered our understanding of the role of frontal and parietal lobes in sequenced movements. The apraxia literature is difficult to disentangle. Although much of the work has focused on the primary role played by the left hemisphere in the production of sequential behavior (e.g., Kimura, 1982), apraxic patients almost always have associated problems with language (Kertesz, 1985), making it difficult to dissociate linguistic deficits from those specifically related to motor control.

Standard tests of apraxia involve asking patients to produce goal-directed movement gestures, which may be single behavioral acts, such as saluting or holding a ball, or a series of behavioral acts, such as those required to light a pipe or slice a piece of bread. Apraxic patients are generally most impaired when asked to pantomime a given action without the assistance of external props, such as the pipe or the bread knife. Performance usually improves when these tools are provided, although the kinematics may remain abnormal (Clark et al., 1994).

As proposed by Heilman et al. (1981), one of the two forms of ideomotor apraxia is caused by lesions to premotor and prefrontal areas of the frontal lobe, which give rise to the typical pattern of impairments in patients asked to produce sequential acts either from memory or with objects they are provided. An important feature of these impairments is that they are evident in movements made with either the contralesional or ipsilesional hand. That a left-sided lesion impairs left-handed movements further underscores that the problem lies in the representation rather than production of a motor act.

Patients with parietal lobe lesions show a similar pattern of problems when asked to produce goal-directed movements (Haaland et al., 2000). A debate dominating the apraxia literature centers on how best to characterize the parietal lobe apraxia syndrome. Drawing parallels with the language comprehension deficits seen in many of such patients, Geschwind (1975) argued that the problem is essentially a disconnection syndrome: The patients have difficulty comprehending the required action and thus cannot convey instructions or intent to motor structures in either the left or right hemispheres. Heilman and Rothi (1993), on the other hand, argued that the posterior left hemisphere is the repository of the spatiotemporal representations of learned, skilled movements and that lesions affecting this brain region disrupt the memories themselves. This hypothesis provides a better account for why apraxic patients continue to move clumsily even when provided with tools to manipulate. It is felt that the tools should convey the desired action without reference to any sort of verbal instructions.

Heilman and colleagues (1981) took a different approach to explore the hypothesis that the left parietal lobe contains the representations of sequential actions. Patients with left-hemisphere lesions were classified into four groups based on two factors: whether the lesion focus was anterior or posterior and whether the patients were apraxic or nonapraxic. These patients were then given a perceptual test in which they were asked to choose the best of three possible examples of a target act. The stimuli were presented in motion picture clips of an arm making gestures such as using a key or hammering. The movements were either three different, well-performed acts, or the same act performed in three different ways. The apraxic patients with posterior lesions made significantly more errors than the two nonapraxic groups on this perceptual task. In contrast, the anterior apraxic patients performed as well as the nonapraxic participants. Thus the posterior lesions that produced apraxia not only disrupted motor performance of sequential gestures, but also led to a corresponding perceptual impairment. It should be noted that this and subsequent studies (Rothi et al., 1985) have neither tested whether these patients' perceptual deficit is specific to sequential movements nor included a control task involving the perception of some other type of stimuli.

Harrington and Haaland (1992) compared apraxic and nonapraxic patients with left-hemisphere strokes in order to discover why apraxic patients fail to produce coordinated sequential actions. The patients were asked to produce a series of gestures involving either push, poke, or clench movements. The sequence could consist of a repetition of a single gesture or could be composed of a heterogeneous set of gestures. In both reaction time and movement time measures, the apraxic participants were disproportionately impaired on the heterogeneous sequences. Harrington and

Haaland proposed that the apraxic participants were unable to chunk the sequence meaningfully (see also Harrington and Haaland, 1991) and that, rather than developing a hierarchic representation of the sequence, they treated each element of the sequence as an independent gesture.

Supplementary Motor Area

More than any other cortical area, the supplementary motor area (SMA) has been hypothesized to be specifically engaged during sequential movements, especially when such movements require the coordinated use of two limbs. In primates, few changes in general motor behavior are found after the SMA is lesioned, a result that contrasts sharply with the devastating effects observed if a lesion is restricted to the primary motor cortex (Brinkman, 1984). For example, although they have some problems in coordinating fine hand movements to retrieve pieces of food, SMA-lesioned animals can produce reach and grasp movements with no noticeable loss of control. These coordination problems become more apparent, however, when the animals are required to produce bimanual movements. Of particular interest here is that SMA-lesioned monkeys tend to produce mirror movements, even in tasks requiring the coordination of separate gestures from the two hands.

Studies of humans with lesions of the supplementary motor area have tended to report more dramatic deficits, with patients in the acute state being akinetic and mute. Whether this complete disruption of movement should be attributed to damage in the supplementary motor area or whether it results from an extension of the pathology into underlying cingulate cortex is unknown. As in the animal studies, patients with chronic supplementary motor lesions have marked problems with bimanual movements (Halsband et al., 1993; Laplane et al., 1977).

In Halsband et al., 1993, SMA-lesioned patients asked to reproduce a series of rhythmic responses, either with one hand or by alternating between the two hands, were severely impaired, producing gross distortions of the rhythmic structure of the sequences. Although this deficit was most dramatic when the responses were made bimanually (for converging EEG evidence, see Lang et al., 1990), these patients showed little impairment in producing the rhythms when an auditory pacing signal was provided, and had no difficulty on a rhythm perception task. From this, Halsband and colleagues concluded that the SMA plays a critical role in the internal generation of sequential activity. It should be noted that, although the deficits were not as marked, similar problems were also found in patients with lesions of lateral premotor cortex.

Halsband and colleagues (1993) suggested that the particular contribution of the SMA in the production of sequential behavior was in the temporal control of movements. However, if this were so, the patients with SMA lesions would also have been expected to be impaired even when the pacing tones were present because the responses tend to anticipate the tones rather than follow them (Mates et al., 1994). An alternative approach, one consistent with the fact that SMA-lesioned patients and animals produce inappropriate mirror-symmetrical movements, would be to focus on the role of the SMA in movement selection, making use of the bimanual rhythm task, which requires that patients not only know when to move, but also which hand to move. The PET data reviewed below indicate that the SMA is bilaterally activated during movement planning. Perhaps this reflects the activation of multiple modes for achieving a goal (e.g., left or right hand) and these candidate actions engage in a competitive process for selection. In normal unimanual processing, only one movement is selected. For bimanual movements, a distinct gesture for each hand is selected in order to produce a coordinated action. With unilateral SMA damage, the intact hemisphere may select a gesture that is applied generically.

Converging evidence for a role of the supplementary motor area in movement selection, especially within a sequential context comes from a study in which transient lesions were produced in normal individuals via high-frequency repetitive transcranial magnetic stimulation (TMS; Gerloff et al., 1997). The participants were trained to produce a difficult 16-element sequence of finger movements at a rate of 2 Hz. Once the pattern could be produced without error, rTMS was applied on some of the trials. When motor cortex was stimulated, errors were limited to the time window during which the rTMS was applied, whereas, when the SMA was stimulated, the errors began a few responses after stimulation onset and extended up to 4 s after stimulation offset. Thus motor cortex stimulation appeared to induce errors in the production of the current movement, errors that the participants reported as feeling as though their fingers would not do what they wanted them to do. SMA stimulation, on the other hand, disrupted the representation of a forthcoming sequence of responses. Indeed, the participants reported having forgotten the end of the sequence or their place within the sequence.

8.5 Brain Activity during the Production of Sequential Movements

Neuroimaging and neurophysiological methods have been employed in many laboratories over the past decade in an effort to identify the neural correlates of sequential behavior. PET and fMRI studies with humans have been used to delineate the network of areas recruited during sequential movement tasks and determine how activity across these networks changes as a function of learning. Single-cell recording studies with primates have sought to determine the functional contribution of different neural areas to sequential movements.

Analysis of Component Operations Involved in Sequential Movements

How do different neural areas get recruited as task demands change from simple movements to complex sequences? In one of the earliest imaging studies of motor control, Roland and his colleagues (1980) compared a condition in which participants made simple finger flexion or extension movements to one in which a complex sequence was produced with all of the fingers. With a rest condition as a baseline, the simple movement condition produced very restricted changes in neural activity, limited to contralateral sensorimotor cortex, whereas the sequence condition produced widespread changes, including contralateral sensorimotor cortex, lateral premotor cortex, and superior parietal lobe, as well as bilateral activation in the supplementary motor area and prefrontal cortex. Subcortically, the sequence condition is associated with bilateral activation in the basal ganglia (caudate, not putamen) and ipsilateral cerebellum (Roland et al., 1982; Shibasaki et al., 1993).

More recent studies have applied more sophisticated analytic techniques. For example, parametric manipulations of sequence length or complexity have allowed researchers to analyze metabolic signals over a range of conditions. Using this approach, Catalan and colleagues (1998) reported that in one of two types of neural responses, all movement conditions exhibited increased activity compared to the rest condition and a further increase when subjects had to perform the movements sequentially. Areas exhibiting this pattern included bilateral sensorimotor cortex, contralateral SMA and premotor cortex, and ipsilateral cerebellum. Given that these areas were more active in various sequence conditions than in simple movement conditions suggests a role in sequence execution. However, none of these areas showed a further increase in activation when the sequence length was manipulated. Rather, this effect was observed in right premotor cortex and bilateral parietal areas, which, Catalan and colleagues suggest, reflects the involvement of spatial working memory in the retrieval of complex movement sequences (see also Sadato et al., 1996).

A different way to manipulate complexity is to vary the number of finger transitions (Harrington et al., 2000). The sequences 23333 and 23233 are both five elements long and involve only two responses, but the latter requires more transitions. Activation in the latter condition was greater in various occipital regions (presumably because more complex analysis was required of the visually cued digit sequences), premotor cortex, and superior and inferior regions of parietal cortex. The premotor and parietal activations would be consistent with those in the apraxia literature. Interestingly, as found in many imaging studies of sequence learning and sequence production, the premotor and parietal activations were bilateral even though all of the responses were made with the right hand. This bilateral activation may reflect the abstract nature with which sequential actions are planned: The representation is of a sequence of goals and the transformation of this goal into a specific set of responses occurs only at late stages in the motor pathways. Another possibility is that the right-hemisphere activation reflects a spatial code used to represent the sequences of responses. An experiment in which the sequences were produced with the left hand would be useful in evaluating these two hypotheses.

Physiological Correlates of Skill Acquisition

Although studies in which the sequence can change from trial to trial have much to tell us about the neural correlates of sequence generation and execution, they have little to say about how sequence-specific learning occurs and how the neural landscape may shift with the development of skill. Imaging studies of the serial reaction time task (see "Neural Correlates of Learning in the Serial Reaction Time Task" in section 8.3) suggest that different associative pathways may be engaged depending on task conditions. With attentional distraction, learning was restricted to a network that encompassed more traditional motor regions of motor cortex, the supplementary motor area, and inferior parietal cortex, whereas, without distraction, the loci of learning shifted to lateral prefrontal cortex, premotor cortex, and more ventral regions of posterior cortex.

The lateral prefrontal/premotor–ventral pathway network may constitute a system involved in extracting regularities between external events ("what" comes next) and then mapping these stimulus expectancies onto the appropriate motor responses (Keele et al., forthcoming). This latter operation would be consistent with the thesis that premotor cortex is essential for establishing stimulus-response associations (Wise et al., 1996). Studies of trial-and-error learning in humans and primates support prefrontal/premotor involvement in sequence learning. Jenkins and colleagues (1994) had participants learn an eight-element pattern. In each trial, participants pressed one of four keys and the pitch of a tone indicated whether that response was correct or not. Lateral premotor and prefrontal cortex were more active when the participants were learning a new sequence than when they were performing a well-learned sequence. In contrast, neural activity has generally been found to increase in the supplementary motor area, putamen, lateral cerebellum, and parietal cortex when participants perform well-learned sequences (reviewed in Hikosaka et al., 1999).

These results have been confirmed in more recent imaging studies with the addition of a new area, the pre–supplementary motor area (pre-SMA), to the list of regions exhibiting more pronounced activity during the early stages of learning (e.g., Sakai et al., 1998). Like premotor cortex, the pre-SMA has been hypothesized to play a role in forming stimulus-response (S-R) associations, although the pre-SMA may learn these associations across a greater context and may even code abstract properties such as the ordinal position of a particular S-R association within the sequence (Clower and Alexander, 1998; Shima and Tanji, 2000).

The lateral-medial distinction within frontal cortex has been characterized in terms of whether responses are externally guided or internally generated (Deiber et al., 1991, 1999; Goldberg, 1985; Mushiake et al., 1991). For example, Mushiake and colleagues (1991) trained monkeys to press a sequence of three buttons under two different instruction sets. For externally guided sequences, three buttons were illuminated in succession and the animals pressed each one in turn. For internally guided sequences, the animals learned a particular sequence and then reproduced it after hearing an auditory signal. Sequence-specific neurons were found both in the SMA and in premotor cortex. That is, the activity of a particular cell would be correlated with a movement, but only when that movement was embedded in a particular sequence. Cells in the SMA were disproportionately active

Table 8.2
Taxonomy of brain regions involved in sequenced movements

Component of sequenced movement	Brain region	Computation
Goal development	Frontal lobes	Strategic planning; memory retrieval
Sequence representation and planning	Parietal cortex	Series of goals expressed as target locations: "Where is response directed?"
	Temporal cortex	Series of goals expressed as stimulus expectancies: "What is the next event?"
Movement selection	Premotor area	Biased to be driven by external inputs
	Supplementary motor area	Biased to reflect internal goals and motivation; consolidation of successive responses into action chunk with practice.
Movement specification	Cerebellum	Temporal patterns and initiation of activation; prediction of consequences
	Basal ganglia	Switching between old state and new state of activation.
Movement execution	Motor cortex	Signal to motor system to implement movement

during internally guided sequences. In contrast, cells in lateral premotor cortex were disproportionately active during externally guided sequences.

Such a shift is consistent with the notion that, as learning progresses, external cues are likely to play a diminishing role in sequence performance. Indeed, in many tasks, there is likely to be a high degree of correspondence between the level of learning and the extent to which a behavior is dependent on external cues. As children learning to write, we must carefully examine the outcome of each stroke; with skill, our handwriting suffers little if visual feedback is removed. A similar decrease in reliance on external cues (and concomitant increase in reliance on internal representations) can be expected to characterize our performance on most sequential actions.

In reviewing issues central to a cognitive neuroscience of sequential behavior, we have provided a hypothesis for each brain region reviewed (see table 8.2) in terms of how it might contribute to the production of coordinated, sequential behavior. Although these hypotheses will almost certainly be replaced by more refined ones, they are offered as heuristic tools to guide future research.

Acknowledgments

We are grateful to Steven Keele for his insightful comments on an earlier draft of this chapter. Our work was funded by National Science Foundation grant GER 9355034 and by National Institutes of Health grants NS30256, NS33504, and NS1778.

References

Agostino, R., Berardelli, A., Formica, A., Accornero, N., and Manfredi, M. (1992). Sequential arm movements in patients with Parkinson's disease, Huntington's disease, and dystonia. *Brain* 115: 481–495.

Aldridge, J. W., and Berridge, K. C. (1998). Coding of serial order by neostriatal neurons: A "natural action" approach to movement sequence. *J. Neurosci.* 18: 2777–2787.

Barlow, G. W. (1977). Modal action patterns. In *How Animals Communicate*, T. A. Sebeok (ed.). Bloomington: Indiana University Press, pp. 98–128.

Baxter, L. R. (1999). Functional imaging of brain systems mediating obsessive-compulsive disorder. In *Neurobiology of Mental Illness*, D. S. Charney, E. J. Nestler, and B. S. Bunney (eds.). New York: Oxford University Press, pp. 534–547.

Beppu, H., Suda, M., and Tanaka, R. (1984). Analysis of cerebellar motor disorders by visually guided elbow tracking movement. *Brain* 107: 787–809.

Berridge, K. C., and Whishaw, I. Q. (1992). Cortex, striatum, and cerebellum: control of serial order in a grooming task. *Exp. Brain Res.* 90: 275–290.

Botvinick, M., Nystrom, L. E., Fissell, K., Carter, C. S., and Cohen, J. D. (1999). Conflict monitoring versus selection-for-action in anterior cingulate cortex. *Nature* 402: 179–181.

Bower, J. M. (1997). Control of sensory data acquisition. *Int. Rev. Neurobiol.* 41: 489–513.

Brainard, M. S., and Doupe, A. J. (2000). Interruption of a basal ganglia-forebrain circuit prevents plasticity of learned vocalizations. *Nature* 404: 762–766.

Brinkman, C. (1984). Supplementary motor area of the monkey's cerebral cortex: Short- and long-term deficits after unilateral ablation and the effects of subsequent callosal section. *J. Neurosci.* 4: 918–929.

Catalan, M. J., Honda, M., Weeks, R. A., Cohen, L. G., and Hallett, M. (1998). The functional neuroanatomy of simple and complex sequential finger movements: A PET study. *Brain* 121: 253–264.

Chun, M. M., and Phelps, E. A. (1999). Memory deficits for implicit contextual information in amnesic subjects with hippocampal damage. *Nat. Neurosci.* 2: 844–847.

Clark, M., Merians, A. A., Kothari, A., and Poizner, H. (1994). Spatial planning deficits in limb apraxia. *Brain* 117: 1093–1106.

Clower, W. T., and Alexander, G. E. (1998). Movement sequence-related activity reflecting numerical order of components in supplementary and presupplementary motor areas. *J. Neurophysiol.* 80: 1562–1566.

Cohen, A., Ivry, R. I., and Keele, S. W. (1990). Attention and structure in sequence learning. *J. Exp. Psychol. Learn. Mem. Cogn.*16: 17–30.

Corkin, S. (1968). Acquisition of motor skill after bilateral medial temporal-lobe excision. *Neuropsychologia* 6: 255–265.

Courchesne, E., and Allen, G. (1997). Prediction and preparation, fundamental functions of the cerebellum. *Learn. Mem.* 4: 1–35.

Cromwell, H. C., and Berridge, K. C. (1996). Implementation of action sequences by a neostriatal site: A lesion mapping study of grooming syntax. *J. Neurosci.* 16: 3444–3458.

Curran, T., and Keele, S. W. (1993). Attentional and nonattentional forms of sequence learning. *J. Exp. Psychol. Learn. Mem. Cogn.* 19: 189–202.

Deiber, M. P., Passingham, R. E., Colebatch, J. G., Friston, K. J., Nixon, P. D., and Frackowiak, R. S. (1991). Cortical areas and the selection of movements: A study with positron-emission tomography. *Exp. Brain Res.* 84: 393–402.

Deiber, M.P., Honda, M., Ibáñez, V., Sadato, N., and Hallett, M. (1999). Mesial motor areas in self-initiated versus externally triggered movements examined with fMRI: Effect of movement type and rate. *J. Neurophysiol.* 81: 3065-3077.

Eibl-Eibesfeldt, I. (1989). *Human Ethology.* Hawthorne, N.Y.: Aldine de Gruyter.

Ekman, P. (1973). Cross-cultural studies of facial expression. In *Darwin and Facial Expression: A Century of Research in Review,* P. Ekman (ed.). New York: Academic Press, pp. 169–220.

Fentress, J. C. (1973). Emergence of pattern in the development of mammalian movement sequences. *J. Neurol.* 23: 1529–1556.

Ferraro, F. R., Balota, D. A., and Connor, L. T. (1993). Implicit memory and the formation of new associations in nondemented Parkinson's disease individuals and individuals with senile dementia of the Alzheimer type: A serial reaction time (SRT) investigation. *Brain Cogn.* 21: 163–180.

Frensch, P. A., Lin, J., and Buchner, A. (1998). Learning versus behavioral expression of the learned: The effects of a secondary tone-counting task on implicit learning in the serial reaction task. *Psychol. Res.* 61: 83–98.

Gellman, R., Gibson, A. R., and Houk, J. C. (1985). Inferior olivary neurons in the awake cat: Detection of contact and passive body displacement. *J. Neurophysiol.* 54: 40–60.

Georgiou, N., Bradshaw, J. L., Iansek, R., and Phillips, J. G. (1994). Reduction in external cues and movement sequencing in Parkinson's disease. *J. Neurol. Neurosurg. Psychiatry* 57: 368–370.

Gerloff, C., Corwell, B., Chen, R., Hallett, M., and Cohen, L. G. (1997). Stimulation over the human supplementary motor area interferes with the organization of future elements in complex motor sequences. *Brain* 120: 1587–1602.

Geschwind, N. (1975). The apraxias: Neural mechanisms of disorders of learned movement. *Am. Scientist* 63: 188–195.

Golani, I. (1992). A mobility gradient in the organization of vertebrate movement: The perception of movement through symbolic language. *Behav. Brain Sci.* 15: 249–308.

Goldberg, G. (1985). Supplementary motor area structure and function: Review and hypotheses. *Behav. Brain Sci.* 8: 567–616.

Gómez-Beldarrain, M., García-Moncó, J. C., Rubio, B., and Pascual-Leone, A. (1998). Effect of focal cerebellar lesions on procedural learning in the serial reaction time task. *Exp. Brain Res.* 120: 25–30.

Grafton, S. T., Hazeltine, E., and Ivry, R. (1995). Functional mapping of sequence learning in normal humans. *J. Cogn. Neurosci.* 7: 497–510.

Grafton, S. T., Hazeltine, E., and Ivry, R. B. (1998). Abstract and effector-specific representations of motor sequences identified with PET. *J. Neurosci.* 18: 9420–9428.

Haaland, K. Y., Harrington, D. L., and Knight, R. T. (2000). Neural representations of skilled movement. *Brain* 123: 2306–2313.

Halsband, U., Ito, N., Tanji, J., and Freund, H. J. (1993). The role of premotor cortex and the supplementary motor area in the temporal control of movement in man. *Brain* 116: 243–266.

Harrington, D. L., and Haaland, K. Y. (1991). Sequencing in Parkinson's disease. *Brain* 114: 99–115.

Harrington, D. L., and Haaland, K. Y. (1992). Motor sequencing with left hemisphere damage. Are some cognitive deficits specific to limb apraxia? *Brain* 115: 857–874.

Harrington, D. L., Rao, S. M., Haaland, K. Y., Bobholz, J. A., Mayer, A. R., Binder, J. R., and Cox, R. W. (2000). Specialized neural systems underlying representations of sequential movements. *J. Cogn. Neurosci.* 12: 56–77.

Hayes, A. E., Davidson, M. C., Keele, S. W., and Rafal, R. D. (1998). Toward a functional analysis of the basal ganglia. *J. Cogn. Neurosci.* 10: 178–198.

Hazeltine, E., Grafton, S. T., and Ivry, R. (1997). Attention and stimulus characteristics determine the locus of motor-sequence encoding a PET study. *Brain* 120: 123–140.

Heilman, K. M., and Rothi, L. J. G. (1993). Apraxia. In *Clinical Neuropsychology,* 3d ed., K. M. Heilman and E. Valenstein (eds.). New York: Oxford University Press, pp. 141–163.

Heilman, K. M., Rothi, L. J., and Valenstein, E. (1981). Two forms of ideomotor apraxia. *Neurology* 32: 342–346.

Helmuth, L. L., Mayr, U., and Daum, I. (2000). Sequence learning in Parkinson's disease: A comparison of spatial-attention and number-response sequences. *Neuropsychologia* 38: 1443–1451.

Henderson, L., and Goodrich, S. J. (1993). Simple reaction time and predictive tracking in Parkinson's disease: Do they converge on a single, fixed impairment of preparation? *J. Mot. Behav.* 25: 89–96.

Hikosaka, O., Nakahara, H., Rand, M. K., Sakai, K., Lu, X., Nakamura, K., Miyachi, S., and Doya, K. (1999). Parallel neural networks for learning sequential procedures. *Trends Neurosci.* 22: 464–471.

Holmes, G. (1939). The cerebellum of man. *Brain* 62: 1–30.

Honda, M., Deiber, M.-P., Ibáñez, V., Pascual-Leone, A., Zhuang, P., and Hallett, M. (1998). Dynamic cortical involvement in implicit and explicit motor sequence learning: A PET study. *Brain* 121: 2159–2173.

Hore, J., Watts, S., Tweed, D., and Miller, B. (1996). Overarm throws with the non-dominant arm: Kinematics of accuracy. *J. Neurophysiol.* 76: 3693–3704.

Imamizu, H., Miyauchi, S., Tamada, T., Sasaki, Y., Takino, R., Pütz, B., Yoshioka, T., and Kawato, M. (2000). Human cerebellar activity reflecting an acquired internal model of a new tool. *Nature* 403: 192–195.

Inhoff, Diener, Rafal, R., and Ivry, R. B. (1989). The role of the cerebellar structures in the execution of serial movements. *Brain* 112: 565–581.

Ivry, R. (1997). Cerebellar timing systems. *Int. Rev. Neurobiol.* 41:555–573.

Ivry, R. (2000). Exploring the role of the cerebellum in sensory anticipation and timing: Commentary on Tesche and Karhu. *Hum. Brain Mapp.* 9: 115–118.

Jackson, G. M., Jackson, S. R., Harrison, J., Henderson, L., and Kennard, C. (1995). Serial reaction time learning and Parkinson's disease: Evidence for a procedural learning deficit. *Neuropsychologia* 33: 577–593.

Jenkins, I. H., Brooks, D. J., Nixon, P. D., Frackowiak, R. S. J., and Passingham, R. E. (1994). Motor sequence learning: A study with positron-emission tomography. *J. Neurosci.* 14: 3775–3790.

Karni, A., Meyer, G., Jezzard, P., Adams, M. M, Turner, R., and Ungerleider, L. G. (1995). Functional MRI evidence for adult motor cortex plasticity during motor skill learning. *Nature* 377: 155–158.

Keele, S. W., Jennings, P., Jones, S., Caulton, D., and Cohen, A. (1995). On the modularity of sequence representation. *J. Mot. Behav.* 27: 17–30.

Keele, S.W., Ivry, R., Mayr, U., Hazeltine, E., and Heuer, H. (in press). The cognitive and neural architecture of sequence representation. *Psychological Review.*

Kertez, A. (1985). Apraxia and aphasia: Anatomical and clinical relationship. In *Neuropsychological Studies of Apraxia and Related Disorders,* E. A. Roy (ed.). New Holland: Elsevier Scientific Publishers, pp. 163–178.

Kimura, D. (1982). Premotor and supplementary motor cortex in rhesus monkeys: Neuronal activity during externally and internally instructed motor tasks. *Exp. Brain Res.* 72: 237–248.

Lang, W., Obrig, H., Lindinger, G., Cheyne, D., and Deecke, L. (1990). Supplementary motor area activation while tapping bimanually different rhythms in musicians. *Exp. Brain Res.* 79: 504–514.

Laplane, D., Talairach, J., Meininger, V., Bancaud, J., and Orgogozo, J. M. (1977). Clinical consequences of corticectomies involving the supplementary motor area in man. *J. Neurol. Sci.* 34: 301–314.

Lashley, K. (1951). The problem of serial order in behavior. In *Cerebral Mechanisms in Behavior*, L. A. Jeffress (ed.). New York: Wiley, pp. 112–136.

Lorenz, K. Z. (1950). The comparative method in studying innate behavior patterns. In *Physiological Mechanisms in Animal Behavior*. New York: Academic Press, pp. 221–254.

MacKay, D. G. (1982). The problems of flexibility, fluency, and speed-accuracy trade-off in skilled behavior. *Psychol. Rev.* 89: 483–506.

Massaro, D. W. (1998). *Perceiving Talking Faces: From Speech Perception to a Behavioral Principle*. Cambridge, Mass.: MIT Press.

Mates, J., Mueller, U., Radil, T., and Poeppel, E. (1994). Temporal integration in sensorimotor synchronization. *J. Cogn. Neurosci.* 6: 332–340.

Milner, A. D., and Goodale, M. A. (1995). *The Visual Brain in Action*. New York: Oxford University Press.

Molinari, M., Leggio, M. G., Solida, A., Ciorra, R., Misciagna, S., Silveri, M. C., and Petrosini, L. (1997). Cerebellum and procedural learning: Evidence from focal cerebellar lesions. *Brain* 120: 1753–1762.

Mushiake, H., Inase, M., and Tanji, J. (1991). Neuronal activity in the primate premotor, supplementary, and precentral motor cortex during visually guided and internally determined sequential movements. *J. Neurophysiol.* 66: 705–718.

Nissen, M. J., and Bullemer, P. (1987). Attentional requirements of learning: Evidence from performance measures. *Cogn. Psychol.* 19: 1–32.

Nissen, M. J., Knopman, D. S., and Schacter, D. L. (1987). Neurochemical dissociation of memory systems. *Neurology* 37: 789–794.

Owen, A. M., Roberts, A. C., Hodges, J. R., Saummers, B. A., Polkey, C. E., and Robbins, T. W. (1993). Contrasting mechanisms of impaired attentional set-shifting in patients with frontal lobe damage or Parkinson's disease. *Brain* 116: 1159–1175.

Pascual-Leone, A., Grafman, J., Clark, K., Stewart, M., Massaguoi, S., Lou, J. S., and Hallet, M. (1993). Procedural learning in Parkinson's disease and cerebellar degeneration. *Ann. Neurol.* 34: 594–602.

Pascual-Leone, A., Grafman, J., and Hallett, M. (1994). Modulation of cortical motor output maps during development of implicit and explicit knowledge. *Science* 263: 1287–1289.

Perrett, S. P., Ruiz, B. P., and Mauk, M. D. (1993). Cerebellar cortex lesions disrupt learning-dependent timing of conditioned eyelid responses. *J. Neurosci.* 13: 1708–1718.

Povel, D.-J., and Collard, R. (1982). Structural factors in patterned finger tapping. *Acta Psychol.* 52: 107–123.

Rand, M. K., Hikosaka, O., Miyachi, S., Lu, X., and Miyashita, K. (1998). Characteristics of a long-term procedural skill in the monkey. *Exp. Brain Res.* 118: 293–297.

Rand, M. K., Hikosaka, O., Miyachi, S., Lu, X., Nakamura, K., Kitaguchi, K., and Shimo, Y. (2000). Characteristics of sequential movements during early learning period in monkeys. *Exp. Brain Res.* 131: 293–304.

Rapoport, J. L. (1989). The biology of obsessions and compulsions. *Sci. Am.* 280: 83–90.

Robertson, C., and Flowers, K. A. (1990). Motor set in Parkinson's disease. *J. Neurol. Neurosurg. Psychiatry* 53: 583–592.

Roland, P. E., Larsen, B., Lassen, N. A., and Skinhoj, E. (1980). Supplementary motor area and other cortical areas in organization of voluntary movements in man. *J. Neurophysiol.* 43: 118–136.

Roland, P. E., Meyer, E., Shibasaki, T., Yamamoto, Y. L., and Thompson, C. J. (1982). Regional cerebral blood flow changes in cortex and basal ganglia during voluntary movements in normal human volunteers. *J. Neurophysiol.* 48: 467–480.

Rothi, L. G., Heilman, K. M., and Watson, R. T. (1985). Pantomime comprehension and ideomotor apraxia. *J. Neurol. Neurosurg. Psychiatry* 48: 207–210.

Roy, E. A., Saint-Cyr, J., Taylor, A., and Lang, A. (1993). Movement sequencing disorders in Parkinson's disease. *Int. J. Neurosci.* 73: 183–194.

Sadato, N., Campbell, G., Ibáñez, V., Deiber, M., and Hallett, M. (1996). Complexity affects regional cerebral blood flow change during sequential finger movements. *J. Neurosci.* 16: 2691–2700.

Sakai, K., Hikosaka, O., Miyauchi, S., Takino, R., Sasaki, Y., and Puetz, B. (1998). Transition of brain activation from frontal to parietal areas in visuomotor sequence learning. *J. Neurosci.* 18: 1827–1840.

Schmidtke, V., and Heuer, H. (1997). Task integration as a factor in secondary-task effects on sequence learning. *Psychol. Res.* 60: 53–71.

Shibasaki, H., Sadato, N., Lyshkow, H., Yonekura, Y., Honda, M., Nagamine, T., Suwazono, S., Magata, Y., Ikeda, A., and Miyazaki, M. (1993). Both primary motor cortex and supplementary motor area play an important role in complex finger movement. *Brain* 116: 1378–1398.

Shima, K., and Tanji, J. (2000). Neuronal activity in the supplementary and presupplementary motor areas for temporal organization of multiple movements. *J. Neurophysiol.* 84: 2148–2160.

Stadler, M. A. (1995). Role of attention in implicit learning. *J. Exp. Psychol. Learn. Mem. Cogn.* 21: 674–685.

Stelmach, C. E., Worringhan, C. J., and Strand, E. A. (1987). The programming and execution of movement sequences in Parkinson's disease. *Int. J. Neurosci.* 36: 55–65.

Tanji, J. (1994). The supplementary motor area in the cerebral cortex. *Neurosci. Res.* 19: 251–268.

Thelen, E. (1984). Learning to walk: Ecological demands and phylogenetic constraints. *Adv. Infancy Res.* 3: 213-250.

Timmann, D., Watts, S., and Hore, J. (1999). Failure of cerebellar patients to time finger opening precisely causes ball high-low inaccuracy in overarm throws. *J. Neurophysiol.* 82: 103–114.

Tulving, E., Kapur, S., Craik, F. I., Moscovitch, M., and Houole, S. (1994). Hemispheric encoding/retrieval asymmetry in episodic memory: Positron-emission tomography findings. *Proc. Natl. Acad. Sci. U.S.A.* 91: 2016–2020.

Willingham, D. B. (1999). Implicit motor sequence learning is not purely perceptual. *Mem. Cognit.* 27: 561–572.

Willingham, D. B., and Goedert-Eschmann, K. (1999). The relation between implicit and explicit learning: Evidence for parallel development. *Psychol. Sci.* 10: 531–534.

Willingham, D. B., and Koroshetz, W. J. (1993). Evidence for dissociable motor skills in Huntington's disease patients. *Psychobiology* 21: 173–182.

Willingham, D. B., Nissen, M. J., and Bullemer, P. (1989). On the development of procedural knowledge. *J. Exp. Psychol. Learn. Mem. Cogn.* 15: 1047–1060.

Willingham, D. B., Greenberg, A. R., and Thomas, R. C. (1997). Response-to-stimulus interval does not affect implicit motor sequence learning, but does affect performance *Mem. Cognit.* 25: 534–542.

Willingham, D. B., Wells, L. A., Farrell, J. M., and Stemwedel, M. E. (2000). Implicit motor sequence learning is represented in response locations. *Mem. Cognit.* 28: 366–375.

Wise, S. P., Di Pellegrino, G., and Boussaoud, D. (1996). The premotor cortex and nonstandard sensorimotor mapping. *Can. J. Physiol. Pharmacol.* 74: 469–482.

Bimanual Action Representation: A Window on Human Evolution

Elizabeth A. Franz

9.1 Introduction

A remarkable feature of humans is our hands. Whether to quench our thirst or to write down our thoughts, our hands readily translate our ideas into action. Indeed, the first species of humans was named "*habilis*" (handy) after its "handmaking" of stone tools (Eccles, 1989, p. 23), which required, at the very least, coordination of both hands.

This chapter describes research by my colleagues and me into bimanual representation, a process critical to human evolution. Focusing on how different forms of abstract spatial coupling may reflect representational processes in the brain, it considers possible links with research using other experimental approaches, with the greater goal of promoting discussion across what appears to be an emerging multidisciplinary area of study.

The timing properties of unimanual movements provided the initial impetus for present-day research on bimanual actions. Studies using the Fitts task (see Fitts, 1954) demonstrated that a highly reliable relationship exists between movement difficulty and movement time in unimanual movements to targets. Whereas the original Fitts task was performed by tapping repetitively between two targets, the relationship generalized reliably to discrete aiming movements (Fitts and Peterson, 1964) as well as to a host of other unimanual tasks (e.g., Langolf et al., 1976; Jagacinski et al., 1978).

In the early 1970s, investigators were beginning to examine the temporal properties of interlimb coordination tasks. For example, Cohen (1971) observed that homologous muscles (identical sequences) and nonhomologous muscles (opposite sequences) often moved with temporal synchrony. Somewhat earlier, Wyke (1967) had begun pioneering work on the effects of brain damage to speed of unimanual and bimanual movements. Adding another interesting twist to history, Kelso and colleagues (1979) combined two Fitts's aiming movements in a bimanual task. When they changed the difficulty of the two tasks by varying distance, target width, or both, they observed that the two hands of subjects initiated and terminated movements in a much more coupled fashion than Fitts's law would have predicted. Kelso and colleagues concluded that in bimanual tasks of this type, the hands operate as a "functional synergy," a term borrowed from the earlier writings of Bernstein (1967).

About the same time as the study by Kelso and colleagues, another influential approach was developed by Klapp (1979) and by Peters (1977), among others. Time patterns were manipulated by requiring subjects to tap in rhythms with simple harmonics or complex nonharmonic relations. Demonstrating that, in the absence of considerable practice, subjects could not produce two distinct timing patterns without interference, Klapp (1979) concluded that the movement system is constrained to produce a single timing pattern. Effects of attention were also found to influence bimanual temporal coupling (Peters, 1981). Numerous studies have now identified specific properties of temporal coupling in bimanual movements (discussion of which is beyond the scope of this chapter). Some compelling evidence comes from tasks of bimanual tapping (Yamanishi et al., 1981), pendula swinging (Turvey et al., 1986), flexion-extension movements of the limbs (Swinnen and Walter, 1991), and continuous drawing of curved trajectories (Semjen et al., 1995). These and other investigations illuminate the importance of temporal compatibility and phase relations as constraining features in bimanual movements.

Studies on temporal coupling led my colleagues and me (Franz et al., 1991) to investigate spatial coupling to determine whether there was a constraint in the spatial domain similar to the one operating in the temporal domain. Subjects asked to draw circles with one hand while drawing lines with the other tend to produce curved lines and linelike circles, which has been taken as evidence of spatial coupling (Franz et al., 1991; Franz, 1997; Chan and Chan, 1995).

Spatial coupling also generalizes to discrete bimanual tasks, such as drawing squares combined with circles. Figure 9.1 shows examples of some bimanual drawing tasks, illustrating the extreme forms of interference that result from spatial coupling of complex shapes. Findings on spatial coupling seemed to reveal constraints that cannot be accounted for by timing or phase relations alone. A task such as drawing circles or squares requires

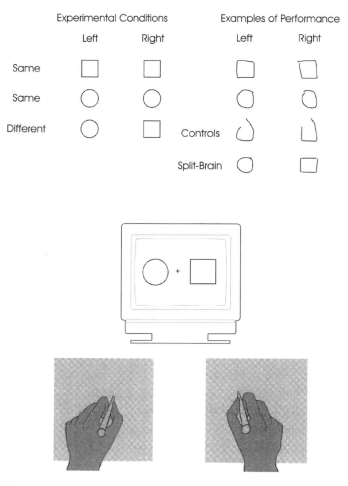

Figure 9.1
(*Bottom*) Basic experimental setup to examine spatial coupling effects in discrete drawing tasks. One stimulus is presented on each side of a visual monitor to instruct what each hand should draw. (*Top*) When identical figures are produced by the two hands, the bimanual task is easy to perform; however, when distinct figures are presented, neurologically normal individuals experience extreme spatial interference of the type shown, whereas split-brain patients do not.

movements with many degrees of freedom that the limb's extremities are specialized to produce. The ability to move in directions and orientations away from the body midline appears to be an evolutionary development unique to primates. This provides one clue that the spatial constraints under investigation are most likely a phylogenetically recent development (for additional evidence, see Franz, 1997).

Accomplished musicians are able to finger a rhythm with one hand while playing a melody with the other (see Shaffer, 1981). What are the mechanisms of learning two tasks at once? Must the whole brain focus on one task at a time? What are the neural mechanisms that make it difficult to produce two different spatial tasks simultaneously?

9.2   Neural Processes of Spatial and Temporal Coupling

For the past nine years or so, I have had the privilege of working daily with people who have rare neurological conditions, and who have educated me about bimanual actions in ways that textbooks or scientific studies could not.[1] These individuals have provided real-life demonstrations of how remarkably resilient people are in their compensatory abilities that often hide in the shadow of deficits. Although I cannot document all of the insights I have gained, I can at least illustrate some that led my colleagues and me to our laboratory studies. The first set of studies examines the neural processes of spatial and temporal coupling in patients with callosotomy (surgical section of the corpus callosum). The initial question was whether the neural processes that underlie spatial planning and temporal coupling of hand actions could be dissociated. If so, it might be possible to perform two different tasks at once, provided certain neural processes of the two tasks are confined to separate cerebral hemispheres. This set of experiments has led to follow-up studies investigating well-learned versus novel bimanual actions in patients with callosotomy and in those with callosal agenesis.

The second set of studies, which focuses on the existence of phantom limb movement after amputation, investigated whether forms of central representation may result in spatial coupling even when no peripheral feedback is possible. Such evidence would suggest that there exist forms of spatial processes that depend on information already within the brain (i.e., a representation), rather than depending on on-line information from the periphery.

The third set of studies focuses on congenital mirror coupling that occurs in the distal extremities of some people. Its findings suggest some intriguing possibilities about development and perhaps even about human evolution. These three sets of studies will be discussed in turn.

Callosotomy Patients

A surgical procedure that severs the corpus callosum, the main commissure between the two cerebral hemispheres, callosotomy ("split brain") is applied in severe cases of uncontrollable epilepsy. The operation is believed to leave subcortical structures intact. An extensive database exists on this topic from decades of influential research by Gazzaniga, Sperry, and others, showing that in the split brain, perceptual, cognitive, and memory processes can be carried out in each cerebral hemisphere separately—without awareness of the other hemisphere (for review, see Gazzaniga and Sperry, 1967). This apparent split in processing led my colleagues and me to wonder whether each hemisphere could operate separately and simultaneously in the processes of motor planning of actions that require *both* hemispheres to act in concert to orchestrate distinct drawing movements of the two hands. We hypothesized that spatial coupling between the limbs would be eliminated with callosotomy, but that temporal coupling would not. These two facets of coupling will be discussed in turn.

Spatial Coupling Because each hemisphere issues motor commands to the opposite hand (Brinkman and Kuypers, 1973), we were able to capitalize on the procedure of visual lateralization (Gazzaniga et al., 1965) by presenting shapes to each hemisphere and asking subjects to draw them. These stimuli could be presented one at a time for unimanual trials, or bilaterally for bimanual trials. Bimanual trials consisted of identical or distinct stimuli. One version of the task presented combinations of curved and straight trajectories similar to those shown in figure 9.1. Another version consisted of three-sided rectangles that were either identically aligned for the tasks of the two hands, or orthogonally oriented (rotated) with respect to one another. The stimuli were presented for a brief duration (<150 ms), and eye movements were monitored. Participants were instructed to draw the stimuli as quickly and accurately as possible. Reaction time and movement properties were recorded and analyzed off-line.

To our delight, callosotomy patients were able to draw two different trajectories simultaneously without the spatial interference demonstrated by

controls with intact callosi. Moreover, the reaction time for patients drawing with both hands was the same when they drew two distinct shapes, as
when they drew identical shapes. In contrast, the reaction time for control
participants was considerably longer when they drew distinct shapes than
when they drew identical shapes, indicating substantial spatial interference.
We inferred from these findings that the corpus callosum provides for interactions in the spatial plans of movements. With callosotomy, each hemisphere appears to be able to separately orchestrate a spatial plan into action,
and the two hemispheres do this simultaneously for motor systems of the
hands (Franz et al., 1996a).

A follow-up study of spatial coupling after each stage of two-stage
callosotomy surgery provided some evidence that spatial coupling was less
affected by anterior surgery than by posterior surgery (Eliassen et al., 1999).
This result might suggest that posterior regions of the corpus callosum produce the interactions that underlie normal spatial coupling processes. Other
studies have shown evidence of a lack of functional disconnection in some
cognitive processes with posterior sparing of the callosum. Findings on
monkeys with partial commissurotomy also support the role of the splenium
in the transfer of visual information associated with limb movements
(Brinkman and Kuypers, 1973).

Little is known about the possible role of other callosal regions in
interlimb coupling. In a study that examined a patient's bimanual performance before and after surgical resection of the center section of the corpus
callosum due to an angioma (Dimond et al., 1977), the bimanual task consisted of drawing repeated semicircles from the top to the bottom of a page
with both hands simultaneously and with mirror symmetry. Unlike in the
aforementioned studies of spatial coupling where the hands were obstructed
from the participant's view, here it appears they were not. Although the
authors reported that the subjects' performance was unimpaired following
the surgery, because the tasks were mirror symmetrical, perfect performance
may indicate complete spatial independence rather than the elimination of
spatial coupling. Future studies on the effects of central callosal section on
bimanual coupling would indeed be valuable in producing convergent
results.

Redundant pathways of spatial information transfer across the corpus
callosum may exist in the normal brain. Indeed, neurons with directional
properties have been found in posterior (parietal) as well as anterior (motor
cortical) regions in reaching tasks performed by a single limb (Georgopoulos

et al., 1982; Kalaska et al., 1983). Through corticocortical pathways, this information may transfer between anterior and posterior regions within each hemisphere, and between hemispheres at more than one possible callosal region. If this is so, partial callosal section would not completely eliminate interhemispheric spatial interactions, whereas complete section would. Testing the effects of partial callosal section with the order of the two-stage callosotomy reversed may be one way to examine this issue. Examining patients with callosal tumors may provide additional information.

Although the above findings consider spatial coupling in direction, coupling in amplitude may also occur. Franz et al., 1996a, manipulated amplitude as well as direction in the task of discrete drawing. Like differences in direction, differences in amplitude between the tasks of the two hands elicited increases, albeit smaller increases, in reaction time and spatial interference in control subjects. Moreover, the effects of spatial coupling in amplitude were much less apparent in the callosotomy patients, suggesting that callosal connections may play a less important role in normal coupling of movement amplitude than of movement direction. In control participants, it appears that when two movements of different amplitudes are paired, the shorter movement becomes slightly longer, and the longer movement becomes slightly shorter (Franz, 1997). Error in endpoint accuracy has also been demonstrated using target aiming tasks to different amplitudes (Martenuik et al., 1984).

It is not clear to what extent amplitude coupling reflects planning versus execution processes. Amplitude accommodation tends to occur when the temporal requirements of bimanual movements demand different movement patterns, as in pairing a single flexion movement with more than one flexion movement performed simultaneously by the opposite limb (Swinnen and Walter, 1991). Spijkers and Heuer (1995) have recently begun to distinguish between programming and execution forms of coupling in amplitude. They demonstrated that amplitude coupling occurs when different but constant amplitudes are assigned to the two limbs. This form of execution coupling becomes more prevalent with increases in movement speed. Spijkers and Heuer also investigated amplitude coupling using movements that alternated between small and large amplitudes, a manipulation believed to reflect programming demands. This manipulation also produced amplitude coupling, but the degree of coupling did not increase with a faster movement speed. Clearly, amplitude coupling effects may reveal operations of complex neural processes that remain to be elucidated.

Temporal Coupling   To investigate whether temporal coordination of the hands is affected by callosotomy, Tuller and Kelso (1989) examined relative phase in semidiscrete tapping movements in callosotomy patients and in two groups of control participants, those with no musical training and skilled musicians. Brief lateralized visual pulses indicated the time to tap each hand, and the relative phase between movements of the two hands was varied across trials. In all groups, performance was least variable when movements were either in phase (0°) or antiphase (180° phase shifted) relative to other nonharmonic phase relations. Because vision was used in this task, Tuller and Kelso concluded that absence of the corpus callosum does not affect visuomotor coordination of the hands. Notably, because there were no explicit spatial demands, the task they employed focused primarily on temporal properties.

Based on Tuller and Kelso, 1989, my colleagues and I had no reason to suspect that temporal coupling would be eliminated after callosotomy. We therefore hypothesized that temporal coupling would be maintained on a version of a continuous drawing task, even though spatial coupling was predicted to be eliminated. Callosotomy patients were asked to draw linear trajectories with each hand in a continuous fashion. The lines were to be drawn either in the same orientation (both horizontal or both vertical) or in an orthogonal orientation (one vertical and the other horizontal). As in the experiment using discrete shapes described above, stimuli were lateralized using a brief duration. In this case, the stimuli were single lines. Subjects were instructed to draw continuous repetitions of the visually presented lines at a preferred pace in the orientation indicated. No specific instructions were given about coupling the hands.

Consistent with the primary findings of Tuller and Kelso (1989), temporal coupling of these movements was no different between the callosotomy patients and the control subjects. In fact, participants from both groups tended to begin and end the cycles of movements of both hands within approximately 20 ms of one another. In addition, there was no evidence of spatial coupling in the trajectories of callosotomy patients, whereas there were severe spatial deviations in the orthogonal trajectories drawn by control subjects. These results led to the inference that the neural mechanisms of spatial and temporal coupling are dissociable. Spatial coupling in the abstract plans for action relies on the corpus callosum. In contrast, temporal coupling of the hands appears not to depend critically on callosal connections (Franz et al., 1996a).

It is possible that temporal coupling, phase locking, or both depend on subcortical circuitry such as the basal ganglia, cerebellum, thalamus, or a combination of these. With respect to the basal ganglia, synchronization could occur between both halves of the basal ganglia, which could result in a coordinated "go" signal to both sides of the cortex (see also Graybiel, 1995). With respect to the cerebellum, coupling between the two sides could be mediated by the cerebellar commissures or the red nucleus. Patients with unilateral cerebellar lesions display a marked increase in timing variance across repetitive cycles of tapping movements by the ipsilesional versus the contralesional hand (Ivry and Keele, 1989), whereas they display a decrease in timing variance in the impaired hand on bimanual tasks, as though movements of the unimpaired hand somehow facilitate performance of the impaired hand (Franz et al., 1996b). It would appear that, although the timing processes themselves may be affected by cerebellar damage, the temporal coupling processes exist outside of the cerebellar circuitry; otherwise, a unilateral lesion might be expected to influence both hands in the same way. Notably, temporal coupling may occur through cerebellar commissures that operate on cerebellar output.

Other possible influences on temporal coupling are the central spinal generators (Grillner, 1985), which may be modulated through cortical and subcortical input (Donchin et al., 1999). If movements consist of a proximal component, coupling between the two sides may be accomplished through contributions of ipsilateral and contralateral projections emanating from the same hemisphere (Gazzaniga and Sperry, 1967).

In summary, results on bimanual coupling tasks in callosotomy patients indicate that spatial coupling in the planning of bimanual actions relies on callosal interactions in the normal brain. Temporal coupling of the limbs appears to rely much less, or not at all, on callosal connections. The next section provides additional evidence that some spatial coupling processes operate on central representations.

Phantom Limbs

Following amputation of a limb, some individuals report experiencing residual sensations of the missing limb. The "phantom limb" phenomenon has been documented since the writings of Descartes (see Corballis, 1991, pp. 6–11). The sensation may range from a light pain to a very vivid sensation of the actual experience of movement, referred to as "phantom limb movement" (Ramachandran and Hirstein, 1998). People with vivid sensation of phantom limb movement often claim that they can elicit the sensation of movement through their own volition. We were interested in whether spatial coupling would occur between an intact limb and a phantom limb.

Franz and Ramachandran (1998) applied an adapted version of the circle-line bimanual task to patients who had one arm amputated, with a stump extending 4–6 inches from the shoulder. We were interested in whether vivid experience of movement associated with a phantom limb would result in bimanual spatial coupling of a form similar to that observed in people with two intact arms. If so, we could conclude that at least one form of residual spatial coupling is a central phenomenon, rather than a result of biomechanics or peripheral sensation.

We asked the amputated patients to draw linear segments in a continuous fashion with the intact arm on a drawing tablet, while performing either a spatially compatible or an orthogonal task with the phantom arm. For the task of the phantom arm, participants were instructed to activate the "arm" in the instructed manner by eliciting the experience of movement. In the parallel (spatially compatible) task, tapping movements of the phantom index finger were to be performed as vividly as possible. These movements were linear-like, just as the line drawing movements of the intact arm. In the orthogonal task, twirling movements of the index finger were to be performed as vividly as possible. This task is similar to the circle-line task that resulted in substantial spatial interference in our previous studies. One can illustrate this form of interference by simply trying the task. If you draw lines with one hand while twirling the index finger of your other hand, you most likely will experience spatial coupling, and neither task will be performed in the instructed manner.

Of note, the insertion of fiber tracts controlling movement of the finger was below the level of the amputation for all participants with a missing arm. Therefore, any residual motor signals through the stump would not be able to directly influence finger movements. Of course, because performance of only the intact arm was directly measurable, comparisons were made on performance of the intact arm across all experimental conditions. The findings from these individuals were clear. An amputee with vivid sensation of phantom limb movement produced spatial coupling in the line drawing tasks when imagined twirling movements were performed by vivid imagery of movement of the phantom. These effects were similar to those observed in control participants with two intact arms during actual bimanual performance. Spatial interference effects of this type were not observed in the direction-compatible parallel tasks performed by either group.

Control participants with single arm amputation but no phantom limb sensation were also tested for imagery effects. When asked to perform the same set of tasks using actual movement of one arm and vivid imagery of the amputated arm, no evidence of spatial interference was observed. That is, vivid imagery without a phenomenal sensation of movement did not produce the degree of spatial coupling that occurred when the sensation of movement was more vivid. This latter finding was verified by asking control participants to perform the same set of tasks using actual movement of one arm combined with vivid imagery of movement of the other. This task also did not produce the degree of spatial coupling demonstrated on the orthogonal task with actual bimanual movements. Notably, there were no apparent differences in mean duration or its standard error across bimanual conditions or between groups. These findings suggest that the phenomenal experience of movement is necessary for spatial coupling to occur.

Given imagery alone did not result in the same degree of spatial interference as the phenomenal experience of movement, it is possible that an efference copy of the movements may mediate spatial coupling effects. Early investigators of visual processes coined the term *efference copy* to refer to a duplicate copy of the motor commands of eye movement sent somewhere else in the brain to be evaluated (von Holst, 1954; Sperry, 1950). Although difficult to directly investigate, it is possible that a form of efference copy of the limb commands may result in spatial coupling effects of the type we observed (Franz and Ramachandran, 1998). Our hope is to investigate this issue further using functional imaging.

Together, the bimanual effects demonstrated in callosotomy patients and in patients with the sensation of phantom limb movement are suggestive of some properties of spatial coupling. First, at least one form of spatial coupling appears to reflect central rather than peripheral influences. Second, because it occurs even when completely different muscle groups are used to perform the tasks, spatial coupling appears to refer to an abstract form of coupling, as opposed to one that is effector specific.

The hypothesis that spatial coupling across the corpus callosum involves abstract, as opposed to muscle-specific, processes gains support from other findings. Direct callosal connections between cortical hand representation areas in the two cerebral hemispheres are believed to be sparse or nonexistent (Weisendanger et al., 1996; for a concise review of relevant studies, see Jakobsen et al., 1994). Perhaps a separate circuit produces coupling between homologous muscles of the distal extremities on both sides of the body. Interoperative recordings of cells in the hand area have demonstrated some evidence of ipsilateral connections from the motor cortex to the index and middle fingers of the hands, in addition to the normally observed contralateral connections (Goldring and Ratcheson, 1972). With respect to coupling in volitional movements, studies on tapping have revealed evidence of coupling between the same fingers of the two hands (Rabbitt and Vyas, 1970). The next subsection explores a neural process that results in homologous finger coupling which appears to be distinct from the callosal processes that result in abstract spatial coupling.

Congenital Mirroring

Suppose a person had an innate neural "wiring" of the hands that resulted in a complete coupling of movements, in apparent contrast to the spatial uncoupling observed in callosotomy patients? There do exist people having congenital mirror movements in their hands and fingers. With each volitional movement of the distal extremities, there is a mirror movement of the respective muscles on the opposite side. Thus volitional movements of the right index finger also result in precisely mirrored left index finger movements, although the mirror movements tend to occur with smaller amplitude than the volitional movements. Although there is some debate as to the cause of this mirroring; one account is that people with congenital mirroring have abnormally dense ipsilateral projections from the brain to the spinal cord that transmit a motor signal not only to the hand contralateral to the stimulated hemisphere (as in normal movement), but also to the hand ipsilateral to the stimulated hemisphere.

Some direct ipsilateral control of the distal extremities appears to be present in the normal population, which may in part account for the difficulties beginning musicians have in producing different sequences of finger movements with their two hands. Moreover, because postures of the distal extremities can be mimicked following lateralized visual presentation to the cerebral hemisphere ipsilateral to the responding hand in callosotomy patients (Trope et al., 1987), it is possible that redundant pathways become active following the surgical procedure.

The extreme form of homologous muscle coupling observed in people with congenital mirroring appears to be abnormal. Cohen and colleagues

(1991) applied transmagnetic stimulation to the hand representation area of one motor cortex of people with normal movement and people with congenital mirror movement. The stimulation in normal controls resulted in localized muscle activation in the hand contralateral to the stimulus. The same stimulation applied to individuals with congenital mirroring resulted in muscle activation of the hand contralateral as well as the hand ipsilateral to the stimulus. These responses occurred at approximately equal latency, which suggests that the signals for movement were not transmitted across the corpus callosum. In addition, an early report of a person with congenital mirror movements who suffered stroke to one motor cortex documented a persistence of movement in the hand contralateral to the damage due to stroke (Haerer and Currier, 1966). These findings suggest that the mirror movements result from extra ipsilateral corticospinal projections emanating from the undamaged hemisphere.

I have had the good fortune of being introduced to a family six of whose members have congenital mirror movements: a father, his two sons, the father's sister, and her son and daughter. Tracing the family tree suggests that the mutation is autosomal dominant. There are no other known neurological disorders associated with this form of congenital mirroring. Moreover, certain tests rule out the possibility that the mirror coupling is due to fusion at the spinal level (a cause of other types of mirroring). Since meeting them, I have met yet another, unrelated family with the same disorder, living across the world in another country. Both families are now part of our research program.

Because the mirroring occurs predominantly in the distal extremities, these subjects afford the opportunity to examine the neural circuitry underlying the vast majority of intricate movements involved in bimanual skilled actions unique to humans. It is known that surgical lesions to descending projections on one side of the spinal cord in primates initially result in paralysis of the limb on that side. Gradual recovery of function is eventually observed in the proximal muscles of the limbs, presumably due to bilateral innervation from interneurons in the ventromedial zone of the spinal cord, although recovery is limited in the distal extremities innervated by contralateral projections whose spinal terminals are not coupled via spinal interneurons (Lawrence and Hopkins, 1976; Tower, 1940).

Figure 9.2 depicts a simple schematic of three types of descending pathways. The normally observed contralateral projections to distal extremities are labeled "contralateral C.S. [corticospinal] tracts." Also shown are

corpus callosum

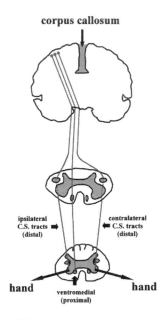

ipsilateral
C.S. tracts ➡
(distal)

contralateral
⬅ C.S. tracts
(distal)

hand   **hand**

ventromedial
(proximal)

Figure 9.2
Schematic diagram of proposed homologous finger coupling process distinct from
the abstract coupling of the corpus callosum. Three descending projections are
shown. The contralateral and ipsilateral projections to the distal extremities are
shown as one possible mechanism of muscle coupling (proposed to be active in
congenital mirroring). The ventromedial projections innervate interneurons at the
spinal level, enabling for bilateral control of proximal muscles. Note that, though
distal projections do not innervate spinal interneurons, distal coupling may occur
due to a common origin. C.S., corticospinal.

the ventromedial pathways that project ipsilaterally to the spinal cord,
where they connect to spinal interneurons, which are known to innervate
proximal muscles bilaterally (Porter and Lemon, 1991). In addition, a pathway labeled "ipsilateral C.S. [corticospinal] tracts" illustrates the proposed
uncrossed projections to distal extremities. Because these proposed projections innervate the same distal extremities as those that are crossed, the
pathways are drawn with the same spinal sites of termination as the crossed
pathways. Note that the diagram shows projections from only one side of
the brain, although they project from both.

In our initial investigations, my colleagues and I asked people with
congenital mirroring to draw circles with one hand and lines with the other,
as in our studies on abstract spatial coupling. Provided the proximal muscles are used to perform the tasks, these individuals produce patterns of be-

havior that are neither better nor worse than those of control subjects, although they are not able to even begin to perform the bimanual task of twirling the finger of one hand and tapping the finger of the other. Mirror coupling of the muscles is so severe that sustained cocontraction tends to occur. Clearly, the processes that result in forms of abstract coupling appear to be intact (corpus callosum), and the mirror coupling produces an additional source of bimanual interaction in movements of the distal extremities. Through their normal compensatory behaviors, these individuals must work to inhibit the unwanted movements.

Interestingly, the corticospinal tract that transmits motor signals to muscles of the distal extremities is a circuitry most phylogenetically recent neural in humans. This circuitry is unique to primates; its density of projections increases throughout phylogeny from monkeys to chimpanzees to humans (Porter and Lemon, 1993, p. 94). The extra density in the human over other species points to neural mechanisms that may have facilitated the emergence of bimanual skills.

Subjects with congenital mirror movements show a remarkable ability to compensate for the mirroring through deliberate control of their actions. For example, the eldest son of one of the families being tested has learned to ride a motorcycle. This skill requires that the fingers of one hand control the throttle at the same time that fingers of the other hand produce an entirely different sequence of actions to control the brake. He would have to be adept at this task, given the cost associated with error. Another member of the same family has taught himself to play a twelve-string guitar marvelously. Is this evidence of extraordinary levels of expertise? One is led to wonder whether, just as advanced forms of compensation may be examples of perturbations in human evolution, so too may deficits. These issues form the basis of ongoing research in our laboratory. One aspect of these investigations is to consider how skilled bimanual actions rely on higher-order representations.

9.3 Representation of Cooperative Bimanual Actions

The aforementioned tasks employed procedures in which a specific task is assigned to each hand, and the processes of coupling between the hands are studied. In this sense, there exist two tasks—one for each hand. Bimanual studies have demonstrated that at least two forms of coupling occur in dual-task procedures of this type: One involves spatial coupling, and the other, temporal coupling. Spatial coupling comes in at least two forms—coupling of direction and coupling of amplitude—both of which appear to rely on the corpus callosum.

This section considers situations in which the two hands cooperate to perform a unified task, such as opening a jar or tying shoes. Little is known about the neural processes underlying these types of bimanual skills and how they are represented in the brain. Interestingly, it may be the case that the task itself defines the binding properties of such bimanual actions.[2]

Effects of Callosotomy on Novel versus Well-Learned Tasks

Given that abstract forms of spatial coupling between the hands appear to rely on interactions provided by callosal connections, it is astonishing that callosotomy patients are so capable of performing coordinated actions, as noted by Zaidel and Sperry (1977) in their comprehensive study of a large group of patients with full or partial callosotomy tested at least five years after surgery. These and other investigators (e.g., Preilowski, 1972) have noted, in particular, the importance of vision in the learning of bimanual actions. Mark and Sperry (1968) examined the performance of split-brain monkeys in a task of retrieving a food pellet by pushing it with one hand through a hole, and catching it with the other. There was some evidence that the monkeys' performance, after extensive practice on this task using vision, was not completely impaired, in some cases, even without vision. Little is known, however, about the storage of already-learned bimanual skills in humans, who have the capacity to utilize symbolic codes for actions (see also Geffen et al., 1994).

In our research, my colleagues and I had the opportunity to test a patient on novel and well-learned bimanual tasks just following callosotomy surgery. During an initial visit to this patient following her recovery from surgery, we observed that she was able to tie her shoes, rather spontaneously, without the use of vision. Indeed, Zaidel and Sperry (1977) reported that a buttoning task performed by a callosotomy patient in full vision took approximately 150% longer than the same task performed by controls, which suggests that vision may actually slow an already-learned task that otherwise might be performed relatively automatically. The patient we observed appeared able to tie her shoes virtually automatically when no vision was used. This observation and helpful comments offered by the patient have led to a series of studies in which we are examining well-learned and novel bimanual actions both with and without vision. A clear result emerged from an initial investigation in this series of experiments.

Two callosotomy patients and a small group of control participants were asked to pantomime certain movements in response to oral commands, while blindfolded. The commands were worded in the form "Please show me how you would . . . ," and the command was completed either by a phrase describing a task requiring one hand ("Reach for a cup"), or a bimanual action ("Peel an orange"). In this study, objects were not shown. Subjects were free to pantomime single-hand actions with whichever hand they preferred (so that apraxia would not be a limiting factor). Given that both hemispheres comprehend speech input, instructions were presented aloud (Gazzaniga and Sperry, 1967). Subjects were queried afterward about the extent of their experience on each task, and family members were consulted to verify these answers when necessary. Results of this study showed a clear difference in the latency to respond and accuracy in performance on well-learned tasks versus tasks never learned before the surgery. Performance on novel tasks was much less accurate than on well-learned tasks in the patients but not in the controls. Similarly, one of the patients produced an increased latency to respond on novel versus well-learned tasks, whereas the second patient responded quickly but incorrectly on novel bimanual tasks. There were no differences in spatial accuracy or response latency on well-learned tasks between patients and controls (Franz et al., 2000).

These findings suggest that well-learned cooperative actions remain intact following callosotomy in humans, and can be performed even without the guidance of vision. Consistent with Zaidel and Sperry, 1977, unfamiliar bimanual actions could not be performed without the aid of vision. One model for these findings is that well-learned tasks are represented in areas of the brain directly accessible to the motor systems of both cerebral hemispheres.

Because verbal codes were used in our study, it seems reasonable to suggest that well-learned behaviors become stored in action codes that no longer require the on-line cross-matching of perceptual information that is necessary during the processes of learning (Franz et al., 2000). Evidence from functional magnetic resonance imaging (fMRI) is consistent with this claim. For example, Karni and colleagues (1995) showed a decrease in activation in the prefrontal cortex in subjects learning a complex motor task. Shadmehr and Holcomb (1997) have shown shifts in neural activation from prefrontal cortical areas to premotor, posterior parietal, and cerebellar areas in subjects after only hours of practice on a motor task.

Synchronous activity across neurons in the striate cortex of cats has been demonstrated during what appears to be binding processes in visual perception (Engel et al., 1991; Gray et al., 1989, 1992). Synchronous activity across visual areas of both cerebral hemispheres, followed by the elimination of interhemispheric synchrony with callosal section, has also been demonstrated in cats (Engel et al., 1991). Based on such findings, it is reasonable to suggest that a similar form of synchronous activity may occur across the corpus callosum in humans during the learning of bimanual tasks.

Andres and colleagues (1999) examined learning-related changes in the coherence of neural activity across sensorimotor systems of the cortex during a bimanual task. They recorded scalp activity using surface electrodes during performance of an 8-key sequence. The sequence was first overlearned in unimanual blocks of trials, with each hand trained separately. The task was then tested under bimanual conditions in which overlearned sequences of the left and right hands were combined so that the key presses alternated to form a 16-key bimanual sequence. The highest coherence between left and right cerebral cortices occurred during bimanual learning. This coupling was higher than in unimanual control trials. After bimanual performance became stable through practice, the level of coherence returned to that observed in unimanual control trials. This evidence strongly suggests that synchronous activity across the corpus callosum occurs with learning of a cooperative bimanual task. After the task is well learned, synchronous activity is reduced.

Given that the motor cortices of both hemispheres must be active to project movement signals to the two hands, how are well-learned cooperative bimanual tasks accessed by both cerebral hemispheres? One possibility is that one hemisphere controls both hands, even if the movements involve the distal extremities to some extent. Accordingly, the codes for action may reside in one hemisphere (probably the left), and movement commands would project from that hemisphere to both the contralateral and ipsilateral hands (Gazzaniga and Sperry, 1967). A second possibility is that action codes of the well-learned bimanual task are stored in subcortical loci, namely, the cerebellum or basal ganglia. These codes would then be accessed by both cerebral hemispheres, each of which channels the appropriate movement commands to the hand it controls. This possibility would be difficult to differentiate from one in which the two cerebral hemispheres each contain action codes of the bimanual task.

Evidence on the functional role of the supplementary motor area (SMA) in bimanual actions may be interpreted as consistent with the hypothesis that duplicate codes become mirrored in the two hemispheres during learning. Early studies on the SMA indicated that this structure is bilaterally organized (Travis, 1955) and connections between the two sides are "callosal" (DeVito and Smith, 1959). Investigating the role of the SMA in an adapted version of the task in Mark and Sperry, 1968, Brinkman (1984) reported that small unilateral SMA lesions produced minor and transient effects on bimanual performance, whereas larger lesions extending into more anterior regions produced an abnormal form of mirror movements during a bimanual task. Specifically, monkeys were trained to obtain a small food reward by pressing the food pellet through a hole in an upright board with one hand, and catching the pellet with the other. Following unilateral lesions of considerable size, the animals attempted to perform the bimanual task by simultaneously pressing the finger of each hand through the hole. Brinkman attributed this mirroring (not related to the type of congenital mirroring described earlier) to the bilateral projections from the SMA to both sides of the motor cortex. It seems possible that the SMA mediates the duplication of action codes to the other hemisphere via intact callosal projections. Given that the basal ganglia are known to project to the SMA, it is possible that action codes in these subcortical structures (i.e., the striatum) mediate the performance of well-learned bimanual actions in humans (Franz et al., 2000). However, recent investigations have reexamined issues related to SMA function in the bimanual performance of monkeys, suggesting that earlier findings may have been a result of compensatory processes (for a thorough study, see Kazennikov, 1998). More evidence of SMA involvement is discussed below.

Egocentric versus Allocentric Influences and the Acallosal Brain

Preilowski (1972) examined performance of patients with anterior callosal section on a bimanual task that required turning a left-hand held knob to control vertical movement of a cursor and a right handheld knob to control horizontal movement of the same cursor. Production of linear movements along a perfect diagonal (45° orientation) required left- and right-hand knob turns at the same rate. Performance of patients revealed a larger degree of spatial deviation for lines slanted more vertically than horizontally with respect to the 45° diagonal. To account for these effects, the investigators suggested that the right-hand (left-hemisphere) contribution is more difficult to inhibit than the left-hand (right-hemisphere) contribution. Thus, there was an alleged left-hemisphere dominance in performing the bimanual task.

My colleagues and I have begun to explore possible hemisphere asymmetries in spatial control on bimanual tasks when instructions are not lateralized. One of our primary issues of interest concerns how the brain organizes bimanual actions into the separate requirements of each hand. We began to address this issue using a drawing task in which the precise assignment to each hand was unspecified. This idea will be described more thoroughly below. First, I will introduce under group of participants who have graciously volunteered to participate in our studies.

When testing callosotomy patients, one cannot help but wonder whether similar behaviors would be observed in people born without a corpus callosum. It seems reasonable to assume that vast forms of neural reorganization may be apparent in them. I recently had the good fortune of being introduced to a family consisting of three females with callosal agenesis. All three are able to run around and kick a ball, throw and catch, carry on normal conversations, and perform the other routine daily activities that most people do. Watching the remarkable ability of these individuals to perform these actions normally, or at least apparently so, one wonders how their brains have compensated for the lack of interhemispheric connections.

In our preliminary studies, my colleagues and I found that all three individuals from this family demonstrated a right-hemisphere dominance in their motor actions, as revealed by standardized tests in which stimuli were presented to both hemispheres simultaneously and errors in responding were recorded. In right-handed callosotomy patients, such tests often reveal evidence of extinction of the stimulus presented to the right hemisphere, indicating a left-hemisphere dominance. Similar (and other) tests performed on our callosal agenesis subjects revealed just the opposite— a right-hemisphere dominance for motor actions. This finding led us to begin a set of studies on bimanual processes in the absence of a corpus callosum in two groups of subjects with opposite cerebral dominance: callosotomy participants with left-hemisphere dominance, and callosal agenesis participants with right-hemisphere dominance.[3]

Our initial experimentation has focused on task selection properties in bimanual actions. Our primary interest is in the way bimanual actions are organized so that each hand is instructed to perform its respective action, especially in tasks that pose more than one possible performance solution. Do there exist asymmetries in control that result in one cerebral hemisphere performing the role of arbiter? If so, do the two hemispheres show biases in the types of information they predominantly process? In our initial investigations of these issues, we chose the task of bimanual circle drawing, a task well studied in neurologically normal individuals, and one used to quantify phase differences between the hands under different movement conditions (Carson et al., 1997; Semjen et al., 1995; Stucchi and Viviani, 1993; Swinnen et al., 1997).

When drawing circles with both hands, there are four different performance solutions that fit into a classification scheme consisting of two basic coordination modes: The first is referred to as "mirror symmetrical" because the two hands draw circles in a mirror-symmetrical fashion with respect to the body midline; and the second, as "parallel" because the two hands draw circles in the same direction with respect to external space. According to Swinnen and colleagues (1997), these two general categories of movement have been used to illustrate, respectively, egocentric and allocentric processing. *Egocentric* refers to movements that occur with respect to a body coordinate frame. Mirror-symmetrical circle drawing tends to be characterized as "egocentric" because the movements do not rely on external information, but only the relative position of the two hands with respect to the body. In contrast, *allocentric* refers to parallel movements, given the two hands must move in the same direction with respect to external space.

To give each hemisphere an equal chance of taking control, rather than lateralizing input, my colleagues and I orally instructed participants. With oral information, both cerebral hemispheres have access to the instructions. People were simply instructed to draw circles with both hands, and data were recorded using digitizer tablets (see figure 9.3). We first thoroughly examined performance of a large group of right-handed participants with intact corpus callosi and no known neurological problems. We recorded kinematics of the circle trajectories, in addition to two other forms of information. The first was to record the probability of selecting the mirror versus parallel coordination mode. We could then compute the conditional probability of selecting either of the two direction modes, given each

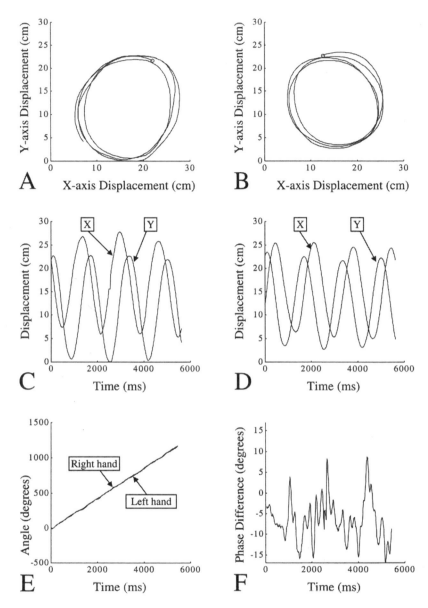

Figure 9.3
Kinematic data in a bimanual symmetrical circle task. (A,B) Displacement data (x-axis versus y-axis) for the left and right hands, respectively. (C,D) Displacement data for each dimension separately for each hand. (E) Accumulated angular distance across time during the trial, for both hands (closely time locked). (F) Instantaneous differences in phase between the two hands through time. Note that the average phase difference is negative, showing that mirror-symmetrical tasks are usually performed with a right-hand lead, and suggesting a left-hemisphere organization.

choice of coordination mode. The second variable was whether one hand tended to lead the other, and if so, which one. The purpose of this second manipulation was to access the degree to which the choice of lead hand was related to the choice of coordination mode.

Our control participants demonstrated an overwhelming bias to select the mirror-symmetrical over the parallel mode (approximately 90% chose the mirror-symmetrical mode). When subsequently instructed to perform the less-chosen parallel mode, approximately half of the control participants chose the clockwise direction, and half chose the counterclockwise mode. Interestingly, clockwise parallel drawing was characterized by a right-hand lead in approximately 80% of the trials, whereas counterclockwise parallel drawing was characterized by a left-hand lead in approximately 80% of the trials.

We applied identical procedures to callosotomy and callosal agenesis participants, with the goal of examining how different cerebral dominance would influence task selection. We were surprised to find that the two groups spontaneously selected different coordination modes. Callosotomy participants chose to draw mirror symmetrical movements, and were unable to draw in the parallel mode without the use of vision. In contrast, callosal agenesis participants selected the parallel mode (counterclockwise), and were unable to draw in the mirror-symmetrical mode without the use of vision. One inference of these findings is that the corpus callosum provides for the flexible allocation of dominance, given that neither group could perform one category of tasks (Franz, 2000a, 2000b; Franz et al., forthcoming).

These findings are also suggestive of biases in the type of spatial information predominantly processed in each cerebral hemisphere. Note that the callosotomy patients with left-hemisphere dominance for motor actions performed only the mirror-symmetrical task. Conversely, the right-hemisphere-dominant acallosal participants performed only the parallel task. Although speculative at this time, our findings may link these two types of the processing to different cerebral hemispheres. Accordingly, in the normal brain, the corpus callosum allows for flexible allocation of dominance to either hemisphere, depending on task demands. It is possible that for this reason, the left hemisphere is usually the dominant hemisphere in speech output. Speech, like mirror-symmetrical movements, requires precise processing of the relative relations among articulators. In contrast, the right hemisphere tends to be more facile at processes related to information from outside of the organism. Of course, because these tentative conclusions are based purely on performance of a bimanual task (Franz, 2000a, 2000b), they remain subject to rigorous experimental testing.

Recent neurophysiological, neuropsychological, and functional imaging evidence indicates that some neurons respond to bimanual related activity. In a single-unit study, Tanji and colleagues (1988) demonstrated changes in neural response patterns of SMA neurons when comparing bimanual to unimanual performance on a task requiring finger flexion movements in monkeys. Donchin and colleagues (1998) recorded neuronal responses of the supplementary motor area (SMA) and primary motor cortex (M1) in homologous sites of the two hemispheres during a bimanual task performed by rhesus monkeys. The task consisted of moving two arm manipulanda to achieve target locations with both arms, which would involve proximal as well as distal muscle contributions. The locations required movements either in the same direction (leftward or rightward) or in mirror-symmetrical directions (one to the left and the other to the right). Movements of the two arms were to be performed simultaneously. Donchin and colleagues presented data of both SMA and M1 neurons firing vigorously for bimanual movements. These findings indicate that both cortical areas contain bimanually sensitive neurons, at least for movements involving some proximal contribution. In a compelling demonstration presented by Donchin and colleagues, a right SMA neuron fired vigorously when both hands moved together in the leftward (parallel) direction, but fired much less vigorously when both moved in the rightward direction, and virtually not at all when the two hands moved in mirror-symmetrical directions. This demonstration is consistent with our own claim that there may be a hemispheric dominance in the organization of bimanual tasks, particularly with respect to mirror-symmetrical versus parallel bimanual movements.

Sadato and colleagues (1997) recorded cerebral blood flow during unimanual and bimanual sequences of finger movements in right-handed subjects. Bimanual movements consisted either of mirror-symmetrical sequences of the two hands, in which homologous fingers moved together, or of parallel sequences in which nonhomologous fingers moved together. These investigators found that both types of bimanual tasks activated areas of the parietal lobe, sensorimotor, and premotor areas, and subcorticol structures of the cerebellum, putamen, and thalamus bilaterally. In addition, the dorsal premotor area and the supplementary motor area of the right hemisphere demonstrated a significantly higher level of activation in parallel compared to mirror-symmetrical tasks. These findings are consistent with our thesis that the right hemisphere plays a dominant role in the organization of parallel movements and the left hemisphere plays a dominant role in the organization of mirror-symmetrical movements.

Other compelling evidence consistent with the proposal of hemispheric asymmetries in the organization of mirror-symmetrical and parallel bimanual movements comes from neurological patient studies. Chan and Ross (1988) reported a patient with a right-hemisphere ischemic infarction that involved a large region of the right hemisphere including anterior cingulate, the medial prefrontal region, and the SMA. This patient presented an inability to perform bimanual tasks that required nonmirror movements, although he was much less impaired in the performance of mirror-symmetrical movements.

In our ongoing studies, my colleagues and I are investigating the properties of reorganization that may influence representation of bimanual actions in people with callosal agenesis. It is not clear whether the right hemisphere dominance we observed in our small group of these participants reflects reorganization. It also remains to be determined whether the hemispheric asymmetries we observed between the two groups of acallosal participants reflect differences in the way space is represented in the two hemispheres (egocentric versus allocentric).

9.4 Conclusions

It seems clear that the representation of bimanual actions can be studied at many levels of the cognitive and motor systems. The hands and fingers are represented in motor representation areas of each cerebral hemisphere, among other areas in the brain. Callosal connections appear to produce abstract forms of spatial coupling between tasks that are lateralized to separate hands (i.e., separate cerebral hemispheres). If a bimanual task is merely assigned to the performer, but contributions of the two hands are not specified as distinct tasks, the brain must organize which action goes with which hand. It appears that higher-order forms of spatial representation may influence this organization, and the intact corpus callosum may enable flexible allocation of cerebral dominance. When cooperative bimanual tasks of the two hands become well learned, the unitary task may become represented in a different form than in the learning stages. Our most recent work examines the way conceptual representations may be used to unify separate tasks of the two hands. The use of such conceptual representations during performance may allow for a reduction in the interference that would otherwise occur in the dual-task situation. This may be one example of how a dual-task becomes a single task (Franz et al., 2001).

Although we are far from understanding either how the human brain manufactures tools or how representations occur there, the representation of bimanual actions may provide a valuable window on the emerging picture of our evolution.

Notes

1. I wish to acknowledge that all participants in these and all our experiments are volunteers who receive no material benefits of any kind. Their generosity and willingness to educate others, while remaining completely anonymous, is indeed a rare find.

2. I borrowed this idea from Daniel Gopher during a discussion at the Attention and Performance XIX meeting in Kloster Irsee, Germany in July 2000.

3. We were surprised to find evidence of right-hemisphere dominance in these individuals. I am not of course suggesting that this is a hallmark of callosal agenesis because any number of factors may be contributing; indeed, our initial findings may provide more clues about cerebral dominance than they do about callosal agenesis per se.

References

Andres, F. G., Mima, T., Schulman, E., Dichgans, J., Hallett, M., and Gerloff, C. (1999). Functional coupling of human cortical sensorimotor areas during bimanual skill acquisition. *Brain* 122: 855–870.

Bernstein, N. (1967). *The Coordination and Regulation of Movements*. Oxford: Pergamon Press.

Berridge, K. C., and Whishaw, I. Q. (1992). Cortex, striatum, and cerebellum: Control of serial order in a grooming sequence. *Exp. Brain Res.* 90: 275–290.

Brinkman, C. (1984). Supplementary motor area of the monkey's cerebral cortex: Short- and long-term unilateral ablation and the effects of subsequent callosal section. *J. Neurosci.* 4: 918–929.

Brinkman, J., and Kuypers, H. G. J. M. (1973). Cerebral control of contralateral and ipsilateral arm, hand, and finger movements in the split-brain monkey. *Brain* 96: 633–674.

Carson, R. G., Thomas, J., Summers, J. J., Walters, M. R., and Semjen, A. (1997). The dynamics of bimanual circle drawing. *Q. J. Exp. Psychol.* 50A(3): 664–683.

Chan, J-L., and Ross, E. D. (1998). Left-handed mirror writing following right anterior cerebral artery infarction: Evidence for nonmirror transformation of motor programs by right supplementary motor area. *Neurology* 38: 59–63.

Chan, T., and Chan, K. (1995). Effect of frequency ratio and environmental information on spatial coupling: A study of attention. *Ecol. Psychol.* 7: 125–144.

Cohen, L. (1971). Synchronous bimanual movements performed by homologous and non-homologous muscles. *Percep. Mot. Skills* 32: 639–644.

Cohen, L. G., Meer, I., Tarka, S., Bierner, S., Leiderman, D. B., Dubinsky, R. M., et al. (1991). Congenital mirror movements. *Brain* 114: 381–403.

Corballis, M. C. (1991). *The Lopsided Ape: Evolution of the Generative Mind.* New York: Oxford University Press.

DeVito, J. L., and Smith, O. A., Jr. (1959). Projections from the mesial frontal cortex (supplementary motor area) to the cerebral hemispheres and brainstem of the *Macaca mulatta. J. Comp. Neurol.* 111: 261–277.

Dimond, S. J., Scammell, R. E., Brouwers, E. Y. M., and Weeks, R. (1977). Functions of the centre section (trunk) of the corpus callosum in man. *Brain* 100: 543–562.

Donchin, O., Gribova, A., Steinberg, O., Bergman, H., and Vaadia, E. (1998). Primary motor cortex is involved in bimanual coordination. *Nature* 395: 274–277.

Donchin, O., de Oliveira, S. C., and Vaadia, E. (1999). Who tells one hand what the other is doing: The neurophysiology of bimanual movements. *Neuron* 23: 15–18.

Eccles, J. C. (1989). *Evolution of the Brain: Creation of the Self.* London: Routledge.

Eliassen, J., Baynes, K., and Gazzaniga, M. S. (1999). Direction information coordinated via the posterior third of the corpus callosum during bimanual movements. *Exp. Brain Res.* 128: 573–577.

Engel, A. K., Konig, P., Kreiter, K., and Singer, W. (1991). Interhemispheric synchronization of oscillatory neuronal responses in cat visual cortex. *Science* 252: 1177–1179.

Fitts, P. M. (1954). The information capacity of the human motor system in controlling the amplitude of movement. *J. Exp. Psychol.* 47: 381–391.

Fitts, P. M., and Peterson, J. R. (1964). Information capacity of discrete motor responses. *J. Exp. Psychol.* 67: 103-112.

Franz, E. A. (1997). Spatial coupling in the coordination of complex actions. *Q. J. Exp. Psychol.* 50A: 684–704.

Franz, E. A. (2000a). A double dissociation in the cerebral dominance of bimanual control: Callosotomy versus callosal agenesis. Paper presented at the international meeting of Attention and Performance XIX, Kloster Irsee, Germany. July.

Franz, E. A. (2000b). A double dissociation between callosal agenesis and callosotomy participants on a bimanual task. Paper presented at the Forum for European Neurosciences, Brighton, England. July.

Franz, E. A., and Ramachandran, V. S. (1998). Bimanual coupling in amputees with phantom limbs. *Nat. Neurosci.* 1: 443-444.

Franz, E. A., Zelaznik, H. N., and McCabe, G. (1991). Spatial topological constraints in a bimanual task. *Acta Psychol.* 77: 137–151.

Franz, E. A., Eliassen, J., Ivry, R. B., and Gazzaniga, M. S. (1996a). Dissociation of spatial and temporal coupling in the bimanual movements of callosotomy patients. *Psychol. Sci.* 7: 306–310.

Franz, E. A., Ivry, R. B., and Helmuth, L. L. (1996b). Reduced timing variability in patients with unilateral cerebellar lesions during bimanual movements. *J. Cogn. Neurosci.* 8: 107–118.

Franz, E. A., Waldie, K. E., and Smith, M. J. (2000). The effect of callosotomy on novel versus familiar bimanual actions: A neural dissociation between controlled and automatic processes? *Psychol. Sci.* 11: 82–85.

Franz, E. A., Zelaznik, H. N., Swinnen, S. P., and Walter, C. (2001). Spatial conceptual influences on the coordination of bimanual actions: When a dual task becomes a single task. *J. Mot. Behav.* 33: 103–112.

Franz, E. A., Rowse, A., and Finlay, D. (forthcoming). Flexible control properties of the corpus callosum: Callosal agenesis and callosotomy.

Gazzaniga, M. S., and Sperry, R. W. (1967). Language after section of the cerebral commissures. *Brain* 90: 131-148.

Gazzaniga, M. S., Bogen, J. E., and Sperry, R. W. (1965). Observations on visual perception after disconnexion of the cerebral hemispheres in man. *Brain* 88: 221–236.

Geffen, G. M., Jones, D. L., and Geffen, L. B. (1994). Interhemispheric control of manual motor activity. *Behav. Brain Res.* 64: 131–140.

Georgopoulos, A. P., Kalaska, J. F., Caminiti, R., and Massey, J. T. (1982). On the relations between the direction of two-dimensional arm movements and cell discharge in primate motor cortex. *J. Neurosci.* 2: 1527–1537.

Goldring, S., and Ratcheson, R. (1972). Human motor cortex: Sensory input data from single neuron recordings. *Science* 175: 1493–1495.

Gray, C. M., Konig, P., Engel, A. K., and Singer, W. (1989). Oscillatory responses in cat visual cortex exhibit inter-columnar synchronization which reflects global stimulus properties. *Nature* 338: 334–337.

Gray, C. M., Engel, A. K., Konig, P., and Singer, W. (1992). Synchronization of oscillatory neuronal responses in cat striate cortex: Temporal properties. *Vis. Neurosci.* 8: 337–347.

Graybiel, A. M. (1995). Building action repertoires: Memory and learning functions of the basal ganglia. *Curr. Opin. Neurobiol.* 5: 733–741.

Grillner, S. (1985). Neurobiological bases of rhythmic motor acts in vertebrates. *Science* 228: 143–149.

Haerer, A. F., and Currier, R. D. (1966). Mirror movements. *Neurology* 16: 757–760.

Ivry, R. B., and Keele, S. (1989). Timing functions of the cerebellum. *J. Cogn. Neurosci.* 1: 136–152.

Jagacinski, R. J., Hartzell, E. J., Ward, S., and Bishop, K. (1978). Fitts' law as a function of system dynamics and target uncertainty. *J. Mot. Behav.* 10: 123–131.

Jakobsen, L. S., Servos, P., Goodale, M. A., and Lassonde, M. (1994). Control of proximal and distal components of prehension in callosal agenesis. *Brain* 117: 1107–1113.

Kalaska, J. F., Caminiti, R., and Georgopoulos, A. P. (1983). Cortical mechanisms related to the direction of two-dimensional arm movements: Relations in parietal area 5 and comparison with motor cortex. *Exp. Brain Res.* 51: 247–260.

Karni, A., Meyer, G., Jezzard, P., Adams, M., Turner, R., and Ungerleider, L. G. (1995). Functional MRI evidence for adult motor cortex plasticity during motor skill learning. *Nature* 377: 155–158.

Kazennikov, O., Hyland, B., Wick, U., Perrig, S., Rouiller, E. M., and Weisendanger, M. (1998). Effects of lesions in the mesial frontal cortex on bimanual co-ordination in monkeys. *Neuroscience* 85: 703–716.

Kelso, J. A. S., Southard, D. L., and Goodman, D. (1979). On the coordination of two-handed movements. *J. Exp. Psychol. Hum. Percept. Perform.* 5: 229–238.

Klapp, S. T. (1979). Doing two things at once: The role of temporal compatibility. *Mem. Cognit.* 7: 375–381.

Langolf, G. D., Chaffin, D. B., and Foulke, J. A. (1976). An investigation of Fitts' law using a wide range of movement amplitudes. *J. Mot. Behav.* 8: 113–128.

Lawrence, D. G., and Hopkins D. A. (1976) The development of motor control in the rhesus monkey: Evidence concerning the role of corticomotoneuronal connections. *Brain* 99: 235–254.

Mark, R. F., and Sperry, R. W. (1968). Bimanual coordination in monkeys. *Exp. Neurol.* 21: 92–104.

Marteniuk, R. G., MacKenzie, C. L., and Baba, D. M. (1984). Bimanual movement control: Information processing and interaction effects. *Q. J. Exp. Psychol.* 36A: 335–365.

Peters, M. (1977). Simultaneous performance of two motor activities: The factor of timing. *Neuropsychologia* 15: 461–465.

Peters, M. (1981). Attentional asymmetries during concurrent bimanual performance. *Q. J. Exp. Psychol.* 33A: 95–103.

Porter, R., and Lemon, L. (1993). *Corticospinal Function and Voluntary Movement.* Oxford: Clarendon Press, pp. 84–96.

Preilowski, B. F. B. (1972). Possible contributions of the anterior forebrain commissures to bilateral motor coordination. *Neuropsychologia* 10: 267–277.

Rabbitt, P. M. A., and Vyas, S. M. (1970). An elementary preliminary taxonomy for some error in laboratory choice RT tasks. *Acta Psychol.* 33: 56–76.

Ramachandran, V. S., and Hirstein, W. (1998). The perception of phantom limbs: The D.O. Hebb Lecture. *Brain* 121: 1603–1630.

Sadato, N., Yonekura, Y., Waki, A., Yamada, H., and Ishii, Y. (1997). Role of the supplementary motor area and the right premotor cortex in the coordination of bimanual finger movements. *J. Neurosci.* 17: 9667–9674.

Semjen, A., Summers, J. J., and Cattaert, D. (1995). Hand coordination in bimanual circle drawing. *J. Exp. Psychol. Hum. Percept. Perform.* 21: 1139–1157.

Shadmehr, R., and Holcomb, H. H. (1997). Neural correlates of motor memory consolidation. *Science* 277: 821–825.

Shaffer, L. H. (1981). Performances of Chopin, Bach, and Bartok: Studies in motor programming. *Cogn. Psychol.* 13: 326–376.

Sperry, R. (1950). Neural basis of the optokinetic response produced by visual inversion. *J. Comp. Physiol. Psychol.* 43: 482–489.

Spijkers, W., and Heuer, H. (1995). Structural constraints on the performance of symmetrical bimanual movements with different amplitudes. *Q. J. Exp. Psychol.* 48A: 716–740.

Stucchi, N., and Viviani, P. (1993). Cerebral dominance and asynchrony between bimanual two-dimensional movements. *J. Exp. Psychol. Hum. Percept. Perform.* 19: 1200–1220.

Swinnen, S. P., and Walter, C. B. (1991). Toward a movement dynamics perspective on dual-task performance. *Hum. Factors* 33: 367–387.

Swinnen, S. P., Jardin, K., Meulenbroek, R., Dounskaia, N., and Hofkens-Van Den Brandt, M. (1997). Egocentric and allocentric constraints in the expression of patterns of interlimb coordination. *J. Cogn. Neurosci.* 9: 348–377.

Tanji, J., Okano, K., and Sato, K. C. (1988). Neuronal activity in cortical motor areas related to ipsilateral, contralateral, and bilateral digit movements of the monkey. *J. Neurophysiol.* 60: 325–343.

Tower, S. (1940). Pyramidal lesion in the monkey. *Brain* 63: 36–90.

Travis, A. M. (1955). Neurological deficiencies following supplementary motor area lesions in *Macaca mulatta. Brain* 78: 174–198.

Trope, I., Fishman, B., Gur, R. C., Sussman, N. M., and Gur, R. E. (1987). Contralateral and ipsilateral control of fingers following callosotomy. *Neuropsychologia* 25: 287–291.

Tuller, B., and Kelso, J. A. S. (1989). Environmentally specified patterns of movement coordination in normal and split-brain patients. *Exp. Brain Res.* 75: 306–316.

Turvey, M. T., Rosenblum, L. D., Kugler, P., and Schmidt, R. C. (1986). Fluctuations and phase symmetry in coordinated rhythmical movements. *J. Exp. Psychol. Hum. Percept. Perform.* 12: 564–583.

von Holst, E. (1954). Relations between the central nervous system and the peripheral organs. *Br. J. Anim. Behav.* 2: 89–94.

Weisendanger, M., Rouiler, E. M., Kazenikov, O., and Perrig, S. (1996). Is the supplementary motor area a bilaterally organized system? *Adv. Neurol.* 70: 85–93.

Wyke, M. (1967). Effect of brain lesions on the rapidity of arm movement. *Neurology* 17: 1113–1120.

Yamanishi, J., Kawato, M., and Suzuki, R. (1981). Studies on human finger tapping neural networks by phase transition curves. *Biol. Cybern.* 33: 199–208.

Zaidel, D., and Sperry, R. W. (1977). Some long-term motor effects of cerebral commissurotomy in man. *Neuropsychologia* 15: 193–204.

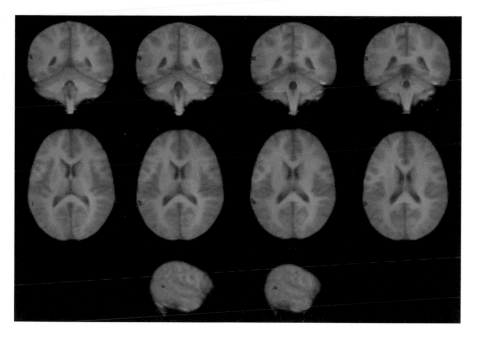

Plate 1

Area (red) in the superior temporal cortex region that seems to be matching a visual description of the action to be imitated with the predicted sensory consequences of a planned imitative action. In this picture the right hemisphere is on the left side. See chapter 4.

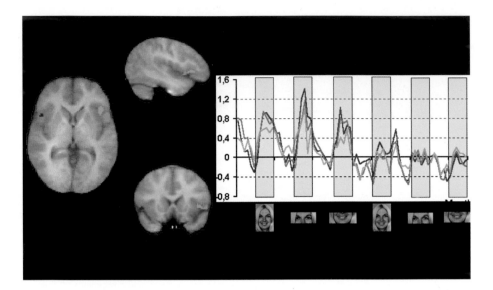

Plate 2
Insula as relay? During imitation of facial emotional expressions, activation occurs in the left frontal operculum (red), in the right frontal operculum (blue), and in the anterior insula (green). Corresponding time series expressed as normalized percent change are shown with corresponding colors. See chapter 4.

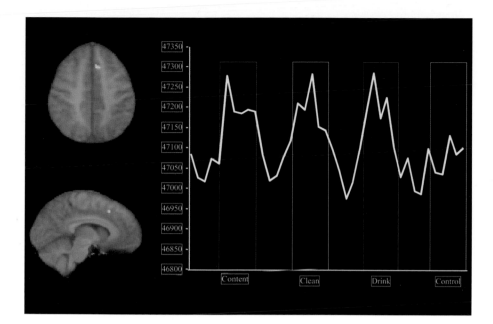

Plate 3

Activity in a caudal area of the anterior cingulate that responds to the presence of the context but not to the explicit request of processing the purpose of the action according to the context. Activity is expressed in raw signal rescaled by the smoothing process. See chapter 4.

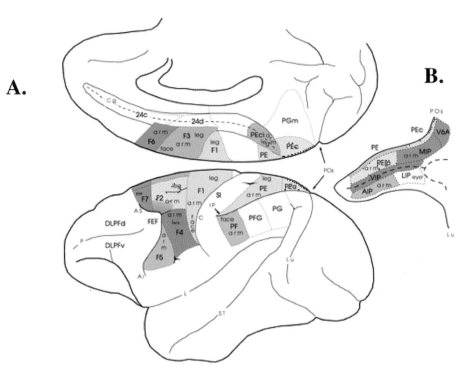

Plate 4
Parietofrontal areas involved in sensorimotor transformations. Parietal and frontal areas that are interconnected are shown in the same colors. Blue denotes areas receiving input from prefrontal cortex. (*A*) Parcellation of the motor, posterior parietal, and cingulate cortices displayed on mesial and lateral surfaces of the monkey brain. (*B*) The intraparietal sulcus unfolded to reveal functionally defined areas. AI, inferior arcuate sulcus; AS, superior arcuate sulcus; C, central sulcus; Cg, cingulate sulcus; DLPFd, dorsolateral prefrontal cortex, dorsal; DLPFv, dorsolateral prefrontal cortex, ventral; L, lateral fissure; Lu, lunate sulcus; P, principal sulcus; Pos, parieto-occipital sulcus; ST, superior temporal sulcus. (Adapted with permission from Rizzolatti and Luppino, 2001.) See chapter 7.

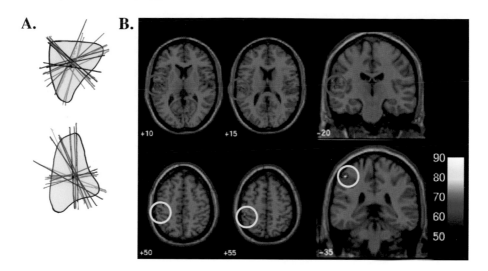

Plate 5

Putative homologue of area AIP of the monkey parietofrontal grasp circuit. (A) Two
of the shapes used in the grasping experiment. Each line represents the opposing
force vectors from two points on the objects' surfaces contacted by the thumb and
forefinger on a given trial. Across four different orientations, subjects consistently
chose grips that caused these opposing forces to cancel through objects' centers
of mass. (B) Approximately 90% of participants showed activation in the anterior
IPs (yellow circles; putative AIP) and secondary somatosensory cortex (blue circles;
SII) during visually guided precision gripping as contrasted with pointing. See
chapter 7.

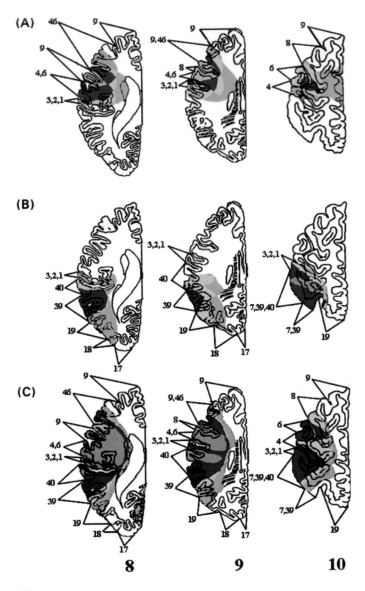

(A)

(B)

(C)

8   **9**   **10**

Plate 6
Lesion overlap in patients with upper-limb apraxia (*A, B,* and *C*) and patients who
are not apraxic (*D, E,* and *F*). Patients are organized according to the location of
their lesions: anterior (*A* and *D*), posterior (*B* and *E*), or both anterior and posterior (*C* and *F*) to the central sulcus. Importantly, for the anterior lesion group with
apraxia there was 100% lesion overlap (yellow) in the middle frontal gyrus (sections
8 and 9). By contrast, there was considerably less overlap in these areas for nonapraxic patients with anterior lesions (*D*). Apraxics with posterior lesions (*B*)
showed maximal overlap (pink) in the parietal areas including the angular and

(D)

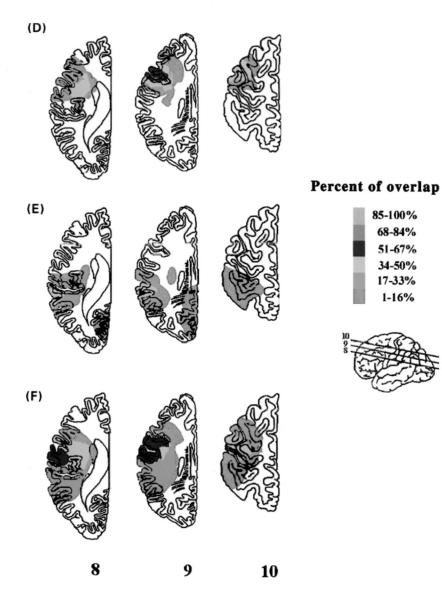

Percent of overlap

	85-100%
	68-84%
	51-67%
	34-50%
	17-33%
	1-16%

(E)

(F)

8   **9**   **10**

Plate 6 (continued)

supramarginal gyri (section 10). Conversely, there was much less overlap (dark blue) in the IPL for nonapraxics with posterior lesions (*E*). Finally, apraxic patients with anterior and posterior lesions (*C*) showed 100% overlap (yellow) in the middle frontal gyrus (section 8), while anterior–posterior lesioned nonapraxics (*F*) showed much less overlap (green) in these regions. Maximal parietal overlap (pink) in the apraxic group was centered in the supramarginal gyrus (section 9), while less overlap (red and green) was observed here in the nonapraxics. (Reprinted with permission from Haaland et al., 2000.) See chapter 7.

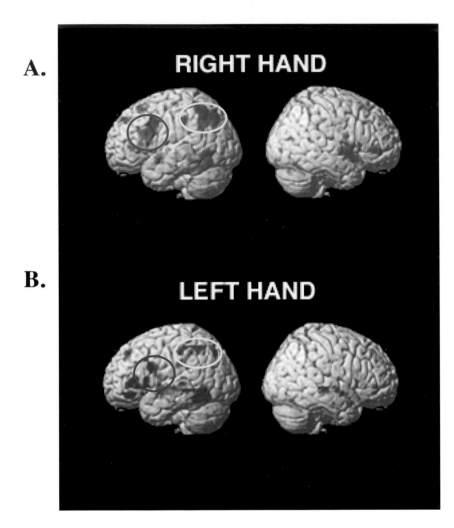

Plate 7
(*A*) Areas involved in preparing tool use gestures for the right hand. Preparing tool use actions is associated with activations in the left IPL (yellow circle) and GFm (blue circle). (*B*) This left lateralized parietofrontal network is also activated when gestures are prepared with the left hand. See chapter 7.

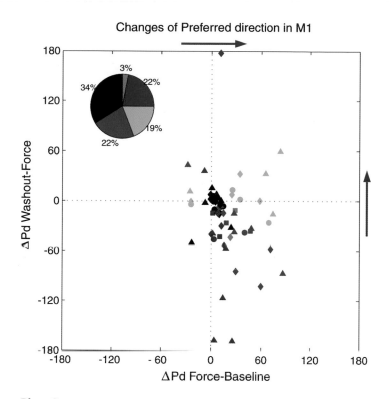

Changes of Preferred direction in M1

Plate 8

Scatter plot of changes in preferred direction (Pd) of M1 neurons. The *x*-axis represents the changes of Pd in the force epoch compared to the baseline. The *y*-axis represents the changes of Pd in the washout compared to the force epoch. For both axes, positive values indicate shifts in the direction of the external force (see red arrows). In the scatter plot, each symbol represents one cell and cells are color-coded according to their classes. Kinematic cells (black) lie close to the origin because their Pd is unchanged across epochs. Dynamic cells (blue) lie on the diagonal through the second and fourth quadrant, because their Pd shifts in one direction in the force epoch (in general, the same direction as the force field) and in the opposite direction in the washout. Memory I cells (green) lie on the *x*-axis; their Pd shifts in the force epoch (in general, in the direction of the external force) and does not shift in the washout. Conversely, memory II cells (red) lie on the *y*-axis; their Pd is unchanged in the force epoch, and shifts in the direction opposite to the previously encountered force field in the washout epoch. "Other cells" (*x-y-z*) are shown in gray. (Reprinted with permission from Li et al., 2001; ©2001 Elsevier Science.) See chapter 11.

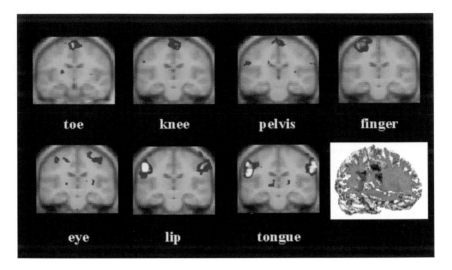

Plate 9
Coronal view of activated areas along the precentral gyrus. Color-coded *p*-values of increased BOLD response for the different motor tasks (labeled by body part) projected on an averaged talairach anatomical background. Results for the grand average of nine subjects. The inset summarizes the individual task activations in a 3D perspective. See chapter 13.

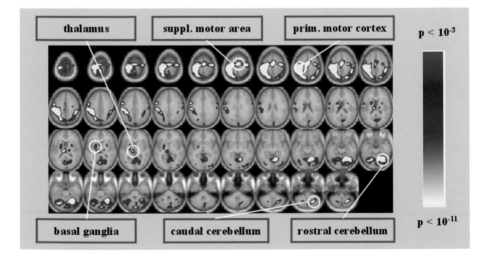

Plate 10
Grand average results for the selective averaging of the right-hand sequential finger exercise. Increased BOLD response in axial view shown by color-coded *p*-values (scale on the right) projected on the anatomical background. Areas of interest are labeled for orientation within a representative slice; right is right to the viewer. See chapter 13.

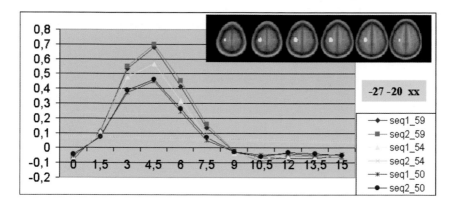

Plate 11

Reconstruction of the BOLD responses for the primary motor cortex with three different talairach coordinates for the z-value (rostral to caudal values 59, 54, and 50). Example for z=54 is shown in the upper left corner. The individual BOLD responses are labeled in the lower right corner, with "seq1" and "seq2" representing sequential finger movements of the right-hand version 1 and version 2, respectively. The y-axis is scaled in percentage of signal change, the x-axis in seconds after stimulus presentation. Because the different sequences showed identical responses, it was reasonable to collapse the results of the study. The different z values did not affect the general shape even though the amplitude varied. See chapter 13.

Plate 12 (overleaf)

Reconstruction of the BOLD responses for eight different areas of interest. Grand average results for right-hand exercise and the BOLD response values during left-hand exercise in the same areas are shown. In the upper left corner are the reconstructed areas of interest in axial view; the right upper corner combines the talairach coordinates and the functional area name with M1, primary motor cortex; SM2, secondary sensorimotor area; PMr, premotor area rostral; PMc, premotor area caudal; THAL, thalamus; BG, basal ganglia; and CEB1 and CEB2, two areas within the cerebellum. The BOLD responses are expressed as percentage signal change values over the time period following the stimulus presentation (in seconds). Although no major differences are notable for the general shape, SM2, BG, CEB1, and CEB2 demonstrate a significant delay of about 1.5 s. See chapter 13.

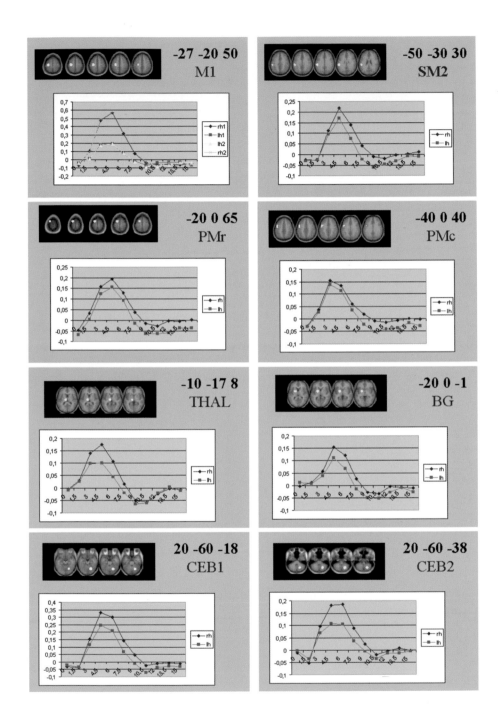

10

Feedback or Feedforward Control: End of a Dichotomy

Michel Desmurget and Scott Grafton

Since the pioneering monograph of Woodworth (1899), the respective contribution of feedforward and feedback processes to movement generation has been a matter of considerable debate. The last century has seen the pendulum swing back and forth repeatedly between two extreme views. Supporters of the feedforward view dominated the field early. They argued that a pattern of muscle activation had to be defined in advance of a movement because the dexterity of the motor system was not dramatically altered when vision was absent and unable to guide an ongoing movement toward a target (Bowditch and Southard, 1880; Woodworth, 1899). Supporters of the feedback view responded quickly to this claim by stressing that vision was not the only source of sensory information and that movement could be guided through proprioceptive feedback. To support their assertion, they provided evidence confirming that monkeys with a deafferented limb were only able to produce erratic movements (Mott and Sherrington, 1895; Lassek, 1953). This result was promptly challenged by two observations showing, first, that monkeys were able to recover relatively normal motor functions within a few weeks provided they were forced to rely exclusively on their deafferented limb (Knapp et al., 1963; Taub and Berman, 1968; Taub, 1976), and second, that delays in sensorimotor loops were too prolonged to allow useful sensory feedback control for fast reaching movements (Hollerbach, 1982). Supporters of the feedback concept fought back, claiming that the ability to generate accurate movements in the absence of any sensory input in no way implied that the motor command was assembled in advance. Their rebuttal originated in the so-called equilibrium point model, which had provided evidence that the pattern of muscle activation could be generated gradually during an ongoing movement in the form of a progressive shift of the equilibrium arm configuration toward the target (Bizzi et al., 1984, 1992; Flanagan et al., 1993; Feldman and Levin, 1995).

Far from concluding the debate, this result provoked a vigorous counter-offensive by supporters of the feedforward view, who pointed out that the equilibrium point hypothesis lacked consistent support, at least for multi-joint movements (for a review, see Desmurget et al., 1998). In other words, although a progressive shift of the equilibrium arm configuration could provide a purely feedback basis for motor control, experimental observations of unrestrained reaching or pointing movements clearly contradicted this idea. This was a strong blow to the feedback view. After almost a century of controversy, then, the feedforward view of motor control prevailed. It provided theoretical underpinnings for most of the studies aimed at understanding how visually directed movements were generated. Its dominant position was further reinforced by the observation that computational models totally ignoring the potential contribution of feedback loops were remarkably successful at capturing the main characteristics of reaching movements, including Fitts's law (Plamondon and Alimi, 1997), the pattern of endpoint errors (Flanders et al., 1992; Vindras et al., 1998; Desmurget et al., 1999a), the typically bell-shaped aspect of velocity profiles (Flash and Hogan, 1985; Uno et al., 1989; Plamondon and Alimi, 1997; Harris and Wolpert, 1998), and the curvature of movement paths (Flash, 1987; Uno et al., 1989; Harris and Wolpert, 1998).

Like the mythical Phoenix, the feedback-feedforward debate has recently risen from its ashes. After two decades of unchallenged stability, the pendulum has swung back, although, this time, it has stopped in a new area somewhere between the feedforward and feedback views. The main aim of this chapter is to delineate this area. Section 10.1 reviews evidence generally presented as establishing the dominant role of feedforward movement control, namely, that accurate movements can be generated in the absence of sensory information and that sensory feedback loops are too slow to allow efficient feedback control during the entire trajectory. Section 10.2 reviews recent evidence showing that on-line control by visual and non-visual information occurs early and smoothly in movement. Section 10.3 provides a framework for understanding the nature of these early corrections; in particular, it shows that feedback mechanisms can rely on much more than sensory inflow, as traditionally thought. Feedback control strategies become viable if the nervous system can infer the instantaneous and future hand location through a "forward model" that integrates efferent and afferent signals to infer, with no delay, the current and upcoming state of the motor system. Section 10.4 shows that the motor command is not generated gradually during the course of the movement on the basis of feedback loops that compare in real time the respective locations of the hand and target. To this end, it provides converging arguments showing that a crude motor plan, subject to subsequent optimization, is assembled before movement onset. Section 10.5 discusses the functional anatomy of movement feedback loops with emphasis on the potential contribution of the posterior parietal cortex and the cerebellum. And section 10.6 summarizes our conclusions.

10.1   Ballistic Reaching Movements: Original Evidence

In computer science, a program describes a fragment of code that is stored on a disk and that specifies a series of actions that are carried out sequentially (Keele, 1968). By analogy, in neuroscience, a motor program defines a series of neural commands that are structured in advance and that unfold sequentially until the completion of the movement (Arbib, 1981). Identifying the existence and the content of a program is quite easy in computer science. All you need to do is examine the source code and launch an executable file. Completion of the executable file without further input demonstrates the existence of the program, although inferring the structure of the source code based on the behavior of an executable file can be difficult. On the other hand, inferring source code from behavior is even more difficult in neuroscience, where the only way to demonstrate the existence of a motor program is to show that all the instructions necessary to bring the hand to the target are available in the system before movement onset. In his now famous monograph, Keele (1968) was the first to translate this premise into a working hypothesis. According to Keele, a movement could be considered as resulting from a motor program if it could be carried out uninfluenced by peripheral feedback. In other words, all you need to prove the existence of a motor program is to show that accurate and structured movements can be performed in the absence of any peripheral information. To support this still widely held hypothesis, four experimental observations are detailed below.

Reaching without Proprioception
Although one might expect the motor behavior of deafferented patients to be consistent, the literature abounds with conflicting observations in both humans and monkeys. The controversy started with the pioneering paper

of Mott and Sherrington (1895, p. 481), who reported that monkeys only produced erratic movements with their numb limb after a unilateral deafferentation: "From the time of performance of the section onwards, the movements of the hand and foot are practically abolished." Although confirmed by subsequent studies (Lassek and Moyer, 1953; Lassek, 1955; Twitchell, 1954), these results were seriously challenged by behavioral observations showing that deafferented animals were able to recover virtually normal motor functions (Munk, 1909; Knapp et al., 1963; Taub and Berman, 1968; Bossom, 1972, 1974; Taub, 1976). In an attempt to reconcile these contradictory results, Knapp and colleagues (1963) showed that motor performance did indeed improve, but only when the animals were forced to use their deafferented limb, and that deafferented monkeys exhibited fewer motor impairments after bilateral than after unilateral rhizotomy.

The main evidence supporting the idea that proprioceptive signals were not critical for movement execution was provided Polit and Bizzi (1979) in a now famous experiment. They trained three monkeys to perform single-joint pointing toward visual targets presented in a dark room. These targets were selected among set of 17 light-emitting diodes (LEDs) distributed every 5° in front of the monkey. They were randomly presented and the animal had to point toward the selected target with an accuracy of about 15°. Following a period of training, intrathecal deafferentation of the arm territory at the dorsal root level (C2–T3) was performed and controlled by a stretch-reflex recording. After recovery from surgery, deafferented monkeys were still able to reach to the targets with sufficient accuracy. When the elbow angle position was unexpectedly modified by transiently loading the arm 150–200 ms before movement onset, neither normal nor deafferented monkeys displayed a significant decrease in movement accuracy. The same was also true when the load was applied during the ongoing elbow movement. From these findings, Polit and Bizzi concluded that joint movements depended mainly on neural patterns specified before movement onset. They also suggested that, through the selection of a muscular equilibrium point, these preprogrammed patterns defined a mechanical attractor that could be reached without knowledge of the initial configuration of the motor apparatus. (We will return to these assertions.)

Generalization of the Polit and Bizzi (1979) experimental results to humans was demonstrated by Kelso and Holt (1980), who required human subjects to reach to a previously learned position with their thumb. A load could be unexpectedly applied during the displacement of the thumb. Results showed that subjects were easily able to perform this task, even when the moving finger was deafferented by applying an inflated strap around the wrist joint. Although this particular result could not be reproduced by Day and Marsden (1982), several observations have since confirmed that deafferented subjects are able to realize a wide range of finger movements with remarkable accuracy (Rothwell et al., 1982; Sanes et al., 1985). Nevertheless, these findings should not be considered a reliable proof that proprioception is not critical for movement control. Indeed, the ability of deafferented subjects to successfully perform simple laboratory tasks frequently obscures their inability to use their hand under real-life conditions, where single-joint movements are the exception. Thus Rothwell and colleagues (1982, p. 515) described a deafferented patient whose "hands were relatively useless to him in daily life . . . despite his success with these laboratory tasks." Likewise, Munk (1909) emphasized that, even if deafferented monkeys were able to recover some impressive level of dexterity, they still performed markedly awkward and unskilled movements when compared to normal monkeys.

If one admits, as suggested by Polit and Bizzi (1979), that it is not necessary to know the state of the motor apparatus to plan accurate movements, then the propensity of deafferented subjects to generate clumsy and ataxic multijoint movements challenges the feedforward view of motor control. On the other hand, Polit and Bizzi's results were never successfully replicated and a vast majority of studies carried out during the past 20 years have shown that estimating the initial state of the motor apparatus has a major influence on the accuracy of movement planning (for a review, see Desmurget et al., 1998). Indeed, evidence supporting this view is even found in Polit and Bizzi, 1979. Although the monkeys trained by these authors were able to compensate for undetected modifications of the arm location in the main experimental condition, they were totally unable to adjust for positional shifts affecting the starting posture of their upper arm: When the center of rotation of the elbow joint was shifted forward, the monkeys were no longer able to reach accurately to the targets. Another line of evidence supporting the idea that defining the initial state of the effector is a necessary step of movement planning was provided by behavioral experiments showing that systematic pointing errors reflect biases in the estimation of the initial hand location. This point was initially identified by Prablanc and colleagues (1979a), who compared the accuracy of visually directed movements performed under two different conditions. In the first, full open loop (FOL) condition, vision of the hand was never allowed. In the second, dynamic open loop (DOL) condition, vision of the hand was allowed only in a static position before movement onset. Results showed that movement accuracy was significantly better in the DOL than in the FOL condition. These data were subsequently reproduced and generalized in several studies (Rossetti et al., 1995; Desmurget et al., 1997; Vindras et al., 1998), which also established that the hand needed to be seen in foveal or perifoveal vision to obtain a significant reduction of the systematic errors. When the arm was seen in the peripheral visual field, the only effect observed was a reduction of variable errors without modification of the mean movement accuracy (Rossetti et al., 1994; Desmurget et al., 1995), which fits well with the idea that foveal vision of the limb at rest optimizes the hand localization process. Peripheral vision does not allow such an improvement because spatial estimations are not accurate in the peripheral visual field (Prablanc et al., 1979b; Bock, 1993). As additional evidence supporting this conclusion, the representation of the hand location is significantly biased in the dark (Vindras et al., 1998; van Beers et al., 1998; Desmurget et al., 2000). Recent data have shown that this bias cannot be related to a tendency of the proprioceptive signal to "drift" in the dark (Desmurget et al., 2000), as had been suggested in the past (Paillard and Brouchon, 1968; Wann and Ibrahim, 1992). Seeing the hand at rest allows the nervous system to reset a systematic bias of the proprioceptive signal with respect to the visual world (Desmurget et al., 1995, 2000).

Thus the inability of deafferented subjects to perform multijoint movements appears to reflect a trajectory-planning impairment rather than a feedback deficit. Evidence supporting this view is provided by tendon vibration experiments: Vibrating the biceps tendon prior to movement onset significantly affects movement accuracy (Larish et al., 1984), whereas applying the vibration during the initial two thirds of the movement has no effect on endpoint errors (Redon et al., 1991). Another, more indirect line of evidence comes from reaching studies showing that electromyographic (EMG) activity varies, in a predictive manner, to offset the influence of interaction torque arising from multijoint dynamics (Sainburg et al., 1995; Flanagan and Wing, 1997; Gribble and Ostry, 1999). Because feedforward compensatory mechanisms require a precise estimation of both the limb geometry and the limb inertial properties, the motor system has to rely on proprioception during movement planning. This point was clearly demonstrated by Sainburg and colleagues (1995), who required two patients having large-fiber sensory neuropathy to make a gesture similar to slicing a loaf of bread. Without vision of the moving limb, the patients were unable to compensate for interaction torque, leading to severe impairments in interjoint coordination. In contrast, when allowed to see their arm at rest before movement, they were able to generate virtually normal movements. As shown by Ghez and colleagues (1995), when these two patients were required to point to visual target with prior vision of the limb (dynamic open loop condition), the movement endpoint error, the final endpoint variability, the path curvature and the number of late secondary movements were optimized.

In summary, the previous results, when considered together, suggest that accurate movements can be performed in the absence of dynamic proprioceptive feedback: Whereas proprioception is critical for movement planning, its absence during the movement itself only produces limited effects. This conclusion is in agreement with the hypothesis that visually directed movements are under the control of a motor program that is modifiable by feedback loops.

Reaching in the Dark

The first experimental contribution to the problem of visual control of movement was provided by Woodworth (1899) in a long monograph published more than a century ago. When he asked human subjects to perform repetitive movements with a handheld pencil, (1) movement accuracy degraded significantly with hand velocity when vision of the movement was allowed; (2) movements executed with visual feedback involved small corrective movements at the end of the trajectory; (3) movement accuracy was not affected by hand velocity when vision of the movement was not allowed, that is, when subjects were required to point with their eyes closed. From these results, it was concluded that the speed-accuracy interaction observed in the presence of visual feedback could be explained by the inability of the subjects to control their movement visually when hand velocity went above a critical threshold. According to Woodworth (1899, p. 42), "the bad effect of speed consists in rendering impossible a delicate current control in preventing those later and finer adjustments by means of which a movement is enabled to approximate more and more closely to its goal." When prevented from exerting this "current control," the subject has to rely on a "first impulse," which may be considered as the direct ancestor of Keele's motor program. In an interesting development,

Woodworth even suggested that motor virtuosity was achieved by progressively eliminating final adjustments to rely exclusively on the "first impulse."

During the last century, many studies have confirmed and generalized Woodworth's conclusions. Carlton (1981) established that vision exerted its influence only at the very end of the movement, when velocity is slow. He required subjects to place circular rods in small holes positioned at various distances. Results showed that viewing the hand during the first half of the trajectory did not improve movement accuracy with respect to a condition where the hand was never visible. Carlton concluded that the initial part of the movement was under the control of a preplanned set of motor commands and that fine movement accuracy was achieved through final intermittent repositioning impulses whose direction and amplitude was given by a retinal error signal. A similar conclusion was reached by Beaubaton and Hay (1986) in a classical reaching task in which subjects were required to point to visual targets under absent, total, or partial visual control. (We will examine alternative interpretations of the data presented in Carlton, 1981, and Beaubaton and Hay, 1986, later in this chapter.)

As noted above, seeing the hand at rest prior to movement onset improves the accuracy of visually directed movements, which might suggest that the usual comparison between total open loop (hand never visible) and total closed loop (hand always visible) overestimates the ability of visual feedback loops to correct erroneous trajectories. Indeed, part of the accuracy deficit observed in the total closed loop situation might not be related to a feedback deficit, but to a planning bias. In agreement with this view, Prablanc and colleagues (1979a) showed that fast reaching movements contained substantial endpoint errors even when vision was available during the movement only. These errors were significantly larger than those observed in a total closed loop condition. A result consistent with this finding was reported by Gentillucci and colleagues (1996), who required subjects to point to the more distant vertex of closed and open configurations of the Muller-Lyer illusion, as well as to the vertex of control lines. Two main conditions were investigated. In the first condition (full vision condition), subjects saw both stimulus and their hand before and during movement. In the second condition (nonvisual feedback condition), they saw the stimulus, but not their hand during movement. The Muller-Lyer illusion dramatically affected pointing kinematics with respect to the control lines. Subjects undershot and overshot the vertex location, respectively, in the closed and open configuration, showing that hand trajectory could not be fully corrected in response to the initial illusion, even when vision was present during the entire trajectory.

Reaching Too Fast for the Peripheral System

The strongest evidence against the use of sensory feedback to control movement trajectory is based on the existence of incompressible physiological delay in sensorimotor loops. Indeed, when the processing of sensory information is long with respect to the movement duration, the position of the hand changes dramatically by the time the feedback signal starts to influence the ongoing motor command, and the implemented correction becomes inappropriate (Hollerbach, 1982; Gerdes and Happee, 1994).

The time necessary for visual information to influence the ongoing movement was first investigated with repetitive movements by Woodworth (1899) and by Vince (1948), who reported delays greater than 400 ms. These values seemed somewhat high with respect to visuomotor reaction times, which are usually well below 400 ms. This finding led Keele and Posner (1968) to investigate discrete pointing movements in a new experiment. They tested two conditions: open loop (only the target was visible) and closed loop (both the hand and the target could be seen). The shortest movement duration for which movements were more accurate in the closed loop condition was 260 ms. No difference was observed for 190 ms movements. Keele and Posner concluded that the minimal delay for visual information to influence the movement was within the range of 190–260 ms. Further data confirmed the validity of this initial estimation (Beggs and Howarth, 1970: 290 ms; Wallace and Newell, 1983: 200 ms; Cordo, 1987: 200 ms). By contrast, other studies provided evidence that 200 ms might still represent an overestimation of the delay inherent to visual feedback loops. Carlton (1981) suggested, for instance, that vision was only used at the end of the trajectory when velocity becomes low; he argued that measuring the entire movement biases the results as an overestimation. To test this hypothesis, he required subjects to point with a stylus to visual targets displayed in the sagittal plane. In a first experiment, five conditions were considered, in which 0%, 25%, 50%, 75%, and 93% of the trajectory, respectively, were occluded by a physical shield. Movement accuracy was found to be no different in the 0% and 50% visual conditions. In a second experiment, Carlton reinvestigated the 75% and 93% occlusion conditions in greater detail, measuring the time elapsed between the appearance of the hand in the visual space and the occurrence of corrective submovements. He found a value of 135 ms. Using a similar protocol, Beaubaton and Hay (1986) showed that movements of 130 ms (total duration) were more accurate when the subjects were allowed to see the second half of the trajectory with respect to a condition where vision was occluded during the entire movement. This finding suggests that visual control of movement can be significantly faster than 100 ms in some circumstances. Using a protocol similar to the one initially developed by Keele and Posner, Zelaznik and colleagues (1983) also reported 100 ms, although they demonstrated that vision was used more quickly in blocked than in randomized experimental sessions. This finding indicates that the nervous system is more efficient at processing visual signals when it knows, in advance, that vision will be available.

The time necessary for proprioceptive information to influence the ongoing movement was first evaluated by Vince (1948), who trained human subjects to make accurate movements while pulling a handle attached to a spring. He observed that the subjects needed 160 ms to adjust their movement and compensate for an unexpected modification of the stiffness of the spring. A slightly shorter delay (120 ms) was subsequently reported by Chernikoff and Taylor (1952), who used a paradigm requiring subjects to react as fast as possible when their arm was suddenly dropped from a passively maintained position. Dewhurst (1967) obtained an even shorter delay (100 ms) using an active maintenance task in which the subjects had to react as fast as possible when the weight of the load they were holding was unexpectedly increased. Although the range of 100–150 ms was subsequently validated in many studies (Higgins and Angel, 1970: 136 ms; Cordo, 1990: 120 ms; Flanders and Cordo, 1989: 150 ms), a few experiments have identified much shorter proprioceptive reaction times. For instance, Crago and colleagues (1976) asked human subjects to hold a handle attached to a motor in a reference position. They observed active corrections after a delay of only 70 ms when the force exerted by the motor was suddenly modified.

Considered together, these data indicate that the minimal delay for a proprioceptive signal to influence movement kinematics is within the range of 70–150 ms, a range whose breadth may be explained by different factors such as the characteristics of the task (arm actively maintained or passively sustained) or the nature of the parameters studied (acceleration, velocity, or position signal). The predictability of the motor perturbation may also be a critical factor, as was the ability to predict the availability of the visual signal (see above). This possibility was demonstrated by Newell and Houk (1983), who reported that, when the direction of the perturbation was consistent from trial to trial, the mean reaction time was significantly shorter (135 ms to 181 ms, depending on the subject) than when the direction of the perturbation was randomized (158 ms to 234 ms, depending on the subject).

To better estimate the proprioceptive reaction time, some authors have proposed considering electromyographic (EMG) activity instead of the overt modifications of the arm kinematics, a fairer approach, they argued, given the delay between the application of the muscle contraction and the actual displacement of the limb. Rather than settling the issue, these electrophysiological studies have raised a series of unexpected questions. Far from replicating behavioral observations, they ended up identifying three levels of proprioceptive regulation, usually designated "M1," "M2," and "M3" (Lee and Tatton, 1975; Evarts and Vaughn, 1978; Marsden et al., 1978; Agarwal and Gottlieb, 1980). M1, thought to represent the spinal functional stretch reflex, appears after only 15–25 ms. M2, classically described as a "long-latency supraspinal stretch reflex" (see Godaux and Cheron, 1989), appears after 40–60 ms. It may be worth noting here that neither M1 nor M2 is of sufficient magnitude to counteract the force generated when the arm is dropped from a passively maintained position or when the weight of an actively sustained object is suddenly increased, which explains why these short latency reflex responses failed to be identified in the behavioral paradigms described in the previous paragraph. M3, which Agarwal and Gottlieb (1980) have designated "postmyotatique" to emphasize its nonreflex origin, appears after 70–80 ms.

Numerous studies were carried out to examine the validity of the reflex versus nonreflex classification proposed to account for the existence of M1, M2, and M3. For instance, Marsden and colleagues (1978) required human subjects to produce a constant isometric contraction of the thumb flexors in response to an external force. When the amplitude of this force was suddenly increased, the subjects were required to let go (H1), flex the thumb as fast as possible (H2), or maintain their position (H3). Results showed that EMG activity recorded in the flexor pollicis longus always presented a double burst (M1, M2), irrespective of the experimental instruction. A supplementary burst (M3) was observed only when the subject was explicitly instructed to react to the perturbation (H2, H3). This indicated that M1 and M2 had a reflex origin, whereas M3 resulted from a voluntary response. Although confirmed by Agarwal and Gottlieb (1980), these observations could not be replicated in several subsequent studies (Hagbarth, 1967; Evarts and Tanji, 1974; Lee and Tatton, 1975; Rack, 1981), leaving the problem largely unresolved. The issue was finally settled by Evarts and Vaughn (1978), whose elegant study recorded biceps activity during a movement requiring a contraction of this muscle (in this case, no reflex activity is present). The subjects held a handle that was mobile around a horizontal axis. When this handle was rotated clockwise, the subjects were instructed to accentuate its movement by performing a quick clockwise rotation of the forearm (suppination). Results revealed a large EMG burst in the biceps muscle 70 ms after the perturbation (M3). No earlier response potentially related to M1 or M2 was observed.

Thus, from the data presented, sensory signals can be processed fairly quickly by the central motor system, although even the smallest value reported (70 ms) is large with respect to movement duration (typically, 400–600 ms). In 70 ms, the hand can travel several centimeters, making it impossible to efficiently use sensory feedback during the fastest part of the trajectory.

Reaching in Two Steps: The Dual Model of Movement Control
The main observations presented thus far can be summarized as follows: (1) Accurate movements can be performed in the absence of a dynamic sensory signal (i.e., vision or proprioception during the movement); (2) removing vision during the first half of the movement trajectory or biasing the proprioceptive signal through tendon vibration during the first two thirds of the movement has no effect on endpoint accuracy; (3) endpoint errors are reduced when a sensory signal is present; and (4) the processing of visual and proprioceptive information is too slow to allow sensory feedback control when the hand location is changing rapidly. Considered together, these observations suggest that sensory feedback loops improve the final accuracy of movement by allowing fine control of the hand displacement at the very end of the trajectory, when velocity is low. Stated more formally, reaching movements are segmented into two components: an *initial ballistic component,* entirely driven by a motor plan and ensuring a fast transport of the hand into the vicinity of the target; and a *final homing component,* dependent on sensory feedback loops and allowing fine corrections at the very end of the trajectory. Classically, these final corrections are viewed as a

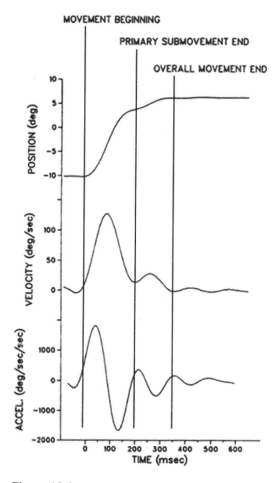

Figure 10.1
Individual position, velocity, and acceleration signals for a single-joint reaching movement performed with the elbow toward a visual target. The trajectory can be divided into two components: a main movement covering more than 80% of the required displacement (from movement beginning to primary submovement end) and a submovement bringing the hand to the target (from primary submovement end to overall movement end). (Adapted with permission from Meyer et al., 1988.)

series of one or more submovements generated at discrete time intervals (Meyer et al., 1988; Milner, 1992; for a review, see Jeannerod, 1988). Supporting this view, it was shown that reaching movements can be represented as a composite of several submovements, each of which represents a scaled version of a prototypic ballistic entity (Milner, 1992). Also, it was found that the first portion of this entity usually covered 80% or more of the total movement distance (Meyer et al., 1988; Milner, 1992). This dual model of movement control is illustrated in figure 10.1. It has long been the prism through which subsequent studies of motor control have been interpreted.

10.2   Continuous Feedback Loops for Fast Reaching Movements: Recent Evidence

To avoid ambiguity, we have divided feedback loops into two categories: *nonsensory*, for which only the efferent information can be used to determine the hand location; and *internal*, for which both sensory (vision or proprioception) and efferent information can be used to determine the hand location. Internal feedback loops are designated "visual" when the subjects can see their hand moving, and "nonvisual" when they cannot. The term *feedback*, by itself, refers to any feedback loop without distinction.

To further distinguish between two different types of feedback, we have divided errors into three different types: *extrinsic*, arising from erroneous localization of the goal of the movement (e.g., overestimating the distance of the target from the body); *intrinsic*, arising from erroneous estimation of the state of the motor apparatus before movement onset (e.g., underestimating the distance of the hand from the body); and *motor*, arising from erroneous estimation of the motor command required to bring the hand from its starting location to the target location (e.g., errors of amplitude or direction during a reach). The following subsection reviews behavioral evidence showing that movement errors can be corrected early, even for fast reaching movements.

Nonsensory Feedback Loops
A displacement of the body with respect to the environment and a displacement of the environment with respect to the body generate the same retinal stimulation. To account for the ability of the nervous system to discriminate between these two situations, von Holst and Mittelstaedt (1950) proposed

that a copy of the motor command was stored somewhere in the brain and used to interpret the perceptual input. This conclusion was extended and generalized leading to the concept of nonsensory feedback loop. According to this view, a copy of the efferent signal sent to the muscle can be used to estimate the current state of the motor apparatus with no delay and thus to prompt efficient path corrections in response to extrinsic errors.

A first line of evidence showing that nonsensory feedback loops can be used to guide biological actuators is found with eye movements. There is now extensive evidence that the oculomotor system uses an efferent signal to control saccadic eye movements. Perturbation experiments indicate that if gaze is shifted during the preparation or the execution of a saccade toward a flashed target, then a compensatory saccade that accurately brings gaze onto the remembered target location is generated (head-fixed saccade; Keller et al., 1996; head-free gaze shifts; Pélisson et al., 1995). Strikingly, because it occurs in full darkness and after surgical deafferentation of extra-ocular proprioception in monkeys, such compensation does not require visual or proprioceptive feedback (Guthrie et al., 1983).

For arm movements, the existence of nonsensory feedback loops was initially suggested in behavioral studies showing that hand trajectory could be amended with a shorter latency than the minimal latency required to process peripheral information. Early evidence supporting this idea was provided by Higgins and Angel (1970), who instructed 11 subjects to hold a lever, which could be displaced to the right or to the left. In the first experimental condition, the subjects were trained to use the lever to displace a line presented, in front of them, on a cathode ray tube. A rightward movement of the lever generated an upward displacement of the line, whereas a leftward movement generated a downward displacement. The subjects were instructed to bring this line in coincidence with a target line stepping from one position to another. In the second experimental condition, the subjects were simply required to hold the lever in a median position and to react as fast as possible to any force that may be generated to move the lever away from its central position. Results showed that subjects sometimes initiated their movement in the wrong direction in the first condition, needing between 83 ms (fastest subject) and 122 ms (slowest subject) to initiate a motor correction. These delays were significantly higher than the ones observed in the proprioceptive reaction time task (between 108 ms and 169 ms). For each subject, the reaction time observed in the first condition was shorter than the reaction time observed in the second condition, supporting the hypothesis that errors in movement initiation can be amended by a central mechanism that operates more rapidly than sensory feedback. A similar conclusion was reached by Jaeger and colleagues (1979), who showed that altering the proprioceptive signal through tendon vibration did not modify the reaction time to a visual perturbation. These data are in agreement with other studies showing the existence of very rapid movement corrections during pointing movements directed at an erroneous target. Cook and Diggles (1984) observed, for instance, successful hand path corrections 45 ms after movement onset, when the initial direction of the motor response was erroneous, a value close to the 30 ms reported by van Sonderen and colleagues (1989) in a double-step task where the initial target location was changed during or after movement initiation. The values of 45 ms and 30 ms are much too fast to be of sensory origin (see above).

The best evidence showing that nonsensory feedback loops can be used to guide the hand toward the target, in response to an initial extrinsic error was provided recently by Bard and colleagues (1999), who required a deafferented patient to look and point to visual targets displayed in the peripheral visual field. Vision of the moving limb was not allowed. In some trials, the target location changed slightly during the course of the ocular saccade. Because of saccadic suppression, this manipulation was not consciously detected by the patient, who was convinced that she pointed to a stationary target (see following subsection for details). The patient was able to correct her movement on-line and to reach to the new target location despite the absence of peripheral feedback, although her corrections were not as accurate as those observed for control subjects, suggesting that under normal conditions the motor outflow is combined with at least some sensory inflow to generate an optimal estimate of hand location. (This point will be addressed in greater detail below.)

Internal Nonvisual Feedback Loops

To an external examiner, the relative coordination of eye, head, and hand during goal-directed reaching appears sequential. When a subject points to a visual target in peripheral space, the eyes move first, followed by the head, and finally the hand. Because eye movement duration is brief, the gaze arrives at the target before or around hand movement onset (Prablanc et al., 1979b, 1986; Prablanc and Martin, 1992; Desmurget et al., 2001). Based on the observation that the extrafoveal visual signal (peripheral vision) does not allow an accurate estimation of the target location (Prablanc et al.,

1979b; Bock, 1993), it was suggested that the delayed hand movement reflected an obligatory requirement to foveate a target before a reliable motor plan for the arm could be constructed (Paillard, 1982). This appealing hypothesis was disproved, however, by further studies showing that the serial organization observed at the behavioral level for the eye, the head, and the arm resulted primarily from inertial factors. When electromyographic activity is considered, the neural command appears to reach the eye, the head, and the arm at nearly the same time, despite the usual external kinematic markers. The arm reaction time is last simply because it has the greatest inertia. If one considers that the onset of the agonist muscle contraction occurs 50–100 ms before the actual arm motion for reaching movements (Biguer et al., 1982; Turner et al., 1995), this result agrees with psychophysical studies showing that the overt arm movement follows generally the saccadic response with a lag of 60–100 ms (Prablanc et al., 1979b, 1986; Prablanc and Martin, 1992; Desmurget et al., 2001).

From the above observations, the initial motor command is issued on the basis of an imperfect estimation of the target location. At the end of the saccadic displacement, when the hand starts moving, the target location is reestimated on the basis of accurate perifoveal information. This updated information can then be used by the nervous system to adjust the ongoing trajectory, as initially demonstrated by Prablanc and colleagues (1986), who required subjects to point without vision of the moving limb "as quickly and accurately as possible" to visual targets presented in their peripheral visual field. In condition 1, the target was turned off just before the end of the ocular saccade preventing the subject from reestimating the target location at the end of the saccadic response. In condition 2, the target was turned off 120 ms after the end of the ocular saccade allowing reestimation of the target location by foveal vision. In condition 3, the target remained illuminated throughout the entire pointing movement. And in condition 4, the target was turned off at hand movement onset; the subject was asked to look at the target first before initiating a reaching movement with the arm. In this fourth condition, the subject had the opportunity to program arm movement on the basis of a perfectly accurate estimation of the target location. Movement error was minimal in condition 3, maximal in condition 1, and intermediate in conditions 2 and 4. These findings confirm that the initial motor program is partially inaccurate because of the existence of an erroneous estimation of the target location (conditions 1 versus 4), and that movements initiated on the basis of accurate foveal information are not necessarily perfectly accurate, with further corrections occurring at movement execution (conditions 3 versus 4). They clearly demonstrate that the motor system can amend the ongoing movement when it has the opportunity to update target location (conditions 1 versus 2).

To investigate in greater detail whether fast reaching movements are the result of a preset pattern of unmodifiable commands, Prablanc and colleagues (Goodale et al., 1986; Pélisson et al., 1986; Prablanc and Martin, 1992) designed a new experimental paradigm in which the initial inaccurate estimation of the target location during movement planning was artificially increased, unbeknownst to the subjects. To achieve their goal, the authors slightly modified the target location during the course of the ocular saccade. This modification has three major advantages: (1) Because of saccadic suppression, the target jump is not perceived consciously by the subject; (2) because saccadic responses to stationary targets involve an initial saccade undershooting the target position and a secondary corrective saccade achieving accurate target acquisition (Becker and Fuchs, 1969; Prablanc and Jeannerod, 1975; Harris, 1995), the target jump does not alter the organization of the oculomotor system; and (3) because pointing movements to stationary targets involve an update of the target location at the end of the saccadic displacement, which is taken into account to amend the ongoing arm trajectory (see above), the target jump does not alter the organization of the manual response. Indeed, one can say that, from a functional point of view, pointing directed at stationary targets is identical to pointing directed at unconsciously displaced targets. The intrasaccadic modification of target location simply increases an error already present in the system.

In a first series of experiments, Prablanc and colleagues (Pélisson et al., 1986; Goodale et al., 1986) required subjects to point "as quickly and accurately as possible" to visual targets presented, at different distances, along a frontoparallel line. Vision of the moving limb was not allowed. In half of the trials, the target remained stationary, whereas in the other half it was slightly displaced to the right or left during the ocular saccade. The magnitude of the target jump represented between 7% and 10% of the initial movement amplitude (e.g., 2 cm for a 30 cm movement; 4 cm for a 40 cm movement). Subjects were fully able to correct the ongoing trajectory in response to the target jump. The observed corrections were surprisingly smooth, as shown by the absence of discontinuities on the wrist velocity curves, which exhibited the same bell-shaped profile for both the perturbed and control movements (figure 10.2, upper panel), thus disproving the

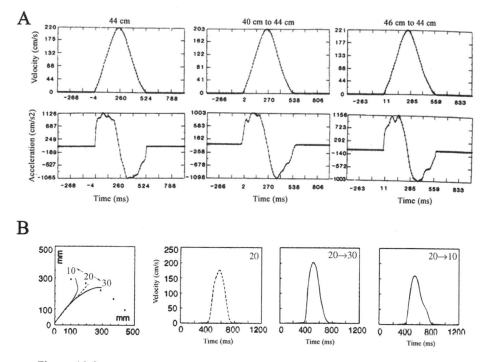

Figure 10.2

Smooth and early path corrections observed during reaching without vision of the limb. (*A*) Initial data by Pélisson et al. (Pélisson et al. 1986) showing that neither the hand velocity profiles nor the hand acceleration profiles were different for reaching movements performed to stationary targets (first column, 44 cm movement amplitude), or to targets that were displaced collinearly to the movement initial direction during the oculomotor response (second and third columns, 40 to 44 cm and 46 to 44 cm movement amplitude). (*B*) Mean hand path performed by one subject (first column) to a stationary target (20°; dashed curve) and to targets that were displaced during the course of the ocular saccades (20° → 30°, 20° → 10°; solid curves), with corresponding velocity profiles (second through fourth columns). (Adapted from Martin and Prablanc, 1991.)

hypothesis that a lack of discontinuity in the velocity curve implies an absence of path correction. Finally, Prablanc and colleagues' results also indicated that path amendments did not involve any increase in movement duration, supporting the hypothesis that the perturbed trials were corrected by adjustments to an existing program rather than the generation of a new motor program. These results were further replicated and generalized by Plablanc and Martin (1992), who initially presented targets at 20°, 30°, and 40° on a circle centered on the hand starting point (radius 30 cm). As a consequence, the target jump (10° to the right or left) implied not simply a modulation of the movement amplitude, as was the case when targets were presented along a line (Pélisson et al., 1986; Goodale et al., 1986), but a complete reorganization of the current motor pattern. Results showed that hand trajectory smoothly diverged from their initial control path (first target) to reach the new target location (figure 10.2, lower panel). Corrections were detectable 110 ms after hand movement onset, showing that hand trajectory was amended very early. Interestingly, Prablanc and Martin also observed that the pattern of path correction, and the reaction time to the perturbation, were similar whether or not vision of the moving limb was available, which suggests that nonvisual feedback loops represent the main process through which extrinsic errors are corrected (see also Komilis et al., 1993).

In contrast to their efficiency in correcting extrinsic errors, nonvisual feedback loops seem quite inefficient in rectifying intrinsic errors. As shown by several studies, final errors in visually directed movements performed without vision of the moving limb reflect, in large part, systematic biases in the estimation of the initial state of the motor apparatus. This finding was initially made by Rossetti and colleagues (1995) in a behavioral experiment where subjects were asked to use their index finger to point toward visual targets without visual reafference from their moving hand. In the first condition, the pointing fingertip was viewed through prisms that created a visual displacement, while the target was presented outside the shifted field and thus was normally seen (no shift). The presence of the proprioceptive-visual mismatch was not detected by the subjects. In the second condition, both the index fingertip and the target were seen normally: The relationship between the hand and the target was not altered. Comparison between these two conditions showed that the visual shift of the fingertip position prior to movement induced a systematic bias of the movement endpoint, in a direction opposite to the visual shift. Interestingly, this shift was already present on the initial movement direction (which was rotated to the left) and on-line feedback loops did not reduce it significantly. The same apparent inability of on-line feedback loops to successfully correct extrinsic errors was also reported by Vindras and colleagues (1998), who tested the performance of human subjects on three sensorimotor tasks. On the first task, where subjects aimed at 48 targets spaced regularly around two starting positions, there was a systematic pattern of errors across targets: A parallel shift of the endpoints accounted, on average, for 49% of the total error. The systematic errors were found to decrease dramatically on the second task, where subjects were allowed to see their hand before movement onset. On the third task, where subjects used a joystick held with their left hand to estimate the location of their (unseen) right hand, the systematic perceptual errors were found to be highly correlated with the motor errors recorded on the first task, supporting the conclusion that systematic pointing errors significantly reflect the erroneous estimation of initial hand position. This result was interpreted as showing the primacy of feedforward control over feedback control. Another interpretation will be proposed below.

Internal Visual Feedback Loops

Based on physiological and psychophysical studies, Paillard (1980, 1996) proposed the existence of two visual feedback channels for movement control: a *static channel,* which operates in central vision, provides accurate position cues, and is essential for the discrete path corrections observed at the end of the movement (see dual model of motor control); and a *kinetic channel,* which operates in peripheral vision, provides motion cues, and is essential for controlling movement initial direction. To test this hypothesis, Bard and colleagues (1985) first investigated a purely directional aiming task. Seated on a chair, subjects held the tip of a pointer that could be rotated on a ball joint fixed to the floor. Four visual targets were presented to them on a strip of Plexiglas at eye level: one directly in front of them, and the others at 10°, 20°, and 30° in the right hemifield. The subjects were instructed to fixate the median target and to move the pointer toward the illuminated target without stopping under it. Directional errors were defined as the angular deviation between the pointer and the target position when the arm crossed the target line. Results showed that directional accuracy was greater when vision was allowed. This was also true for rapid movements as brief as 110 ms. Strikingly, this positive effect of vision was still present when the second half of the movement was occluded by a physical board, suggesting that visual error could be processed in much less than 110 ms. The potential role of peripheral vision for controlling movement direction was further documented in subsequent studies carried out by the same group. Blouin and colleagues (1993a, 1993b) established that early visual control of movement direction was present even when the subjects were not able to see their hand at rest (a light was turned on at movement onset), a critical point that had not been made clear in Bard et al., 1985. Blouin and colleagues (1993a; see also Teasdale et al., 1991) also established that the directional component of aiming movements could be significantly improved when the experimental instruction required the subjects to stop below the target, that is, to control both movement direction and movement amplitude, as is the case in classical reaching tasks.

Based on these observations, several hypotheses can be put forward to account for the inability of previous studies to identify a positive effect of early visual corrections on the accuracy of fast reaching movements (see Paillard, 1996, for a detailed discussion). A first possibility is that the early studies investigated sagittal (Carlton, 1981) or parasagittal movements (Beaubaton and Hay, 1986), which did not favor the occurrence of directional errors. Bard and colleagues (1990) failed, for instance, to observe any positive effect of peripheral vision for sagittal movements. Another factor may be that the error parameters studied in earlier studies were not sufficiently "sensitive." Carlton measured, for instance, the number of "hits" (a "miss or touch" score); Beaubaton and Hay considered the distance between the hand and the target, probably the worst parameter to detect a potential effect of peripheral vision on early path corrections. Indeed, as Paillard (1996) points out, distance error does not vary with directional errors: If subjects point to a target presented on a vertical screen, distance error will be the same whether they reach 1 cm to the right or 1 cm to the left. Finally, the absence of a difference between a condition where vision is always present and a condition where it is only present during the second half of the trajectory need not mean only that early visual control is ineffective. It could also mean that later visual control (during the second half of the movement) is powerful enough to correct any errors not amended by initial feedback loops.

Progressive Recruitment of the Primary Arm Movers

The idea that limb transport is ballistic and under preprogrammed control was originally supported by behavioral studies on the organization of muscle activity during goal-directed movements. Rapid reaching movements generally exhibit a typical triphasic pattern of activation, in which the initial agonist burst is followed first by an antagonist activation and then by a small agonist burst at the end of the hand displacement (Jeannerod, 1988). Because this pattern is still observed when proprioceptive information is absent (Rothwell et al., 1982; Jeannerod, 1988), it was concluded that the triphasic electromyographic (EMG) activation has a central origin. Although this idea was never directly challenged, a series of experiments carried out by Flanders and colleagues (1996) suggest that a preprogrammed triphasic pattern of EMG activity may evolve within a larger motor repertoire. These authors recorded EMG activity from nine superficial elbow and shoulder muscles while human subjects made rapid arm movements. Finding that the different muscles were recruited gradually and that the pattern of activation varied as a function of movement direction, they proposed that this gradual recruitment represented a neuromuscular control strategy in which burst timing contributed to the specification of movement direction. On this basis, it may be tempting to speculate that the ongoing trajectory might be controlled, to a certain extent, by adjusting the temporal pattern of muscle activation. This hypothesis fits well with a second study (Herrmann and Flanders, 1998), carried out by the same group and aimed at determining the pattern of activation of single motor units recruited in the biceps and deltoid during the production of an isometric force. The best directions of the single motor units, determined by measuring their firing rate and threshold force, were found to change gradually with their position in the muscle (best directions vary gradually with location in the muscle rather than clustering into separate groups). Based on this organization, Herrmann and Flanders proposed that various units could be recruited, at different points in the movements, according to their mechanical action. They suggested that a large flexibility of the hand trajectory could be achieved through a gradual recruitment and derecruitment of the units ideally suited for the production of the required force vector at any given time. This remarkable result identifies a potential neuromuscular substrate where the muscle pattern of activation may be smoothly adjusted during the ongoing movement.

10.3   Forward Modeling Allows Feedback Control for Fast Reaching Movements

Sections 10.1 and 10.2 have shown that (1) purely sensory loops cannot be used to control fast reaching movements (Hollerbach, 1982; Gerdes and Happee, 1994); (2) hand trajectory can be updated early and smoothly in response to extrinsic errors (Pélisson et al., 1986; Prablanc and Martin, 1992); and (3) early and smooth corrections of the hand trajectory can occur in the absence of any sensory information (Bard et al., 1999), although these corrections are not as accurate as in control subjects. Considered together, these findings suggest that the motor system is able to combine both different and afferent signals to control fast reaching movements during their time course. The nature of this combination has been formalized under the concept of a "forward model," whose central idea is that the motor system can progressively learn to estimate its own behavior in response to a given command (efferent signal). During the movement, this prediction can be used to estimate the current state of the motor apparatus and to predict what the final state will be. In parallel to this predictive activity, the system can also "store" its successive predictions in a "delayed buffer." If the delay is equivalent to the time necessary to process sensory information then the predicted and sensory estimated states can be compared directly. This comparison can be used to update the current estimation (Miall et al., 1993). To make this "predictive scheme" clear, let us consider a simplified, purely illustrative example. Imagine that a motor command is produced at the time $t_0 = 0$ ms. After 100 ms (t_1), the motor system can estimate the distance already traveled by the hand, based on the command that was generated. This information can be used to correct the current hand path when an extrinsic error is detected (e.g., when the target location has been updated at the end of the ocular saccade). At 100 ms after t_1 ($t_2 = 200$ ms), a sensory signal is finally processed, although this signal is related, not to the current hand position ($t_2 = 200$ ms), but to the position that the hand had 100 ms earlier ($t_1 = 100$ ms). If the stored predicted position (for $t_1 = 100$ ms) and the actually observed sensory position (delivered at $t_2 = 200$ ms but related to $t_1 = 100$ ms) matches, then everything is fine and the current prediction ($t_2 = 200$ ms) is validated (note that this mechanism of comparison can of course involve other parameters such as the predicted and actual proprioceptive reafferences). In contrast, if a discrepancy is detected, the motor system can use the mismatch information to update its current estimation.

With such a model, the probable position and velocity of the effector can be estimated with negligible delays, and even predicted in advance, thus making feedback strategies possible for fast reaching movements.

One way forward modeling might allow on-line motor control is illustrated in figure 10.3. When required to reach a target, subjects first elaborate a motor plan based on the initial movement conditions (respective locations of the hand an target). During the realization of the movement, a forward model of the arm's dynamics is generated. In its simplest version, this model receives as input a copy of the motor outflow (figure 10.3A). In a more general form, this model receives as input a copy of the motor outflow and an error signal defined by comparing a stored estimate of the motor state with the delayed sensory estimate (see figure 10.3B for details). The output of this forward model is a prediction of the movement endpoint. This prediction can be compared continuously with the target location. In case of discrepancy, an error signal is generated, triggering a modulation of the motor command.

Convincing evidence suggesting that a reliable estimation of the current state of the motor apparatus can only be obtained by combining efferent and afferent signals was reported by Wolpert and colleagues (1995), who required subjects to move their hand along a line while holding a lever. Vision of the hand was allowed for 2 s prior to movement onset. The lever was connected to a torque motor that induced resistive or assistive force to the movement. At the end of the trial, subjects estimated the location of their hand using a visual spot controlled by the other hand. The temporal propagation of measured errors exhibited by the subjects could be fully accounted for by assuming that the motor control system integrates both the motor outflow and the sensory inflow to estimate the hand location. Models based exclusively on either the sensory inflow or the motor outflow were unable to predict the observed pattern of error. Hoff and Arbib (1993) came to a similar conclusion in a simulation study, where they showed that a control model for reaching movements that combined efferent signals and afferent information to estimate the current hand location and to adjust the planned pattern of muscle activation successfully captured the kinematic characteristics of visually directed reaching. In particular, this model, which used a look-ahead predictor to compensate for delays in sensorimotor loops, was able to account for the trajectory corrections observed in double-step trials (Pélisson et al., 1986; Goodale et al., 1986).

Further indirect arguments supporting the position that efferent and afferent signals are combined to generate a reliable forward estimation of

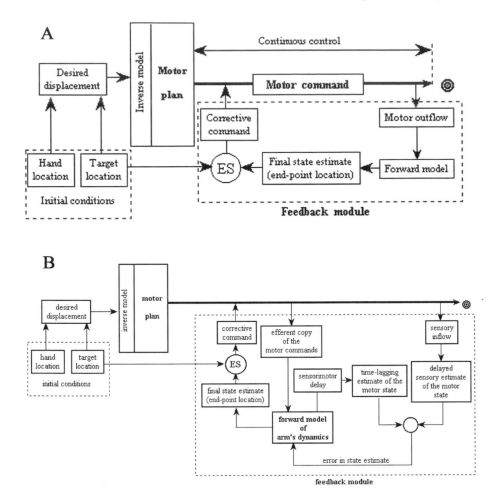

Figure 10.3

Potential motor circuits making use of a forward model of the arm's dynamics for controlling hand movements. (*A*) Purely efferent model, where a motor plan is initially defined based on the respective locations of the hand and target. During the movement a forward model of the arm's dynamics is generated. This model receives as inputs the motor outflow, and generates as output an estimate of the movement endpoint location, which is then compared to the target location. In case of discrepancy, an error signal (ES) is generated triggering a modulation of the ongoing motor command. The movement stops when the hand reaches the target estimated location (bull's-eye). (*B*) Efferent and afferent model. A motor plan is initially defined; during the movement, a forward model of the arm's dynamics is generated, which model receives as input the motor outflow and error signal obtained by comparing the estimated and observed state estimate (Smith predictor; Miall et al., 1993). This comparison can involve parameters such as the predicted and proprioceptively inferred hand location. It can also involve the predicted and observed proprioceptive reafferences. Because of delays in peripheral loops, the

the arm dynamics were provided by recent studies on interjoint coordination. To understand the nature of these arguments it is necessary to remember that movement torques arise not only from the muscles acting on the joints but also from interactions among all the moving segments. As initially demonstrated by Hollerbach and Flash (1982), these torque interactions are significant for multijoint arm movements, and they have to be compensated one way or another. It was first proposed that the compensation was achieved "mechanically" through springlike properties of muscle and reflex activity (Flash, 1987; Bizzi et al., 1992). This proposal was challenged by Kawato and colleagues (Katayama and Kawato, 1993; Gomi and Kawato, 1996), who provided computational evidence that a failure to integrate explicit compensations for limb dynamics in the initial motor command would lead to erratic and maladapted trajectories. To investigate the controversy in greater detail, Gribble and Ostry (1999) studied a reaching task in which muscle activity was directly measured. Human subjects were required to perform single- and multijoint pointing involving shoulder and elbow motion; movement parameters related to the magnitude and direction of interaction torques were manipulated in a systematic way. Gribble and Ostry found that the central control signals sent to the elbow and shoulder muscles were adjusted, in a predictive manner, to compensate for interaction torques arising from multijoint dynamics. Such anticipatory adjustments suggest that the nervous system is able to use a forward model to predict and offset the kinematic consequences of intersegmental dynamics. Interestingly, recent results have indicated that sensory information is critical to parameterize and update this forward model. When, for example, Sainburg and colleagues (1995) required two patients with large-fiber sensory neuropathy to make a gesture similar to slicing a loaf of bread without vision of the moving arm, these patients were unable to compensate for interaction torque, leading to severe impairments in interjoint coordination.

As noted in section 10.2, internal nonvisual feedback loops are apparently quite inefficient in rectifying intrinsic errors; final errors in visually

◀ current estimated state has to be delayed by a duration equal to the sensorimotor delay to be compared to the afferent signal. The forward model generates as output an estimate of the movement endpoint location, which is then compared to the target location. In case of discrepancy, an error signal (ES) is generated triggering a modulation of the ongoing motor command. The movement stops when the hand reaches the target estimated location (bull's-eye). (Adapted and extended with permission from Desmurget and Grafton 2000.)

directed movements performed without vision of the moving limb seem to reflect systematic biases in the estimation of the initial state of the motor apparatus. At first sight, this observation seems to contradict the thesis that movement trajectory is controlled on-line by powerful feedback loops. A close look at the data, however, shows that this impression is misleading. Indeed, the findings on forward modeling clearly indicate that the estimation of the current hand location will be affected in a systematic manner if either the proprioceptive signal (Rossetti et al., 1995; Vindras et al., 1998) or the inverse model that transforms the desired displacement into a motor command (Vindras and Viviani, 1998) is biased. A study performed by Desmurget and colleagues (1995) illustrates this point. Subjects were required to point to a visual target without vision of their moving limb. Pointing accuracy was measured in two conditions where the hand was either never visible ("never" condition) or visible only in the static position before movement onset ("static" condition). Viewing the hand before movement greatly decreased endpoint variability ("static") when compared to never viewing it ("never"). This effect was associated with a significant modification of the movement kinematics: The "static" condition induced a shortened acceleration phase with a corresponding lengthened deceleration phase when compared to the "never" condition. These results were consistent with the hypothesis that viewing the hand before movement onset allowed a decrease of pointing variability through a feedback process. To test this hypothesis, Desmurget and colleagues (1995) performed an additional experiment identical to the first one except that the target was turned off during the deceleration phase of the movement. Turning the target off had no effect upon the "never" condition but induced a significant increase of pointing variability in the "static" condition. This result shows that vision of the static hand decreases movement endpoint variability, not only by improving movement planning, but also by optimizing feedback control: When the noise attached to the estimation of the hand location is reduced, the noise contained in the forward model decreases, and movement variability declines.

10.4 Internal Feedback Loops Are Not Used to Generate the Motor Command in Real Time

The "equilibrium point" model provides a powerful conceptual framework for understanding how visually directed movements might be generated in the absence of any a priori specification of the motor command. To make this point clear, let us present briefly the theoretical foundations of the equilibrium point model. Consider a mass (M) placed on a table and attached to two horizontal springs (S_1 and S_2). The magnitude of the two opposite forces (F_1 and F_2) exerted on M depends on both the stiffness (k) and the length (L) of S_1 and S_2 ($F = kL$). When F_1 equals F_2, M is in equilibrium. If one modifies suddenly the stiffness of one of the springs, M moves to reach a new equilibrium state. As a consequence, a simple way to control the position of the mass is to adjust the relative stiffness of the springs acting on it. By analogy, based on the springlike properties of biological actuators, a simple way to move the hand to a given spatial position would be to set the length-tension curves of all the muscles acting on the upper limb in such a way that the torques exerted by agonist and antagonist muscles nullify each other when the hand is at the desired position (for review, see Feldman, 1986; Bizzi et al., 1992; Desmurget et al., 1998).

In its original formulation, the equilibrium point hypothesis suggested that visually directed movements were achieved, "in one step," by suddenly shifting the equilibrium configuration of the arm to its terminal state (Polit and Bizzi, 1979; Feldman, 1986). This view was challenged by the observation that point-to-point movements followed roughly straight hand paths in the task space, irrespective of the experimental conditions (Morasso, 1981; for review, see Desmurget et al., 1998). To account for this observation, it was suggested that the equilibrium configuration of the arm, rather than shifting in one step, was gradually displaced toward the target (Bizzi et al., 1992; Feldman and Levin, 1995). Evidence supporting this view was initially provided by Bizzi and colleagues (1984) in the context of single-joint movements. These authors trained three monkeys to perform forearm movements toward a visual target presented in a dark room. The performance of the animals was tested before and after a bilateral dorsal rhizotomy in two conditions: arm held in the initial position ("held") and arm displaced toward the target at movement onset ("displaced"). As would have been expected if the nervous system had programmed a gradual shift of the arm equilibrium position, Bizzi and colleagues observed for both the intact and deafferented animals that (1) the initial acceleration of the hand increased gradually with the duration of the holding period in the "held" condition; (2) the forearm moved back in the direction of movement starting point in the "displaced" condition, before reversing its displacement to return to the target. Further evidence supporting a generalization of the "continuous equilibrium point shift" hypothesis to multijoint movements was provided by modeling studies that combined experimental observations and computer simulations and that proceeded from two different approaches: In the first, the series of equilibrium points to be followed was determined in advance (Flash, 1987; Bizzi et al., 1992; Hatsopoulos, 1994); in the second, the arm equilibrium configuration was shifted in real time based on a negative feedback loop aimed at nullifying the hand-target distance (Flanagan et al., 1993; Feldman and Levin, 1995). Approached in the second way, the "continuous equilibrium point shift" hypothesis is quite appealing for at least three reasons: (1) It does not require the computation of a motor plan before movement onset, which greatly simplifies the mechanism of movement generation by removing the need for complex nonlinear inverse transforms; (2) it provides a unified framework within which movement generation and movement control need not be segregated; and (3) it powerfully captures the kinematic features of visually directed movements directed at stationary and jumping targets.

Notwithstanding the attractiveness and computational power of the "continuous equilibrium point shift" hypothesis, however, recent experimental findings clearly establish that the upcoming motor command is at least partially defined before movement onset. The first evidence sustaining this conclusion comes from the identification of fine predictive compensatory adjustments during reaching movements (the kinematic consequences of an upcoming motor command can only be anticipated and canceled if the motor command is known in advance). Several examples of such anticipated compensations can be found in the literature. Gribble and Ostry (1999), for example, showed that electromyographic activity in the shoulder and elbow joints varied in a predictive manner to offset interaction torque arising from multijoint dynamics (see above). In the same vein, Flanagan and Wing (1997) reported the occurrence of fine predictive grip force adjustment during vertical arm movements performed with a handheld load. Likewise, De Wolf and colleagues (1998) described subtle anticipated postural compensations in the case of rapid arm movements.

The second evidence revealing the existence of a preplanning process comes from a recent transcranial magnetic stimulation (TMS) study carried out by our group (Desmurget et al., 1999b). The experimental protocol was similar to that of Prablanc and Martin, 1992. Subjects were instructed to point to visual targets. Vision of the arm was not allowed during the movement. In some trials, the target location was displaced during the sac-

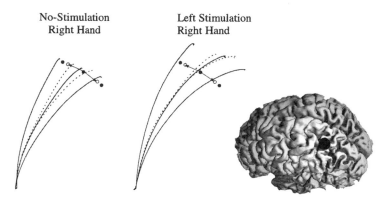

No-Stimulation
Right Hand

Left Stimulation
Right Hand

Figure 10.4
Role of the posterior parietal cortex for on-line movement corrections. Mean hand paths performed by one subject, with (*left*), and without (*middle*) transcranial magnetic stimulation (TMS). The continuous curves represent the mean paths directed at stationary targets (20°, 30°, 40°). The dashed curves represent the mean paths directed at jumping targets (30° → 22.5°, 30° → 37.5°). Filled circles indicate stationary target locations; open circles represent jumping target locations. TMS site (*right*) determined by three-dimensional magnetic resonance imaging (MRI). When TMS is applied, path corrections that normally occur in response to the target jump are disrupted; movements directed at stationary targets become less accurate, although not erratic. (Adapted and extended with permission from Desmurget et al., 1999b.)

cadic response, whereas, in other trials, it remained stationary. Two conditions were tested for each hand. In the first condition, the TMS coil was placed over the left posterior parietal cortex of the subject but no pulse was delivered. In the second condition, the coil was placed over the same location and single TMS pulse was applied at hand movement onset. We observed that (1) path corrections normally occurring in response to the target jump were disrupted by the stimulation when the subjects were required to use the right hand (contralateral to the stimulation site); (2) movements directed at stationary targets remained fairly accurate despite feedback disruption (right-hand session); and (3) there was no feedback disruption for movements performed with the left hand, ruling out that the effect observed for the right hand was related to a visual or oculomotor deficit (figure 10.4). Considered together, these results show that disrupting the continuous control loops that compare the relative locations of the hand and target does not give rise to erratic and totally maladjusted trajectories, as would be expected if negative internal feedback loops were used to generate the motor command in real time.

10.5　Functional Anatomy of Internal Feedback Loops

The past two decades have been dominated by the hypothesis that reaching movements were primarily under preprogrammed control and that sensory feedback loops exerted only a limited influence at the very end of the trajectory. As a consequence, functional investigations have focused chiefly on the cerebral structures participating in motor preparation and execution, yielding few insights into the functional anatomy of on-line movement guidance, which was first investigated only recently by Inoue and colleagues (1998). Using positron emission tomography (PET), these authors examined the functional anatomy of internal visual feedback loops. A target board with six red light-emitting diodes (LEDs) arrayed in a circle around a green LED (fixation point) was placed in front of the subjects. The fixation point and one of the six targets were switched on and off alternatively during the scans. Three tasks were considered. In the control task, (C), subjects were instructed to "look" at the lit LED. In the reaching with visual feedback task (V), and on the reaching without visual feedback task (W), the subjects had to "look and point" to the lit red LED with their right index fingers. The V minus C and V minus W contrasts revealed common significant increase in regional cerebral blood flow (rCBF) in a large set of areas including the supramarginal cortex, the premotor cortex, and the posterior cingulate cortex of the left hemisphere (contralateral to the reaching hand), the caudate nucleus and the thalamus of the right hemisphere and the right cerebellar cortex and vermis. The V minus W contrast identified specific additional activations in the right prefrontal cortex, the right lateral occipital and occipitotemporal cortex, the right superior parietal cortex, the right insula, the left premotor cortex, the left posterior cerebellum and the brainstem. The existence of such an extended network for processing visual feedback of hand movements may appear surprising at first glance, especially because many of the areas identified by Inoue and colleagues have been linked to movement preparation in the past (Grafton et al., 1992, 1996; Deiber et al., 1996; Lacquaniti et al., 1997; Turner et al., 1998; Winstein et al., 1997). A close look at the experimental protocol adopted by Inoue and colleagues sheds some light on this point. To present the targets, the authors used a head-mounted display that permitted vision of the hand only in "the later stages" of the movement. As we have already noted, initial and late visual corrections seem to rely on different neural networks and to involve different processes (Paillard, 1980, 1996). The terminal corrections investigated by Inoue and colleagues have been shown to engage a series of one or more submovements generated at discrete time intervals on the basis of a retinal error signal. This finding indicates that the large cerebral network identified by the authors reflects not only the areas integrating terminal visual feedback of the hand but also the areas processing retinal errors, planning corrective submovements, and estimating final accuracy (this estimation was not possible in the W condition), which might explain, for instance, the unexpected medial prefrontal activation reported by the authors in the V minus W contrast.

A second functional study of movement guidance was recently carried out by our group (Desmurget et al., 2001). Unlike Inoue and colleagues (1998), we investigated reaching movement performed without vision of the moving limb. This choice was based on the observation that internal nonvisual feedback loops represent the primary process allowing early corrections of extrinsic errors (see above). Seven subjects were required to "look at" ("eye") or "look and point to" ("eyearm") visual targets whose location either remained stationary or changed undetectably during the ocular saccade. Functional anatomy of nonvisual feedback loops was identified by comparing the reaching condition involving large corrections ("jump") with the reaching condition involving small corrections ("stationary"), after subtracting the activations associated with saccadic movements and hand movement planning: ("eyearm-jumping" minus "eye-jumping") minus ("eyearm-stationary" minus "eye-stationary"). Statistically, this double difference amounted to an interaction inasmuch as the areas identified were the areas that increased their responsiveness when larger corrections had to be performed. Behavioral data showed, in agreement with earlier studies (Prablanc and Martin, 1992; Desmurget et al., 1999b), that the subjects were both accurate at reaching to the stationary targets and able to update their movement smoothly and early in response to the target jump. PET difference images showed that these corrections were mediated by a restricted network involving the parietal cortex, the frontal cortex, and the cerebellum (figure 10.5). The parietal activation was located in the left intraparietal sulcus, in a region that is generally considered the rostral part of the posterior parietal cortex (PPC). The cerebellar activation was found in the right anterior parasagittal cerebellar cortex, in a region associated with the production of arm movements. The frontal activation was located in the arm-related area of the primary motor cortex. The potential role of these structures is discussed below.

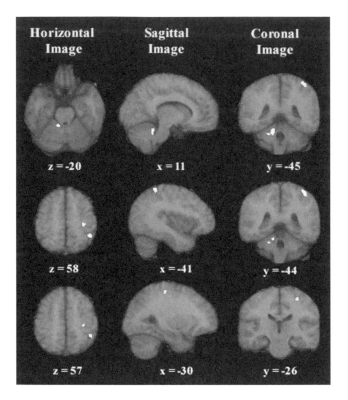

Figure 10.5
Functional anatomy of nonvisual feedback loops, addressed by positron-emission tomography (PET). In these horizontal, sagittal, and coronal difference images, activations are shown superimposed on a mean functional magnetic resonance image (fMRI) in talairach coordinates. On the horizontal and coronal images, the anatomic right side is shown on left side. On the sagittal images, positive values of *x* designate the right hemisphere (ipsilateral to the reaching arm); negative values, the left hemisphere (contralateral to the reaching arm). Images in the upper row are centered on the cerebellar activation site; those in the middle row, on the posterior parietal activation site; and those in the lower row, on the precentral activation site. (Adapted with permission from Desmurget et al., 2001.)

In addition to the PET data reported above, other recent evidence now links the posterior parietal cortex to the process of movement guidance. Among this evidence, the TMS results (Desmurget et al., 1999b) described in section 10.4 is indisputably the most compelling: When the normal functioning of the PPC was perturbed after hand movement onset, internal nonvisual feedback loops allowing correction of the ongoing movement were disrupted. This deficit was recently replicated in clinical studies of a patient having bilateral ischemic lesions of the PPC (Pisella et al., 2000). The patient was asked to "look and point" to visual targets presented in front of her on a computer screen. In some trials, the target remained stationary, whereas, in others, it jumped at movement onset to a new location. Whereas the patient was able to reach the target properly in the stationary condition, she displayed a dramatic inability to correct her ongoing movements in the perturbed condition, generally pointing to the initial target location before initiating a second movement to the final target position. Control subjects exhibited early modifications of the hand path, as expected from earlier studies (Pélisson et al., 1986; Prablanc and Martin, 1992; Desmurget et al., 1999b).

Functionally, it has been suggested that a major role of posterior parietal cortex in movement guidance might be to determine whether and to what extent the current motor response is inadequate (Desmurget et al., 1999b; Desmurget and Grafton, 2000). This hypothesis is based on the observation that PPC displays three main properties that would be expected from an error detection module. First, it modulates its neural activity as the hand approaches the target, that is, as the motor error varies (MacKay, 1992). Second, it has access to a representation of the target and current hand location through afferent information coming from many sensory modalities (visual, proprioceptive, vestibular) and from the main motor structures (Andersen et al., 1997; Brodal and Bjaalie, 1997). Third, it plays a critical role in establishing stable relationships between heterogeneous data merging arm- and target-related signals into a common frame of reference (Clower et al., 1996; Colby, 1998; Xing and Andersen, 2000). To make this latter point clear it is necessary to emphasize that the dynamic motor error (DME) is not an absolute parameter, as implied, for the sake of simplicity, in the initial sections of this chapter. The DME can be computed in various reference frames for goal-directed movements. For instance, it may be defined in a retinal reference frame as the spatial vector joining the retinal projections of the hand and targets (Paillard, 1980, 1996). Also, it may be defined in an egocentric reference frame centered on either the head (McIntyre et al., 1997), the trunk (Yardley, 1990), the hand (Gordon et al., 1994; Vindras and Viviani, 1998), or the shoulder (Flanders et al., 1992). In this case, the error may be defined in extrinsic (or Cartesian) coordinates (Prablanc and Martin, 1992; Hoff and Arbib, 1993) or in intrinsic coordinates (e.g., difference between the current posture and the postural state to be reached; Desmurget and Prablanc, 1997; Gréa et al., 2000). DME may also be represented in an allocentric frame of reference (moving a cursor on a screen using a mouse), or in an object-centred reference frame (grasping a cup of coffee requires locating both the cup in an egocentric frame of reference and the handle in relation to the cup). As emphasized above, neurophysiological and clinical studies have demonstrated that the construction and maintenance of these multiple frames of reference depended critically on the posterior parietal cortex. For instance, Carey and colleagues (1997) reported the case of a patient with a so-called magnetic misreaching, who slavishly reached straight to the fixation point at which she was looking when required to reach to a target presented in her extrafoveal visual field. More recently, Binkofski and colleagues (1999) defined two new clinical syndromes termed *mirror agnosia* and *mirror ataxia* in patients with lesions of the PPC. The patients were asked to reach to and grasp a small ball attached to a stick held by the examiner. When the patients saw the ball under direct vision, they could readily perform this task, whereas, when they saw the ball as a reflection in a mirror, they could not make accurate reaches. The mirror agnosia patients with larger lesions always reached toward the mirror, rather than toward the object. The mirror ataxia patients, with smaller lesions, could reach in the general direction of the target but had difficulty locating it using vision. A critical step necessary to perform these types of reaching movements is the coregistration of multiple frames of reference.

Computation of a dynamic motor error value by the posterior parietal cortex might be achieved through forward modeling. According to this view, a forward model of the arm's dynamics, maintained within the PPC, would predict the final state of the system (e.g., hand position, posture). This prediction would then be compared to the reference state to reach (e.g., target location, target posture). A discrepancy between these two values would give rise to an error signal, as detailed in section 10.4 (figure 10.3). Although there is no direct evidence that PPC generates a prediction of the final state to be reached by the motor system, several arguments suggest that this assumption is not totally unfounded. As expected from the structure allowing forward estimation of the arm dynamics, the PPC integrates sensory signals from many modalities (visual, proprioceptive, auditory, vestibular), as well as efferent copy signals from motor structures (Andersen et al., 1997). In addition, recent studies have provided evidence that the PPC is involved in motor tasks requiring state prediction. Eskandar and Assad (1999) trained monkeys to use a joystick to guide a visual spot to a target. Sensory and motor aspects of this task were experimentally dissociated by occluding the spot transiently and by varying the relationship between the direction of the joystick and spot movements. The authors observed that neurons in the lateral intraparietal area did not respond to either visual input or motor output, but rather encoded a predictive representation of the movement of the stimulus. In agreement with this result, Sirigu and colleagues (1996, 1999) showed that patients with PPC lesions were not able to predict, through mental imagery, the time necessary to perform visually guided pointing gestures. Also, during the execution of finger movements, these patients were unable to decide whether a hand shown on a screen placed in front of them was their own hand or an alien hand. From this finding, one can hypothesize that complex motor disorders such as ideomotor apraxia are due to an inability to create a stable internal model of a gesture or action rather than a disturbance of a motor memory or retrieval.

Once defined in task coordinates (e.g., spatial or joint vector), the dynamic motor error needs to be converted into an actual corrective command. In the case of reaching movements, a primary candidate for this function is the cerebellum. This structure receives abundant input from posterior parietal cortex via the pontine nuclei (Brodal and Bjaalie, 1997; Middleton and Strick, 1998). In addition, converging evidence has demonstrated that inverse models were represented within the cerebellum (Wolpert et al., 1998; Kawato, 1999; Imamizu et al., 2000) and that patients with cerebellar lesions displayed a chronic inability to accurately define the pattern of muscle activation required to direct the hand along a specific path (Bastian et al., 1996; Day et al., 1998). Although on-line trajectory adjustments are not suppressed after extensive lesions of the cerebellum in human (Day et al., 1998), path corrections generated by cerebellar patients are characterized by excessive deviations and ill-turned muscle activation patterns. Such inappropriate compensations are also observed in manual tracking tasks (Haggard et al., 1995).

The previous observations suggest that the cerebellar contribution to on-line movement guidance may be to convert the dynamic motor error signal computed by posterior parietal cortex into an appropriate corrective command. Ultimately, this corrective command needs to interfere with the ongoing motor command. In light of the PET study carried out by our group (Desmurget et al., 2001) and reported above, this interference may be achieved by modulating the neural signal issued by the primary motor cortex. In agreement with this view, it has been shown that the primary motor cortex (M1) receives substantial input from the cerebellum via the ventrolateral thalamus (Asanuma et al., 1983; Brodal and Bjaalie, 1997; Hoover and Strick, 1999). On the other hand, the motor system may be organized in a relative hierarchy such that the primary motor cortex is mainly involved in the low-level aspects of motor control. Consistent with this view, it was shown that purely kinematic and dynamic aspects of the movement are more commonly represented in the motor cortex than, for instance, in the parietal or premotor areas, which seem to encode more abstract variables (Alexander and Crutcher, 1990; Scott et al., 1997; Shen and Alexander, 1997; Turner et al., 1998).

Given this hypothetical scheme for updating a motor command, is there evidence that the posterior parietal cortex cerebellum and motor cortex are working as a functionally connected network? One way to answer this question is to test the PET imaging data reported above (Desmurget et al., 2001) for functional connectivity. We used the partial least squares (PLS) technique to identify brain areas in which there was a strong correlation with activity measured within the intraparietal sulcus of posterior parietal cortex that was specific to the eye-hand tasks (McIntosh, 1996). To do this, the PPC activity was cross-correlated with activity from every other voxel in the brain, for all four tasks (eye, eye-hand, eye-jump, eye-hand-jump). This large correlation matrix was evaluated with singular value decomposition, and reliable latent variables were identified by permutation testing (for methodological details, see McIntosh, 1999). Of particular interest was the second latent variable, which identified interactions between posterior parietal cortex, the rest of the brain, and the task where the eye-hand tasks scaled inversely to the eye-only tasks. The results shown in figure 10.6 show strong, eye-hand-related correlations of PPC activity with left superior parietal and motor cortex, left supplementary motor area, left putamen, and right anterior cerebellum. Stated differently, during on-line control of eye-hand reaching, neural and synaptic activity

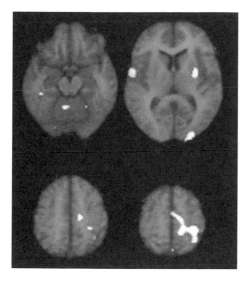

Figure 10.6
Functional connectivity of parietal cortex during on-line error correction. Brain areas showing strong, task-specific correlation (eye-hand movements) with activity in intraparietal cortex (using data from Desmurget et al., 2001) are shown in white. For both stationary and jump conditions of the eye-hand task (and inversely the eye-only tasks), activity of the left superior parietal and motor cortex, left supplementary motor area, left putamen, and right anterior cerebellum correlated with that in the intraparietal sulcus. Significance of the brain salience images was determined by bootstrap testing of latent images, with a standard error cutoff of 2 (for method, see McIntosh, 1996). Anatomic right side is shown on left side.

in these areas scale with the PPC. This finding supports the basic model linking posterior parietal cortex, cerebellum, and motor cortex as a functional unit for on-line control, and it implicates the basal ganglia in this process as well.

Thus there is considerable support for the hypothesis that parietal-cerebellar circuits are critical for hand movement guidance. Based on recent neurophysiological and clinical observations, we hypothesize that posterior parietal cortex computes a dynamic motor error value by comparing, through forward modeling, the updated location of the visual target and the estimated movement endpoint. This value is then sent to the cerebellum, which converts it into a corrective motor command, which modulates the neural signal issued by the primary motor cortex. Of course, this model does not imply that other areas, such as the premotor cortex, the colliculus, or the basal ganglia cannot be involved in movement guidance. In agreement with this observation, recent evidence has suggested that basal ganglia play a critical role in the regulation of movement force during the movement (Turner et al., 2000; Grafton et al., 2001), a possibility that may have been overlooked in the PET study described above (Desmurget et al., 2001) inasmuch as the correction was almost exclusively directional in this case. It is clear that further studies need to be performed to fully understand the functional anatomy of movement guidance.

10.6   Conclusion

Because accurate movements can be achieved in absence of sensory information, reaching movements were thought to be primarily under preprogrammed control and sensory feedback loops to exert only a limited influence at the very end of a trajectory. The present chapter challenges this view. As we have demonstrated, ongoing movement unfolds under the constant supervision of powerful internal feedback loops, which rely on a forward model integrating sensory inflow and motor outflow to evaluate the consequences of motor commands sent to the arm. With such a model, the probable position and velocity of the effector can be estimated with negligible delays, and even predicted in advance, thus making feedback strategies possible for fast reaching movements. The parietal lobe and cerebellum play a critical role in this process.

Acknowledgments

The work described in this chapter was funded by grant NS33504 and National Institutes of Health and by the McDonnell Foundation.

References

Agarwal, G. C., and Gottlieb, G. L. (1980). Electromyographic responses to sudden torques about the ankle joint in man. In *Tutorials in Motor Behavior*, G. E. Stelmach and J. Requin (eds.). Amsterdam: North-Holland, pp. 213–229.

Alexander, G. E., and Crutcher, M. D. (1990). Neural representations of the target (goal) of visually guided arm movements in three motor areas of the monkey. *J. Neurophysiol.* 64: 164–178.

Andersen, R. A., Snyder, L. H., Bradley, D. C., and Xing, J. (1997). Multimodal representation of space in the posterior parietal cortex and its use in planning movements. *Annu. Rev. Neurosci.* 20: 303–330.

Arbib, M. A. (1981). Perceptual structures and distributed motor control. In *Handbook of Physiology*. Sect. 1, *The Nervous System*. Vol. 2, *Motor Control,* W. B. Brooks (ed.). Baltimore: Williams and Wilkins, pp. 1449–1480.

Asanuma, C., Thach, W. R., and Jones, E. G. (1983). Anatomical evidence for segregated focal groupings of efferent cells and their terminal ramifications in the cerebellothalamic pathway of the monkey. *Brain Res.* 286: 267–297.

Bard, C., Hay, L., and Fleury, M. (1985). Role of peripheral vision in the directional control of rapid aiming movements. *Can. J. Psychol.* 39: 151–161.

Bard, C., Paillard, J., Fleury, M., Hay, L., and Larue, J. (1990). Positional versus directional control loops in visuomotor pointing. *Cah. Psychol. Cogn.* 10: 145–156.

Bard, C., Turrell, Y., Fleury, M., Teasdale, N., Lamarre, Y., and Martin, O. (1999). Deafferentation and pointing with visual double-step perturbations. *Exp. Brain Res.* 125: 410–416.

Bastian, A. J., Martin, T. A., Keating, J. G., and Thach, W.T. (1996). Cerebellar ataxia: Abnormal control of interaction torques across multiple joints. *J. Neurophysiol.* 76: 492–509.

Beaubaton, D., and Hay, L. (1986). Contribution of visual information to feedforward and feedback processes in rapid pointing movements. *Hum. Mov. Sci.* 5: 19–34.

Becker, W., and Fuchs, A. E. (1969). Further properties of the human saccadic system: eye movements and correction saccades with and without visual fixation points *Vision Res.* 19: 1247–1258.

Beggs, W. D., and Howarth, C. I. (1970). Movement control in a repetitive motor task. *Nature* 225: 752–753.

Biguer, B., Jeannerod, M., and Prablanc, C. (1982). The coordination of eye, head and arm movements during reaching at a single visual target. *Exp. Brain Res.* 46: 301–304.

Binkofski, F., Buccino, G., Dohle, C., Seitz, R. J., and Freund, H. J. (1999). Mirror agnosia and mirror ataxia constitute different parietal lobe disorders. *Ann. Neurol.* 46: 51–61.

Bizzi, E., Accornero, N., Chapple, W., and Hogan, N. (1984). Posture control and trajectory formation during arm movement. *J. Neurosci.* 4: 2738–2744.

Bizzi, E., Hogan, N., Mussa-Ivaldi, F. A., and Giszter, S. (1992). Does the nervous system use the equilibrium point control to guide single and multiple joint movements. *Behav. Brain Sci.* 15: 603–613.

Blouin, J., Teasdale, N., Bard, C., and Fleury, M. (1993a). Directional control of rapid movements: The role of the kinetic visual feedback system. *Can. J. Physiol. Pharmacol.* 47: 678–696.

Blouin, J., Bard, C., Teasdale, N., and Fleury, M. (1993b). On-line versus off-line control of rapid aiming movements. *J. Mot. Behav.* 25: 275–279.

Bock, O. (1993). Localization of objects in the peripheral visual field. *Behav. Brain Res.* 56: 77–84.

Bossom, J. (1972). Time of recovery of voluntary movement following dorsal rhizotomy. *Brain Res.* 45: 247–250.

Bossom, J. (1974). Movement without proprioception. *Brain Res.* 71: 285–296.

Bowditch, H. P., and Southard, W. F. (1880). A comparison of sight and touch. *J. Physiol. Lond.* 3: 232–245.

Brodal, P., and Bjaalie, J. G. (1997). Salient anatomic features of the cortico-ponto-cerebellar pathway. *Prog. Brain Res.* 114: 227–249.

Carey, D. P., Coleman, R. J., and Della Sala, S. (1997). Magnetic misreaching. *Cortex* 33: 639–652.

Carlton, L. G. (1981). Processing visual feedback information for movement control. *J. Exp. Psychol.* 7: 1019–1030.

Chernikoff, R., and Taylor, F. (1952). Reaction time to kinaesthetic stimulation resulting from sudden arm displacement. *J. Exp. Psychol.* 43: 1–8.

Clower, D. M., Hoffman, J. M., Votaw, J. R., Faber, T. L., Woods, R. P., and Alexander, G. (1996). Role of posterior parietal cortex in the recalibration of visually guided reaching. *Nature* 383: 618–621.

Colby, C. L. (1998). Action-oriented spatial reference frames in cortex. *Neuron* 20: 15–24.

Cooke, J. D., and Diggles, V. A. (1984). Rapid error correction during human arm movements: Evidence for central monitoring. *J. Mot. Behav.* 16: 348–363.

Cordo, P. J. (1987). Mechanisms controlling accurate changes in elbow torque in humans. *J. Neurosci.* 7: 432–442.

Cordo, P. J. (1990). Kinesthetic control of a multijoint movement sequence. *J. Neurophysiol.* 63: 161–172.

Crago, P. E., Houk, J. C., and Hasan, Z. (1976). Regulatory actions of human stretch reflex. *J. Neurophysiol.* 39: 925–935.

Day, B. L., and Marsden, C. D. (1982). Accurate repositioning of the human thumb against unpredictable dynamic loads is dependent upon peripheral feedback. *J. Physiol. Lond.* 327: 393–407.

Day, B. L., Thompson, P. D., Harding, A. E., and Marsden, C. D. (1998). Influence of vision on upper limb reaching movements in patients with cerebellar ataxia. *Brain* 121: 357–372.

Deiber, M. P., Ibáñez, V., Sadato, N., and Hallett, M. (1996). Cerebral structures participating in motor preparation in humans: A positron-emission tomography study. *J. Neurophysiol.* 75: 233–247.

Desmurget, M., and Grafton, S. (2000). Forward modeling allows feedback control for fast reaching movements. *Trends Cogn. Sci.* 4: 423–431.

Desmurget, M., and Prablanc, C. (1997). Postural control of three-dimensional prehension movements. *J. Neurophysiol.* 77: 452–464.

Desmurget, M., Rossetti, Y., Prablanc, C., Stelmach, G. E., and Jeannerod, M. (1995). Representation of hand position prior to movement and motor variability. *Can. J. Physiol. Pharmacol.* 73: 262–272.

Desmurget, M., Rossetti, Y., Jordan, M., Meckler, C., and Prablanc, C. (1997). Viewing the hand prior to movement improves accuracy of pointing performed toward the unseen contralateral hand. *Exp. Brain Res.* 115: 180–186.

Desmurget, M., Pélisson, D., Rossetti, Y., and Prablanc, C. (1998). From eye to hand: Planning goal-directed movements. *Neurosci. Biobehav. Rev.* 22: 761–788.

Desmurget, M., Prablanc, C., Jordan, M. I., and Jeannerod, M. (1999a). Are reaching movements planned to be straight and invariant in the extrinsic space: Kinematic comparison between compliant and unconstrained motions. *Q. J. Exp. Psychol.* 52A: 981–1020.

Desmurget, M., Epstein, C. M., Turner, R. S., Prablanc, C., Alexander, G. E., and Grafton, S. T. (1999b). Role of the posterior parietal cortex in updating reaching movements to a visual target. *Nat. Neurosci.* 2: 563–567.

Desmurget, M., Vindras, P., Gréa, H., Viviani, P., and Grafton, S. T. (2000). Proprioception does not quickly drift during visual occlusion. *Exp. Brain Res.* 134: 363–377.

Desmurget, M., Gréa, H., Grethe, J. S., Prablanc, C., Alexander, G. E., Grafton, S. T. (2001). Functional anatomy of nonvisual feedback loops during reaching: A positron-emission tomography study. *J. Neurosci.* 21: 2919–2928.

Dewhurst, D. J. (1967). Neuromuscular control system. *IEEE Trans. Biomed. Eng.* 14: 167–171.

De Wolf, S., Slijper, H., and Latash, M. L. (1998). Anticipatory postural adjustments during self-paced and reaction time movements. *Exp. Brain Res.* 121: 7–19.

Eskandar, E. N., and Assad, J. A. (1999). Dissociation of visual, motor and predictive signals in parietal cortex during visual guidance. *Nat. Neurosci.* 2: 88–93.

Evarts, E. V., and Tanji, J. (1974). Gating of motor cortex reflexes by prior instruction. *Brain Res.* 71: 479–494.

Evarts, E. V., and Vaughn, W. J. (1978). Intended arm movements in response to externally produced arm displacements in man. In *Cerebral Motor Control in Man: Long Loop Mechanisms*, J. E. Desmedt (ed.). Basel: Karger, pp. 178–192.

Feldman, A. G. (1986). Once more on the equilibrium-point hypothesis (L model) for motor control. *J. Mot. Behav.* 18: 17–54.

Feldman, A. G., and Levin, M. F. (1995). The origin and use of positional frames of reference in motor control. *Behav. Brain Sci.* 18: 723–806.

Flanagan, J. R., and Wing, A. M. (1997). The role of internal models in motion planning and control: Evidence from grip force adjustments during movements of handheld loads. *J. Neurosci.* 17: 1519–1528.

Flanagan, J. R., Ostry, D. J., and Feldman, A. G. (1993). Control of trajectory modifications in target-directed reaching. *J. Mot. Behav.* 25: 140–152.

Flanders, M., and Cordo, P. J. (1989). Kinesthetic and visual control of a bimanual task: Specification of direction and amplitude. *J. Neurosci.* 9: 447–453.

Flanders, M., Helms-Tillery, S. I., and Soechting, J. F. (1992). Early stages in sensorimotor transformations. *Behav. Brain Sci.* 15: 309–362.

Flanders, M., Pellegrini, J. J., and Geisler, S. D. (1996). Basic features of phasic activation for reaching in vertical planes. *Exp. Brain Res.* 110: 67–79.

Flash, T. (1987). The control of hand equilibrium trajectories in multi-joint arm movements. *Biol. Cybern.* 57: 257–274.

Flash, T., and Hogan, N. (1985). The coordination of arm movements: An experimentally confirmed mathematical model. *J. Neurosci.* 5: 1688–1703.

Gentilucci, M., Chieffi, S., Deprati, E., Saetti, M. C., and Toni, I. (1996). Visual illusion and action. *Neuropsychologia* 34: 369–376.

Gerdes, V. G., and Happee, R. (1994). The use of internal representation in fast goal-directed movements: A modeling approach. *Biol. Cybern.* 70: 513–524.

Ghez, C., Gordon, J., and Ghilardi, M. F. (1995). Impairments of reaching movements in patients without proprioception: 2. Effects of visual information on accuracy. *J. Neurophysiol.* 73: 361–372.

Godaux, E., and Cheron, G. (1989). *Le mouvement.* Paris: Medsci/McGraw-Hill.

Gomi, H., and Kawato, M. (1996). Equilibrium-point control hypothesis examined by measured arm stiffness during multijoint movement. *Science* 272: 117–120.

Goodale, M. A., Pélisson, D., and Prablanc, C. (1986). Large adjustments in visually guided reaching do not depend on vision of the hand and perception of target displacement. *Nature* 320: 748–750.

Gordon, J., Ghilardi, M. F., and Ghez, C. (1994). Accuracy of planar reaching movements: 1. Independence of direction and extent variability. *Exp. Brain Res.* 99: 97–111.

Grafton, S. T., Mazziotta, J. C., Woods, R. P., and Phelps, M. E. (1992). Human functional anatomy of visually guided finger movements. *Brain* 115: 565–587.

Grafton, S. T., Fagg, A. H., Woods, R. P., and Arbib, M. A. (1996). Functional anatomy of pointing and grasping in humans. *Cereb. Cortex* 6: 226–237.

Grafton, S. T., Desmurget, M., Grea, H., and Turner, R. S. (2001). Pointing errors in Parkinson's disease reflect feedback inaccuracy. Paper presented at fifty-third annual meeting of the American Academy of Neurology, Philadelphia. May 5–11.

Gréa, H., Desmurget, M., and Prablanc, C. (2000). Postural invariance in three-dimensional reaching and grasping movements. *Exp. Brain Res.* 134: 155–162.

Gribble, P. L., and Ostry, D. J. (1996). Origins of the power law relation between movement velocity and curvature: Modeling the effects of muscle mechanics and limb dynamics. *J. Neurophysiol.* 76: 2853–2860.

Gribble, P. L., and Ostry, D. J. (1999). Compensation for interaction torques during single- and multijoint limb movement. *J. Neurophysiol.* 82: 2310–2326.

Guthrie, B. L., Porter, J. D., and Sparks, D. L. (1983). Corollary discharge provides accurate eye position information to the oculomotor system. *Science* 221: 1193–1195.

Hagbarth, K. E. (1967). EMG studies of stretch reflexes in man. *Electroencephalogr. Clin. Neurophysiol. Suppl.* 25: 74–79.

Haggard, P., Miall, R. C., Wade, D., Fowler, S., Richardson, A., Anslow, P., and Stein, J. (1995). Damage to cerebellocortical pathways after closed head injury: A behavioural and magnetic resonance imaging study. *J. Neurol. Neurosurg. Psychiatry* 58: 433–438.

Harris, C. M. (1995). Does saccadic undershoot minimize saccadic flight-time? A Monte Carlo study. *Vision Res.* 35: 691–701.

Harris, C. M., and Wolpert, D. M. (1998). Signal-dependent noise determines motor planning. *Nature* 394: 780–784.

Hatsopoulos, N. G. (1994). Is a virtual trajectory necessary in reaching movements? *Biol. Cybern.* 70: 541–551.

Herrmann, U., and Flanders, M. (1998). Directional tuning of single motor units. *J. Neurosci.* 18: 8402–8416.

Higgins, J. R., and Angel, R. W. (1970). Correction of tracking errors without sensory feedback. *J. Exp. Psychol.* 84: 412–416.

Hoff, B., and Arbib, M. A. (1993). Models of trajectory formation and temporal interaction of reach and grasp. *J. Mot. Behav.* 25: 175–192.

Hollerbach, J. M. (1982). Computers, brains and the control of movement. *Trends Neurosci.* 5: 189–192.

Hollerbach, J. M., and Flash, T. (1982). Dynamic interaction between limb segments during planar arm movements. *Biol. Cybern.* 44: 67–77.

Hoover, J. E., and Strick, P. L. (1999). The organization of cerebellar and basal ganglia outputs to primary motor cortex as revealed by retrograde transneuronal transport of herpes simplex virus type 1. *J. Neurosci.* 19: 1446–1463.

Imamizu, H., Miyauchi, S., Tamada, T., Sasaki, Y., Takino, R., Putz, B., Yoshioka, T., and Kawato, M. (2000). Human cerebellar activity reflecting an acquired internal model of a new tool. *Nature* 403: 192–195.

Inoue, K., Kawashima, R., Satoh, K., Kinomura, S., Goto, R., Koyama, M., Sugiura, M., Ito, M., and Fukuda, H. (1998). PET study of pointing with visual feedback of moving hands. *J. Neurophysiol.* 79: 117–125.

Jaeger, R. J., Agarwal, G. C., and Gottlieb, G. L. (1979). Directional errors of movement and their correction in a discrete tracking task. *J. Mot. Behav.* 11: 123–133.

Jeannerod, M. (1988). *The Neural and Behavioural Organization of Goal-Directed Movements.* Oxford: Clarendon Press.

Katayama, M., and Kawato, M. (1993). Virtual trajectory and stiffness ellipse during multijoint arm movement predicted by neural inverse models. *Biol. Cybern.* 69: 353–362.

Kawato, M. (1999). Internal models for motor control and trajectory planning. *Curr. Opin. Neurobiol.* 9: 718–727.

Keele, S. W. (1968). Movement control in skilled motor performance. *Psychol. Bull.* 70: 387–403.

Keele, S. W., and Posner, M. I. (1968). Processing of visual feedback in rapid movements. *J. Exp. Psychol.* 77: 155–158.

Keller, E. L., Gandhi, N. J., and Shieh, J. M. (1996). Endpoint accuracy in saccades interrupted by stimulation in the omnipause region in monkey. *Vis. Neurosci.* 13: 1059–1067.

Kelso, J., and Holt, K. G. (1980). Explorating a vibratory systems analysis of human movement production. *J. Neurophysiol.* 43: 1186–1196.

Knapp, H. D., Taub, E., and Berman, A. J. (1963). Movements in monkeys with deafferented forelimbs. *Exp. Neurol.* 7: 305–315.

Komilis, E., Pélisson, D., and Prablanc, C. (1993). Error processing in pointing at randomly feedback-induced double-step stimuli. *J. Mot. Behav.* 25: 299–308.

Lacquaniti, F., Perani, D., Guigon, E., Bettinardi, V., Carrozzo, M., Grassi, F., Rossetti, Y., and Fazio, F. (1997). Visuomotor transformations for reaching to memorized targets: A PET study. *NeuroImage* 5: 129–146

Larish, D. D., Volp, C. M., and Wallace, S. A. (1984). An empirical note of attaining a spatial target after distorting the initial conditions of movement via muscle vibration. *J. Mot. Behav.* 15: 15–83.

Lassek, A. M. (1953). Inactivation of voluntary motor function following rhizotomy. *J. Neuropath. Exp. Neurol.* 12: 83–87.

Lassek, A. M. (1955). Effect of combined afferent lesions on motor functions. *Neurology* 5: 269–272.

Lassek, A. M., and Moyer, E. K. (1953). An ontogenic study of motor deficits following dorsal brachial rhizotomy. *J. Neurophysiol.* 16: 247–251.

Lee, R. G., and Tatton, W. G. (1975). Motor responses to sudden limb displacements in primates with specific CNS lesions and in human patients with motor system disorders. *Can. J. Neurol. Sci.* 2: 285–293.

MacKay, W. A. (1992). Properties of reach-related neuronal activity in cortical area 7A. *J. Neurophysiol.* 67: 1335–1345.

Marsden, C. D., Merton, P. A., Morton, H. B., Adam, J. E. R., and Hallett, M. (1978). Automatic and voluntary responses to muscle stretch in man. In *Cerebral Motor Control*, J. E. Desmedt (ed.). Basel: Karger, pp. 167–177.

Martin, O., and Prablanc, C. (1991). Two-dimensional control of trajectories towards unconsciously detected double step targets. In *Tutorials in Motor Neuroscience*, J. Requin and G. E. Stelmach (eds.). Amsterdam: Kluwer Academic, pp. 581–598.

McIntosh, A. R., Bookstein, F. L., Haxby, J. V., and Grady, C. L. (1996). Spatial pattern analysis of functional brain images using partial least squares. *NeuroImage* 3: 143–157.

McIntosh, A. R., Rajah, M. N., and Lobaugh, N. J. (1999). Interactions of prefrontal cortex in relation to awareness in sensory learning. *Science* 284: 1531–1533.

McIntyre, J., Stratta, F., and Lacquaniti, F. (1997). Viewer-centered frame of reference for pointing to memorized targets in three-dimensional space. *J. Neurophysiol.* 78: 1601–1618.

Meyer, D. E., Abrams, D. A., Kornblum, S., Wright, C. E., and Smith, J. E. K. (1988). Optimality in human motor performance: Ideal control of rapid aimed movements. *Psychol. Rev.* 95: 340–370.

Miall, R. C., Weir, D. J., Wolpert, D. M., and Stein, J. F. (1993). Is the cerebellum a Smith predictor? *J. Mot. Behav.* 25: 203–216.

Middleton, F. A., and Strick, P. L. (1998). The cerebellum: An overview. *Trends Neurosci.* 21: 367–369.

Milner, T. E. (1992). A model for the generation of movements requiring endpoint precision. *Neurosci.* 49: 487–496.

Morasso, P. (1981). Spatial control of arm movements. *Exp. Brain Res.* 42: 223–227.

Mott, F. W., and Sherrington, C. S. (1895). Experiments upon the influence of sensory nerves upon movement and nutrition of the limbs. *Proc. R. Soc. Lond. Biol. Sci.* B57: 481–488.

Munk, H. (1909). *Über die Folgen Sensibilitätverlustes der Extremität für deren Motilität.* In *Über die Funktionen von Hirn und Rückenmark: Gesammelte Mitteilungen*, Berlin: Hirschwald, pp. 247–285.

Newell, K. M., and Houk, J. C. (1983). Speed and accuracy of compensatory responses to limb disturbances. *J. Exp. Psychol. Hum. Percept. Perform.* 9: 58–74.

Paillard, J. (1980). The multichanneling of visual cues and the organization of a visually guided response. In *Tutorials in Motor Behavior,* G. E. Stelmach and J. Requin (eds.). Amsterdam: North-Holland, pp. 259–279.

Paillard, J. (1982). The contribution of peripheral and central vision to visually guided reaching. In *Analysis of Visual Behavior,* D. J. Ingle, M.A. Goodale, and R. J. W. Mansfield (eds.). Cambridge, Mass.: MIT Press, pp. 367–382.

Paillard, J. (1996). Fast and slow feedback loops for the visual correction of spatial errors in a pointing task: A reappraisal. *Can. J. Physiol. Pharmacol.* 74: 401–417.

Paillard, J., and Brouchon, M. (1968). Active and passive movements in the calibration of position sense. In *The Neuropsychology of Spatially Oriented Behavior,* S. J. Freedman (ed.). Homewood, Ill.: Dorsey Press, pp. 35–56.

Pélisson, D., Prablanc, C., Goodale, M. A., and Jeannerod, M. (1986). Visual control of reaching movements without vision of the limb: 2. Evidence of fast unconscious processes correcting the trajectory of the hand to the final position of a double step stimulus. *Exp. Brain Res.* 62: 303–311.

Pélisson, D., Guitton, D., and Goffart, L. (1995). On-line compensation of gaze shifts perturbed by micro-stimulation of the superior colliculus in the cat with unrestrained head. *Exp. Brain Res.* 106: 196–204.

Pisella, L., Grea, H., Tilikete, C., Vighetto, A., Desmurget, M., Rode, G., Boisson, D., and Rossetti, Y. (2000). An "automatic-pilot" for the hand in human posterior parietal cortex: Toward reinterpreting optic ataxia. *Nat. Neurosci.* 3: 729–736.

Plamondon, R., and Alimi, A. M. (1997). Speed-accuracy trade-offs in target-directed movements. *Behav. Brain Sci.* 20: 1–21.

Polit, A., and Bizzi, E. (1979). Characteristics of motor programs underlying arm movements in monkeys. *J. Neurophysiol.* 42: 183–194.

Prablanc, C., and Jeannerod, M. (1975). Corrective saccades: Dependence on retinal reafferent signals. *Vision Res.* 15: 465–469.

Prablanc, C., and Martin, O. (1992). Automatic control during hand reaching at undetected two-dimensional target displacements. *J. Neurophysiol.* 67: 455–469.

Prablanc, C., Echallier, J. F., Jeannerod, M., and Komilis, E. (1979a). Optimal response of eye and hand motor systems in pointing at visual target: 2. Static and dynamic visual cues in the control of hand movement. *Biol. Cybern.* 35: 183–187.

Prablanc, C., Echallier, J. F., Komilis, E., and Jeannerod, M. (1979b). Optimal response of eye and hand motor system in pointing at visual target: 1. Spatio-temporal characteristics of eye and hand movements and their relationships when varying the amount of visual information. *Biol. Cybern.* 35: 113–124.

Prablanc, C., Pélisson, D., and Goodale, M. A. (1986). Visual control of reaching movements without vision of the limb: 1. Role of extraretinal feedback of target position in guiding the hand. *Exp. Brain Res.* 62: 293–302.

Rack, P. M. H. (1981). Limitations of somatosensory feedback in control of posture and movement. In *Handbook of Physiology.* Sect. 1, *The Nervous System.* Vol. 2, *Motor Control,* V. B. Brooks (ed.). Baltimore: Williams and Wilkins, pp. 229–256.

Redon, C., Hay, L., and Velay, J. L. (1991). Proprioceptive control of goal-directed movements in man studied by means of vibratory muscle tendon stimulation. *J. Mot. Behav.* 23: 101–108.

Rossetti, Y., Stelmach, G. E., Desmurget, M., Prablanc, C., and Jeannerod, M. (1994). The effect of viewing the static hand prior to movement onset on pointing kinematics and accuracy. *Exp. Brain. Res.* 101: 323–330.

Rossetti, Y., Desmurget, M., and Prablanc, C. (1995). Vectorial coding of movement: Vision proprioception or both? *J. Neurophysiol.* 74: 457–463.

Rothwell, J. C., Traub, M. M., Day, B. L., Obeso, J. A., Thomas, P. K., and Marsden, C. D. (1982). Manual motor performance in a deafferented man. *Brain* 105: 515–542.

Sainburg, R. L., Ghilardi, M. F., Poizner, H., and Ghez, C. (1995). Control of limb dynamics in normal subjects and patients without proprioception. *J. Neurophysiol.* 73: 820–835.

Sanes, J. N., Mauritz, K. H., Dalakas, M. C., and Evarts, E. V. (1985). Motor control in human with large-fiber sensory neuropathy. *Hum. Neurobiol.* 4: 101–114.

Scott, S. H., Sergio, L. E., and Kalaska, J. F. (1997). Reaching movements with similar hand paths but different arm orientations: 2. Activity of individual cells in dorsal premotor cortex and parietal area 5. *J. Neurophysiol.* 78: 2413–2426.

Shen, L., and Alexander, G. E. (1997). Preferential representation of instructed target location versus limb trajectory in dorsal premotor area. *J. Neurophysiol.* 77: 1195–1212.

Sirigu, A., Duhamel, J. R., Cohen, L., Pillon, B., Dubois, B., and Agid, Y. (1996). The mental representation of hand movements after parietal cortex damage. *Science* 273: 1564–1568.

Sirigu, A., Daprati, E., Pradat-Diehl, P., Franck, N., and Jeannerod, M. (1999). Perception of self-generated movement following left parietal lesion. *Brain* 122: 1867–1874.

Taub, E. (1976). Motor behavior following deafferentation in the developing and motorically immature monkey. In *Neural Control of Locomotion*, R. M. Herman, S. Grillner, D. G. Stein, and D. G. Stuart (eds.). New York: Plenum Press, pp. 675–705.

Taub, E., and Berman, A. J. (1968). Movement and learning in the absence of sensory feedback. In The Neurophysiology of Spatially Oriented Behavior, S. J. Freedman (ed.). Homewood; Ill.: Dorsey Press, pp. 173–192.

Teasdale, N., Blouin, J., Bard, C., and Fleury, M. (1991). Visual guidance of pointing movements: Kinematic evidence for static and kinetic feedback channels. In *Tutorials in Motor Neuroscience*, J. Requin and G. E. Stelmach (eds.). Amsterdam: Kluwer Academic, pp. 463–475.

Turner, R. S., Owens, J. W., Jr., and Anderson, M. E. (1995). Directional variation of spatial and temporal characteristics of limb movements made by monkeys in a two-dimensional work space. *J. Neurophysiol.* 74: 684–697.

Turner, R. S., Grafton, S. T., Votaw, J. R., DeLong, M. R., and Hoffman, J. M. (1998). Motor subcircuits mediating the control of movement velocity: A PET study. *J. Neurophysiol.* 80: 2162–2176.

Turner, R. S., Desmurget, M., Grea, H., and Grafton, S. T. (2000). Pointing errors in Parkinson's disease. *Soc. Neurosci. Abstr.* 590: 1577. Paper presented at the thirtieth annual meeting of the Society for Neuroscience, New Orleans. November 4–9.

Twitchell, T. E. (1954). Sensory factors in purposive movements. *J. Neurophysiol.* 17: 239–252.

Uno, Y., Kawato, M., and Suzuki, R. (1989). Formation and control of optimal trajectory in human multijoint arm movement: Minimum torque-change model. *Biol. Cybern.* 61: 89–101.

van Beers, R. J., Sittig, A. C., and van der Gon, J. J. D. (1998). The precision of proprioceptive position sense. *Exp. Brain Res.* 122: 367–377.

van Sonderen, J. F., Gielen, C. C. A. M., and van der Gon, J. J. D. (1989). Motor programs for goal-directed movements are continuously adjusted according to changes in target location. *Exp. Brain Res.* 78: 139–146.

Vince, M. A. (1948). Corrective movements in a pursuit task. *Q. J. Exp. Psychol.* 1: 85–106.

Vindras, P., and Viviani, P. (1998). Frames of reference and control parameters in visuomanual pointing. *J. Exp. Psychol. Hum. Percept. Perform.* 24: 569–591.

Vindras, P., Desmurget, M., Prablanc, C., and Viviani, P. (1998). Pointing errors reflect biases in the perception of the initial hand position. *J. Neurophysiol.* 79: 3290–3294.

von Holst, E., and Mittelstaedt, H. (1950). Das Reafferenzprinzip: Wechselwirkung zwischen Zentralnervensystem und Peripherie. *Naturwissenschaften* 37: 464–476.

Wallace, S. A., and Newell, K. M. (1983). Visual control of discrete aiming movements. *Q. J. Exp. Psychol.* 35A: 311–321.

Wann, J. P., and Ibrahim, S. F. (1992). Does limb proprioception drift? *Exp. Brain Res.* 91: 162–166.

Winstein, C. J., Grafton, S. T., and Pohl, P. S. (1997). Motor task difficulty and brain activity: Investigation of goal-directed reciprocal aiming using positron-emission tomography. *J. Neurophysiol.* 77: 1581–1594.

Wolpert, D. M., Ghahramani, Z., and Jordan, M. I. (1995). An internal model for sensorimotor integration. *Science* 269: 1880–1882.

Wolpert, D. M., Miall, R. C., and Kawato, M. (1998). Internal models in the cerebellum. *Trends Cogn. Sci.* 2: 338–347.

Woodworth, R. S. (1899). The accuracy of voluntary movement. *Psychol. Rev. Monogr. Suppl.* 3.

Xing, J., and Andersen, R. A. (2000). Models of the posterior parietal cortex which perform multimodal integration and represent space in several coordinate frames. *J. Cogn Neurosci.* 12: 601–614.

Yardley, L. (1990). Contribution of somatosensory information to perception of the visual vertical of the body tilt and rotating visual field. *Percept. Psychophys.* 48: 131–134.

Zelaznik, H. N., Hawkins, B., and Kisselburgh, L. (1983). Rapid visual feedback processing in single-aiming movements. *J. Mot. Behav.* 15: 217–236.

V

Learning and Movement

Acquiring a new action involves altering both internal representations and the neural substrates in which they are realized. Bridging these two levels of analysis presents a formidable challenge, yet one that is at the very core of cognitive neuroscience. Padoa-Schioppa and Bizzi (chapter 11) work from a computational perspective to show that primary motor cortex contributes both to action production and learning: When monkeys acquire a new internal model of arm dynamics, neuronal activity in primary motor cortex undergoes a striking reorganization.

That children and adults throughout the world play games that involve catching and throwing objects belies the remarkably complex set of sensorimotor transformations the brain must solve in order for a hand to intercept a moving target. In their elegant analyses of neurophysiological data, Kruse and colleagues (chapter 12) document the dynamic temporal relationships between target movement, hand movement, and the intervening sensorimotor transformations that take place in motor cortical neurons during this complex act.

Beginning with the electrical mapping studies of Penfield and colleagues in the 1950s, it became apparent that human primary motor cortex is organized in a roughly topographical fashion. Noninvasive neuroimaging techniques have enabled us to explore the details of this topography and the functional relationships between primary motor cortex and other sensorimotor centers. Rotte (chapter 13) considers how these techniques can be used to resolve ongoing questions about the functional localization of and interactivity between areas within the motor system, and how the findings of this work might apply to disorders that affect action production.

11

Neuronal Plasticity in the Motor Cortex of Monkeys Acquiring a New Internal Model

Camillo Padoa-Schioppa and Emilio Bizzi

11.1 Introduction

When we reach for a glass of wine at the dinner table, our central nervous system (CNS) engages in a number of mental processes. It interprets the signals that arrive to our retinas, locates the glass on the table, and makes the decision to reach for the glass. Then, the CNS must design the trajectory (kinematics) that will bring our hand to the glass and compute the forces (dynamics) needed to implement the desired movement. Finally the CNS must activate the muscles to execute the reaching. Exactly what computations the CNS engages in and how and where they take place are fundamental questions in neuroscience.

The present chapter, in reviewing recent advances in our understanding of how the cortex controls movements, concentrates on neuronal activity that reflects the computation of movement kinematics and dynamics. Examining the activity of single cells, it shows that the neuronal activity in primary motor cortex (M1) undergoes a remarkable reorganization (plasticity) when monkeys learn new movement dynamics.

Sections 11.2 and 11.3 review a computational framework of motor control, focusing on the transformations the CNS must compute when producing movement, and on the concept of the internal model. Section 11.4 introduces the experimental paradigm used to dissociate neuronal activity related to movement kinematics from that related to movement dynamics, and that related to motor performance from that related to motor learning. Sections 11.5–11.8 present evidence for neuronal plasticity in M1 associated with the development of a new internal model of the dynamics. And section 11.9 summarizes our conclusions from the results presented.

11.2   Sensorimotor Transformations

One influential view in motor control is that the sensorimotor transformations occurring during sensory-guided movements are processed in
subsequent computational stages. With respect of the actual control of
movements, Alexander and Crutcher (1990a) proposed the scheme illustrated in figure 11.1. Their scheme includes processing (1) the goal (target),
(2) the hand trajectory, (3) the inverse kinematics, (4) the inverse dynamics,
and (5) the activation of muscles. Each of these five processing levels corresponds to a computed (motor) variable, together with a coordinate system.
For example, level 1, processing the goal (processing level) corresponds to
computing the location of the target (motor variable) in real space (coordinate system). Likewise, level 4, processing the inverse dynamics (processing
level) corresponds to computing the torques and their time derivatives (motor variables) in joint space (coordinate system).

From a theoretical perspective, the scheme of figure 11.1 is a *proposal*
of the transformations that the central nervous system *might* be computing.
In reality, the sequence of operations the CNS actually undertakes might
be either simpler or more complicated. For instance, the proposal that the
CNS might control movements by setting the stiffness of the appropriate
muscles (the equilibrium point hypothesis; for review, see Bizzi, 1988)
would greatly simplify the computation of the inverse kinematics and inverse dynamics. At the opposite extreme, no study to our knowledge has
truly tested the one-to-one correspondence between motor variables and

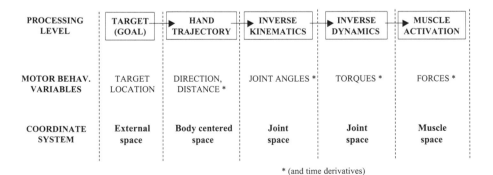

Figure 11.1
Scheme of sensorimotor transformations. (Reprinted with permission from Alexander and Crutcher, 1990a.)

coordinate system outlined in figure 11.1. For all we know, the transformation of the hand trajectory (in extrinsic coordinates) into the inverse kinematics (in intrinsic coordinates) might require two computational steps, not just one.

In defense of the scheme diagrammed in figure 11.1, we shall stress that evidence *against* it is, to date, inconclusive. The scheme is quite general and relatively comprehensive. In other words, researchers generally believe that the CNS operates simpler transformations than that outlined in figure 11.1, not more complicated or tortuous ones. However, alternative computational schemes for the control of voluntary movements still lack convincing support.

From the physiological perspective, it should be noted that the computational stages outlined in figure 11.1 do not simply map onto the neuronal activity of different cortical areas. In fact, several studies showed that different areas of the brain do not process different stages in a rigorously serial and independent manner. For example, Alexander and Crutcher (1990a, 1990b; Crutcher and Alexander, 1990) found that different neurons within the same area (e.g., the supplementary motor area, or SMA) can process different computational stages (e.g., goal and inverse dynamics), and that neurons in different areas (e.g., M1 and SMA) can process the same computational stage (e.g., inverse dynamics).

Nevertheless, we view the scheme of figure 11.1 as a valuable framework for understanding the control of voluntary movements, one that underlies many experimental studies, including ours. It highlights three points central to the purpose of this chapter: First, conceptually, a sensory-instructed movement requires a sequence of processing stages and related transformations. Second, the central nervous system needs, in particular, to transform the desired kinematics into suitable dynamics. And third, this transformation needs to solve an *inverse dynamics* problem. As will become clear in the section 11.3, this is a challenging computation.

11.3 Internal Models

In Newtonian mechanics, forces cause movements, according to the classical equation $\mathbf{f} = \mathbf{ma}$. In the case of a reaching movement, the contraction of muscles (forces) causes the movement of the hand (trajectory). Students of physics are typically asked to solve a "direct dynamics problem": How to compute the trajectory $\mathbf{q}$ (where $\partial_t^2\, \mathbf{q} = \mathbf{a}$), given a set of forces $\mathbf{f}$? In contrast, the central nervous system is faced with an "inverse dynamics problem": How to generate the appropriate muscle forces $\mathbf{f}$, given a desired trajectory $\mathbf{q}$?

For a realistic model of the human arm, the inverse dynamics problem is computationally challenging, for several reasons. First, because of the interacting degrees of freedom, the simple equation $\mathbf{f} = \mathbf{ma}$ assumes a much longer (several pages) and more complicated form. Second, the inverse dynamics problem (considered together with the inverse kinematics problem) is associated with a transformation from extrinsic to intrinsic coordinates. Third, the musculature of the arm is highly redundant; the same set of forces can be produced with very different sets of muscle contractions. Thus, quite apart from the actual implementation of the computed dynamics, the inverse dynamics problem is intrinsically ill posed. (Moreover, because many joint kinematics produce the same hand path, the inverse kinematics problem is also intrinsically ill posed.) Although several hypotheses have been proposed to explain how the central nervous system might simplify and solve these problems, the search for a convincing and comprehensive theory continues.

One emerging concept in motor control is that of the internal model (for reviews, see Wolpert and Ghahramani, 2000; Mussa-Ivaldi and Bizzi, 2000; Kawato, 1999). Specifically, the literature refers to feedforward internal models and feedback internal models. Of interest here are feedforward internal models, which, as internal representations of the dynamic properties of the limbs, represent the transformation of motor commands into movements. According to this view, the central nervous system uses internal models of the dynamics when planning and executing movements, simplifying the inverse dynamics problem by reducing the number of degrees of freedom. It is important to emphasize that internal models are models used by the central nervous system itself to execute movements, *not* models used by researchers to describe the CNS (Wolpert and Ghahramani, 2000).

For our purposes, the most important recent findings are that new internal models can be learned through experience (Shadmehr and Mussa-Ivaldi, 1994), consolidated in the hours following that learning (Brashers-Krug et al., 1996), and kept in long-term memory for later use (Li et al., 2001). In addition, internal models of the dynamics are learned independently of other internal models, for instance, internal models of the kinematics (Krakauer et al., 1999). Section 11.4 reviews some of these findings in greater detail.

11.4   Learning New Internal Models

Studies on the learning of new internal models of the dynamics generally submit human subjects to perturbing forces as they perform reaching movements. In our experiments, we used a monkey version of a paradigm originally designed for human studies. The psychophysics describing the development of a new internal model for the dynamics in monkeys closely parallel those found in humans and first described by Shadmehr and Mussa-Ivaldi (1994).

In our experiments, monkeys grasp the handle of a low-friction robot having two degrees of freedom and perform planar reaching movements from a central location to one of eight peripheral targets. Two torque motors, mounted at the base of the robot and connected independently to each joint, can apply perturbing forces to the handle. A computer monitor placed in front of the monkey displays the targets of the reaching movements and a cursor representing the position of the handle. The perturbing forces are described by "force fields."

Each experimental session is divided into three behavioral epochs: a "baseline" epoch, in which the monkey performs the task without a force field; a "force" epoch, in which a force field is applied; and a "washout" epoch, in which the force field is removed. The force fields are vector fields $\mathbf{F} = \mathbf{BV}$, where $\mathbf{V}$ is the hand velocity vector in Cartesian coordinates, and $\mathbf{B}$ is a constant 2×2 matrix. For $\mathbf{B}$, we chose the antidiagonal rotation matrix $[0, b; -b, 0]$, which defines a viscous, curl force field. The force field is "viscous" in that the magnitude of the applied forces is proportional to the hand velocity. It is "curl" in that the force direction is orthogonal to the direction of the hand velocity. Depending on the sign of "b," the curl is either clockwise or counterclockwise.

The course of a typical experimental session is shown in figure 11.2. During the baseline epoch (figure 11.2a, bottom left), the trajectories are essentially straight. When a counterclockwise force field is introduced in the early force epoch (figure 11.2a, top center), the performance deteriorates; the trajectories are deviated by the perturbing force. As the

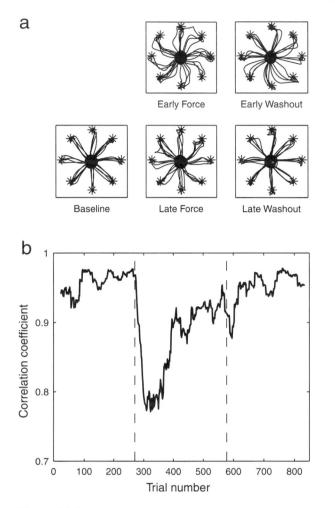

Figure 11.2
Psychophysics of motor adaptation. (*a*) Trajectories in real space roughly follow a straight line in the baseline epoch (*bottom left*), when no perturbation is present. In the early force epoch (*top center*), a counterclockwise force is introduced, and trajectories are initially deviated by the force field. As the monkeys continue in the task, however, the trajectories straighten out. After adaptation (late force, *bottom center*), the trajectories are indistinguishable from those in the baseline epoch. When the force field is removed, the monkeys show an aftereffect (early washout, *top right*); their trajectories are deviated in a way that mirrors that seen in the early force epoch. As monkeys readapt to the nonperturbing conditions, however, trajectories again straighten out in the late washout epoch (*bottom right*). In the analysis of neurons, we compared the activity recorded during trials with comparable kinematics, corresponding to the three bottom panels of the figure. (*b*) Correlation coefficient, plotted against the trial number, highlights the adaptation occurring during the force epoch, and the aftereffect. (Reprinted with permission from Gandolfo et al., 2000; © 2000 by the National Academy of Sciences.)

monkey continues to perform, however, the trajectories gradually straighten out. In other words, the monkey adapts to the perturbation. During the late force epoch (figure 11.2a, bottom center), the trajectories are essentially indistinguishable from those of the baseline epoch. When the force field is removed, we observe an aftereffect, as the trajectories deviate in a way that mirrors the early force epoch; after a brief readaptation phase, trajectories again straighten out in the late washout epoch (bottom right).

The adaptation process can also be seen by inspection of the correlation coefficient (CC; figure 11.2b), a measure of similarity between the actual trajectory and an ideal trajectory (for details, see Shadmehr and Mussa-Ivaldi, 1994). The CC ranges between −1 and 1, and is close to 1 for actual trajectories close to ideal. In the baseline epoch, the CC is close to 1. Early in the force epoch, the CC drops. As the adaptation occurs, the CC recovers, and gradually reaches a steady state. In the washout epoch, there is a brief drop of the CC, corresponding to the aftereffect. The monkey readily readapts to the nonperturbed conditions, and the correlation coefficient recovers its original high values.

The psychophysics illustrated in figure 11.2 highlight two important points. First, as the monkeys adapt to the perturbing force fields (in the force epoch), the kinematics of their movement gradually converge to that observed in the baseline. This convergence is evidence of a kinematic plan. Second, to adapt to the force field, the monkey must learn to transform the desired kinematics into new, adapted dynamics. In other words, the monkey must develop a new internal model of the dynamics.

11.5   Neuronal Plasticity in Primary Motor Cortex: Tune-in and Tune-out Cells

The experimental paradigm illustrated in figure 11.2 was specifically designed to study the neuronal correlates of motor adaptation. We wished to compare the neuronal activity recorded in trials with similar kinematics, corresponding to the three bottom panels of figure 11.2a. Whereas the kinematics of the movement are the same across behavioral epochs (baseline, force, and washout), the dynamics vary. More precisely, the dynamics are the same in the baseline and washout epochs and different in the force epoch (where the monkeys compensate for the external force field). This paradigm thus dissociates the neuronal activity related to kinematics from that related to the dynamics of the movement. Most important, the paradigm also dissociates neuronal activity related to motor performance (kinematics and dynamics) from that related to motor learning. This dissociation is obtained comparing the activity in the washout epoch with that in the baseline epoch. In the washout epoch, both the kinematics and the dynamics of the movement are the same as in the baseline. The only difference is that in the washout epoch the monkeys have recently adapted to the perturbing force field, having developed a new internal model of the dynamics. Thus differences in cell activity between these two epochs correlate with the *memory* of such experience.

Using this paradigm, we recorded the activity of 162 neurons in the primary motor cortex (M1) of two *Macaca nemestrina* monkeys performing the task. We analyzed the movement-related activity (from 200 ms before the movement onset up to the end of movement), separately in the three epochs (baseline, force, and washout). In general, we observed two phenomena of neuronal plasticity associated with the development of a new internal model. First, as the monkeys adapted to the perturbation, some cells developed a new directional tuning (see below). Second, neurons in general transformed their activity following the adaptation (see section 11.6).

Regarding the first phenomenon, we observed that cells not directionally tuned in the baseline epoch became tuned in the force epoch. In many cases, these cells maintained their tuning in the washout epoch; we named them "tune-in cells" (Gandolfo et al., 2000). The activity of one tune-in cell is plotted in figure 11.3a. Whereas the cell has low activity and no directional tuning in the baseline epoch, in the force epoch, it develops a directional tuning. In other words, the cell becomes committed to the task, entering the pool of active cells. As the monkey returns to the nonperturbed conditions (washout), the cell maintains its newly acquired tuning. Its activity thus seems to maintain a trace of the learning experience: It expresses some *memory*.

We also found some cells that lost their tuning as a consequence of the adaptation. The activity of one such "tune-out" cell is plotted in figure 11.3b. As the monkey adapts to the perturbation, the cell loses its tuning. Note that the cell is not just "lost": Its waveform (i.e., the signal of the cell) remains unchanged across epochs. We found that, of the 143 cells tuned in at least one epoch, 35 cells (24%) became tuned after adaptation

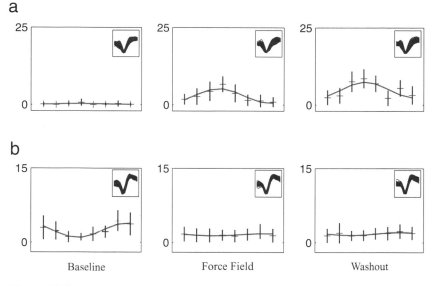

Figure 11.3

Neuronal plasticity: tune-in and tune-out cells. (*a*) Activity of tune-in cell plotted in linear coordinates. Although the cell has a low activity and no significant tuning in the baseline epoch (*left*), as the monkey adapts to the perturbing force, the cell acquires a directional tuning: It becomes committed to the task (*middle*). After removal of the perturbation, the activity of the cell remains directionally tuned (*right*). This plasticity underlies the development of a new internal model of the dynamics. Note that the "signal" of the cell is stable throughout the session, as can be seen from the waveforms plotted in the upper right of each graph. (*b*) Activity of tune-out cell plotted in linear coordinates. Initially tuned in the baseline epoch, this cell loses its tuning in the force epoch, as the monkey adapts to the force field. In the washout epoch, the cell remains untuned, as in the force epoch. Again, the waveforms of the cell were stable throughout the session. (Reprinted with permission from Gandolfo et al., 2000; © 2000 by the National Academy of Sciences.

to the force, and 19 cells (13%) lost their tuning after adaptation to the force (for details, see Gandolfo et al., 2000).

11.6   Constraints on the New Dynamics

For the purpose of investigating the neuronal correlates of the new internal models of the dynamics, the paradigm illustrated in figure 11.2 has two main advantages. First, as discussed in the previous section, the paradigm allows us to dissociate the neuronal activity related to the movement kinematics from that related to the movement dynamics, and that related to motor performance from that related to motor learning. Second, the specific dynamic perturbation used (i.e., curl, viscous force fields) imposes predictable changes on the electromyographic activity of muscles.

The electromyographic (EMG) activity of muscles as a function of the direction of the movement can be described by tuning curves. Furthermore, a preferred direction can be defined, as the direction of movement for which the muscle would contribute maximally. The choice of curl force fields imposes on the preferred directions of muscles a consistent shift in the force epoch, as compared to the baseline epoch. The shift occurs for all the muscles in the same direction, namely, the direction of the external force (i.e., clockwise or counterclockwise, depending on the field used). The point is illustrated in figure 11.4b (see also Li et al., 2001; Thoroughman and Shadmehr, 1999). Consider a muscle whose preferred direction in the baseline epoch is oriented toward 12 o'clock. When the monkey performs in the force epoch, with a clockwise force field, two forces are exerted upon the hand of the monkey: the force of the muscles and that of the external force field. When the muscle under consideration is maximally active (i.e., when the direction of movement corresponds to the preferred direction of the muscle), the two sets of forces (muscular and perturbing) sum vectorially. Whereas, in absence of the perturbing force, the hand of the monkey would move toward 12 o'clock, in its presence, the hand of the monkey actually moves toward a direction shifted clockwise. As a result, the preferred direction of the muscle under consideration is now also shifted clockwise. Most important, the shift of preferred direction occurs in the same direction for each muscle (clockwise for a clockwise force field, counterclockwise for a counterclockwise force field), independently of the original preferred direction.

These predictions (which assume a linear response of the muscles on the external perturbation) are confirmed by empirical evidence in both humans (Thoroughman and Shadmehr, 1999) and monkeys (Li et al., 2001), as shown in figure 11.4c. It can be seen that the preferred directions of all the muscles shift in the direction of the external force in the force epoch (mean shift $18.8°$, $p < 10^{-4}$, t test), and shift back in the opposite direction in the washout epoch (mean shift $-21.7°$, $p < 10^{-7}$, t test).

The shifts of preferred direction observed for muscles across epochs provide a framework for interpreting the activity of single cells. For muscles, the shift of preferred direction is directly imposed by the perturbing force

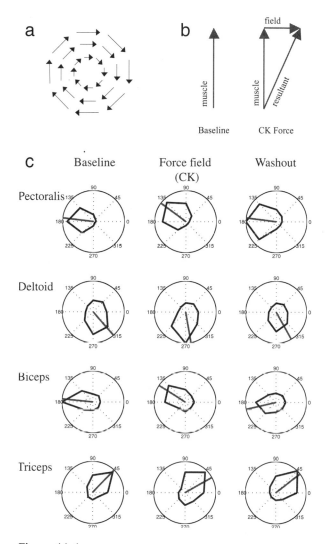

Figure 11.4

Tuning curves of muscles. (*a*) The clockwise force field plotted in velocity space. (*b*) Predicted effects of a clockwise force field on the preferred directions of muscles. Because the force exerted by the muscles and that of the force field sum in the force epoch, the preferred directions of all the muscles shift in the direction of the external force (here, clockwise). (*c*) Tuning curves of four muscles recorded with a clockwise force field. The movement-related activity of the muscles, rectified and integrated, is plotted in polar coordinates together with the preferred direction. For all the muscles the preferred direction shifts in the direction of the force field (clockwise) in the force epoch. In the washout epoch, the preferred directions shift in the opposite direction, back to those in the baseline epoch. (Reprinted with permission from Li et al., 2001; © 2001 by Elsevier Science.)

fields. Reflected in the activity of neurons, the shift of preferred direction is a fingerprint of the new dynamics.

11.7   Neuronal Plasticity in Primary Motor Cortex: Several Classes of Cells

In section 11.5, we showed that cells become tuned (tune-in cells) or lose their tuning (tune-out cells) as a consequence of the learning experience. In this section, we describe other changes of neuronal activity that—together with those of the tune-in and tune-out cells—encode the memory of the new internal model. As the monkeys acquired a new internal model of the dynamics, the activity of cells in M1 changed. We defined three parameters to characterize the tuning curves of cells: the preferred direction (Pd), the average firing frequency (Avf), and the tuning width (Tw). For each parameter, we analyzed changes across behavioral epochs (baseline, force, and washout). The changes of preferred direction are of particular interest and will be described in greater detail.

We classified neurons depending on how their activity changed across epochs with respect to each parameter separately (preferred direction, average firing frequency, and tuning width). Neurons that remained unchanged across the three epochs (x-x-x) were classified as "kinematic cells" because their activity appeared to be correlated with the kinematics of the movement. Neurons whose activity was modulated in the force epoch (x-y-x) were classified as "dynamic cells." With respect to the shift of preferred direction dynamic cells generally shifted their preferred direction in the direction of the external force in the force epoch, and in the opposite direction in the washout epoch. Most important, we found some cells whose activity changed in the force epoch, but did not return to the original pattern in the washout, where their activity resembled that observed in the force epoch more than that observed in the baseline epoch (x-y-y). We classified these (x-y-y) neurons as "memory cells" because they appeared to maintain a memory trace of the previous adaptation. Another group of neurons whose activity did not change in the force epoch but did change in the washout epoch (x-x-y) were also classified as "memory cells," because their activity in the washout epoch was different from that in the baseline epoch. Neurons classified as "memory I cells" (x-y-y) generally shifted their preferred direction in the direction of the external force field in the force epoch, and maintained their new preferred direction in the washout epoch. Those classified as "memory II cells" (*x-x-y*) generally shifted their preferred direction in complementary fashion: not at all in the force epoch, and in the direction *opposite* to that of the previously experienced force field in the washout epoch. Other neurons (*x-y-z*) were modulated in the force epoch and again in the washout epoch.

Figures 11.5a–d show examples of kinematic, dynamic, and memory cells, classified according to the changes of preferred direction (Pd). Because the Pd of the cell shown in figure 11.5a remained essentially unchanged across the three behavioral epochs, it was classified as a "kinematic cell." Because the Pd of the cell shown in figure 11.5b, recorded with a clockwise force field, shifted in the clockwise direction in the force epoch, returning in the washout epoch to essentially the same direction as in the baseline epoch, it was classified as a "dynamic cell." The shift of Pd of dynamic cells closely paralleled the shifts of Pd observed for single muscles (see figure 11.4c). The cell shown in figure 11.5c was classified as a "memory I cell": Although its Pd shifted in the force epoch in the direction of the external force (clockwise), in the washout epoch, it did not shift back, remaining essentially the same as in the force epoch. Thus, this cell seemed to maintain a trace of the recently developed internal model. The Pd of the neuron classified as a "memory II cell" and shown in figure 11.5d changed in an altogether complementary manner: In the force epoch, it remained unchanged compared to the baseline epoch, shifting in the washout epoch in the counterclockwise direction, namely, the direction opposite to the previously experienced force field.

Changes across epochs occurred for all three parameters, preferred direction, average firing frequency, and tuning width (Pd, Avf, and Tw). For instance, the cell shown in figure 11.5b was classified as "dynamic" with respect to both Pd and Tw. Likewise, the cell shown in figure 11.5e was classified as "class I memory" with respect to both Pd and Avf. In contrast, the activity of the cell shown in figure 11.5f, recorded in a control session where there was no force field, was essentially stable across epochs (in this case, arbitrarily defined epochs of approximately 200 trials).

A comprehensive plot of the shifts of preferred direction observed in the primary motor cortex across epochs is shown in figure 11.6 and plate 8. The scatter plot shows the shift of preferred direction in the force epoch compared to that of the baseline epoch (*x*-axis) versus that in the washout epoch compared to that in the force epoch (*y*-axis). All neurons are shown and color-coded according to their class. Kinematic cells (black)

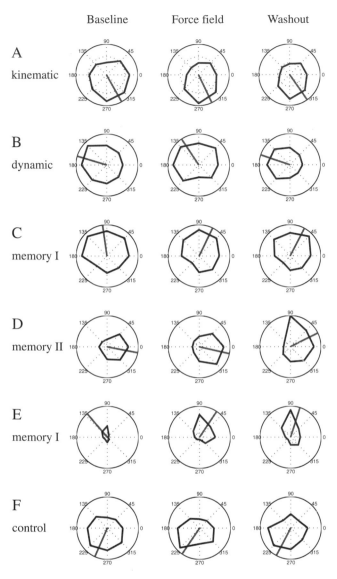

Figure 11.5
Classes of cells in primary motor cortex (M1). For each cell, the three plots represent the movement-related activity in the baseline (*left*), force (*center*), and washout (*right*) epochs; all cells were recorded with a clockwise force field. (*A, B, C, D*) Kinematic (*x-x-x*), dynamic (*x-y-x*), memory I (*x-y-y*), and memory II (*x-x-y*) cells, respectively, classified in terms of the changes of preferred direction. A cell neuron can show changes in more than one parameter. For instance, the neuron in (*B*) is classified as dynamic in terms of both preferred direction and tuning width. Likewise, the neuron in (*E*) has memory properties in terms of both average firing frequency and preferred direction. (*F*) For this neuron collected in a control experiment where no force was ever introduced, the preferred direction remains unchanged across the three (arbitrarily divided) epochs. (Reprinted with permission from Li et al., 2001; © 2001 by Elsevier Science.)

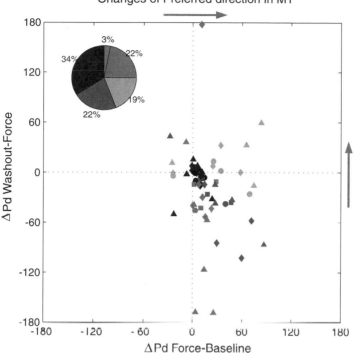

Figure 11.6

Scatter plot of changes in preferred direction (Pd) of primary motor cortex (M1) neurons. The *x*-axis represents the changes of Pd in the force versus baseline epochs. The *y*-axis represents the changes of Pd in washout versus force epochs. For both axes, positive values indicate shifts in the direction of the external force (see red arrows). In the scatter plot, each symbol represents one cell and cells are color-coded according to their classes. Kinematic cells (black) lie close to the origin because their Pd is unchanged across epochs. Dynamic cells (blue) lie on the diagonal through the second and fourth quadrant, because their Pd shifts in one direction in the force epoch (in general, the same direction as the force field) and in the opposite direction in the washout epoch. Memory I cells (green) lie on the *x*-axis; their Pd shifts in the force epoch (in general, in the direction of the external force) and does not shift in the washout epoch. Conversely, memory II cells (red) lie on the *y*-axis; their Pd is unchanged in the force epoch, and shifts in the direction opposite to the previously encountered force field in the washout epoch. "Other cells" (*x-y-z*) are shown in gray. (Reprinted with permission from Li et al., 2001; © 2001 by Elsevier Science.) See plate 8 for color version.

show no significant shifts of preferred direction in either x or the y measure, thus lie close to the origin. Dynamic cells (blue) show shifts of Pd in both measures, but in opposite directions; they lie on the diagonal crossing the second and fourth quadrant. Memory I cells (green) shifting their preferred direction in the x but not in the y measure, thus lie close to the x-axis. Memory II cells (red), shifting their preferred direction in the y but not in the x measure, lie on the y-axis.

Considering the entire neuronal population of the primary motor cortex in the movement-related time window, we observed a significant shift of preferred direction in the direction of the external force in the force epoch compared to the baseline (mean shift 16.2°, $p < 10^{-5}$, t test). In the washout epoch, the preferred direction of the neuronal population shifted in the direction *opposite* to the previously experienced force field, by a comparable amount (mean shift 14.3°, $p < .0003$, t test). As a result, there was no significant shift of preferred direction between washout and baseline epochs (mean shift $-2.2°$, $p = .6$, t test). Thus, the activity of M1 neurons *as a population* matched the activity of muscles.

11.8   Neuronal Correlates of Motor Performance and Motor Learning

In sections 11.5–11.7, we have shown how the neuronal population of the primary motor cortex reorganizes when monkeys acquire a new internal model of the dynamics. Single neurons initially not part of the active pool become committed to the task. Other neurons leave the pool. Yet other neurons that are tuned throughout the recordings change their activity to accommodate the novel internal model of the dynamics. Often, the changes that occur during the adaptation *outlast* the exposure to the perturbation. In other words, considering single cells, the development of a new internal model leaves long-lasting traces. Consistent with other studies (Donoghue, 1995; Wise et al., 1998; Laubach et al., 2000; Nudo et al., 1996; Dorris et al., 2000; Classen et al., 1998), we conclude that the primary motor cortex is involved in *motor learning*.

But this is certainly not all the primary motor cortex (M1) does. When there is nothing to learn (for instance, in our baseline epoch), neurons in M1 are still active, committed to the task, and directionally tuned. Their activity correlates with the parameters of the movement (Evarts, 1968; Georgopoulos et al., 1982; Kalaska et al., 1989; Moran and Schwartz, 1999;

Todorov, 2000). Moreover, the activity of neurons in M1 varies depending on the posture of the monkey (Scott and Kalaska, 1995, 1997). Furthermore, acute lesions of M1 result in severe motor deficits. As many studies have shown, independently of learning, the primary motor cortex participates in the control of movements; in other words, it is involved in *motor performance.*

How can the same neuronal population support both motor performance and motor learning? In our view, two findings reported here speak directly to this question. First, we found that two classes of memory cells balanced each other in the washout epoch with respect to the changes of preferred direction. Second, across the entire population, the changes of preferred direction matched the changes observed for muscles. Considered together, these two findings suggest that, although single cells modify their activity when the monkeys develop a new internal model (motor learning), the neuronal population reorganizes to transmit a global signal appropriate for the behavioral goal (motor performance).

As shown in section 11.7, the curl force field imposed predictable and consistent shifts on the preferred directions of all muscles. In the force epoch, the preferred directions of muscles shifted in the direction of the external force, whereas in the washout epoch, they shifted in the opposite direction. With respect of the neuronal activity in primary motor cortex, we found several classes of cells. In particular, memory cells had different preferred directions in the washout and baseline epochs. Thus, although single cells did not simply match the activity of muscles, the *neuronal population* did. The preferred directions of neurons shifted in the direction of the applied force field in the force epoch and shifted back in the opposite direction in the washout. Notably, we found comparable magnitudes for the shifts of the preferred direction of the neuronal population (mean shifts 16.2° and −14.3° in the "force-baseline" and "washout-force" measures, respectively) and of the muscles (mean shifts 18.8° and −21.7° in the "force-baseline" and "washout-force" measures, respectively).

The match between the neuronal population and the muscles is due to the presence of both memory I and memory II cells. On the one hand, the preferred directions of memory I cells (x-y-y) generally shifted in the direction of the external force field in the force epoch and retained that shift in the washout. On the other hand, the preferred directions of memory II cells (x-x-y) did not change in the force epoch, whereas, in the washout, they shifted in the direction *opposite* to the previously experienced force field. Thus the shifts in the preferred directions of memory I and memory II cells canceled each other in the washout epoch. For the entire population, the shifts of preferred direction between the washout and baseline epochs effectively averaged to zero. Notably, the percentages of memory I and memory II cells were similar (19% versus 22%).

To conclude, we view memory I and memory II cells as complementary correlates of motor performance and motor learning. After readaptation to the nonperturbed condition (washout), the neuronal population regains a state statistically indistinguishable from the initial state (baseline). Accordingly, the motor performance—dictated by the activity of the neuronal population—is similar in terms of both the kinematics and the dynamics of the movement. Considering single cells, however, the activity of neurons after readaptation still reflects the previous adaptation to the force field. For single cells, the final state is different from the initial state. Such neuronal plasticity parallels the development of a new internal model.

11.9   Conclusions

In reporting recent work in our laboratory on the neuronal plasticity of the primary motor cortex (M1) with respect to a new internal model of the inverse dynamics in monkeys, we presented two main results. First, as the monkeys develop a new internal model, new cells become committed to the task. Second, the activity of neurons in the primary motor cortex is modified by the learning experience. Changes in neuronal activity outlast the exposure to the perturbing forces, indicating that M1 is involved in motor learning. Combined across epochs, these changes indicate that primary motor cortex supports both functions of motor performance and motor learning.

Acknowledgment

Our research was funded by National Institutes of Health grant 2-P50MH48185.

References

Alexander, G. E., and Crutcher, M. D. (1990a). Preparation for movement: Neural representations of intended direction in three motor areas of the monkey. *J. Neurophysiol.* 64: 133–150.

Alexander, G. E., and Crutcher, M. D. (1990b). Neural representations of the target (goal) of visually guided arm movements in three motor areas of the monkey. *J. Neurophysiol.* 64: 164–178.

Bizzi, E. (1988). Arm trajectory planning and execution: the problem of coordinate transformation. In *Neurobiology of Neocortex*, P. Rakic and W. Singer (eds.). New York: Wiley, pp. 373–383.

Brashers-Krug, T., Shadmehr, R., and Bizzi, E. (1996). Consolidation in human motor memory. *Nature* 382: 252–255.

Classen, J., Liepert, J., Wise, S. P., Hallett, M., and Cohen, L. G. (1998). Rapid plasticity of human cortical movement representation induced by practice. *J. Neurophysiol.* 79: 1117–1123.

Crutcher, M. D., and Alexander, G. E. (1990). Movement-related neuronal activity selectively coding either direction or muscle pattern in three motor areas of the monkey. *J. Neurophysiol.* 64: 151–163.

Donoghue, J. P. (1995). Plasticity of adult sensorimotor representations. *Curr. Opinion Neurobiol.* 5: 749–754.

Dorris, M. C., Pare, M., and Munoz, D. P. (2000). Immediate neural plasticity shapes motor performance. *J. Neurosci.* RC52: 1–5.

Evarts, E. V. (1968). Relation of pyramidal tract activity to force exerted during voluntary movement. *J. Neurophysiol.* 31: 14–27.

Gandolfo, F., Li, C.-S. R., Benda, B. J., Padoa-Schioppa, C., and Bizzi, E. (2000). Cortical correlates of learning in monkeys adapting to a new dynamic environment. *Proc. Natl. Acad. Sci. U. S. A.* 97: 2259–2263.

Georgopoulos, A., Kalaska, J., Caminiti, R., and Massey, J. (1982). On the relations between the direction of two-dimensional arm movements and cell discharge in primate motor cortex. *J. Neurosci.* 2: 1527–1537.

Kalaska, J. F., Cohen, D. A. D., Hyde, M. L., and Prud'homme, M. (1989). A comparison of movement direction-related versus load direction-related activity in the primate motor cortex, using a two-dimensional reaching task. *J. Neurosci.* 9: 2080–2102.

Kawato, M. (1999). Internal models for motor control and trajectory planning. *Curr. Opin. Neurobiol.* 9: 718–727.

Krakauer, J. W., Ghilardi, M. F., and Ghez, C. (1999). Independent learning of internal models for kinematic and dynamic control of reaching. *Nat. Neurosci.* 2: 1026–1031.

Laubach, M., Wessberg, J., and Nicolelis, M. A. (2000). Cortical ensemble activity increasingly predicts behaviour outcomes during learning of a motor task. *Nature* 40: 567–571.

Li, C.-S. R., Padoa-Schioppa, C., and Bizzi, E. (2001). Neural correlates of motor performance and motor learning in the primary motor cortex of monkeys adapting to an external force field. *Neuron* 30: 593–607.

Moran, D. W., and Schwartz, A. B. (1999). Motor cortical representation of speed and direction during reaching. *J. Neurophysiol.* 82: 2676–2692.

Mussa-Ivaldi, F. A., and Bizzi, E. (2000). Motor learning through the combination of primitives. *Philos. Trans. R. Soc. Lond. B Biol. Sci.* 355: 1755–1769.

Nudo, R. J., Milliken, G. W., Jenkins, W. M., and Merzenich, M. M. (1996). Use-dependent alterations of movement representations in primary motor cortex of adult squirrel monkeys. *J. Neurosci.* 16: 785–807.

Shadmehr, R., and Mussa-Ivaldi, F. A. (1994). Adaptive representation of dynamics during learning of a motor task. *J. Neurosci.* 14: 3208–3224.

Scott, S. H., and Kalaska, J. F. (1995). Changes in motor cortex activity during reaching movements with similar hand paths but different arm postures. *J. Neurophysiol.* 73: 2563–2567.

Scott, S. H., and Kalaska, J. F. (1997). Reaching movements with similar hand paths but different arm orientations: 1. Activity of individual cells in motor cortex. *J. Neurophysiol.* 77: 826–852.

Thoroughman, K. A., and Shadmehr, R. (1999). Electromyographic correlates of learning an internal model of reaching movements. *J. Neurosci.* 19: 8573–8588.

Todorov, E. (2000). Direct cortical control of muscle activation in voluntary arm movements: a model. *Nat. Neurosci.* 3: 391–398.

Wise, S. P., Moody, S. L., Blomstrom, K. J., and Mitz, A. R. (1998). Changes in motor cortical activity during visuomotor adaptation. *Exp. Brain Res.* 121: 285–299.

Wolpert, D. M., and Ghahramani, Z. (2000). Computational principles of movement neuroscience. *Nat. Neurosci.* 3S: 1212–1217.

Neural Mechanisms of Catching: Translating Moving Target Information into Hand Interception Movement

Wolfgang Kruse, Nicholas L. Port, Daeyeol Lee, and
Apostolos P. Georgopoulos

12.1   Introduction

The neural mechanisms underlying the visuomotor coordination of arm
movements have been intensely investigated over the past 20-odd years
(Georgopoulos, 1990; Kalaska and Crammond, 1992; Caminiti et al., 1996;
Schwartz, 1994b). Most of the tasks used have involved movement of the
arm toward stationary targets. Because the visual information about the
target in such tasks is static, consisting simply of the target's location in
space, the key corresponding movement parameters are the direction and
amplitude of the movement. In real life, however, the visual target may
change location, involving a dynamic aspect of visuomotor coordination.
Previous studies addressed this issue partially by shifting the target location
at various times during the reaction or movement time (Georgopoulos et
al., 1981, 1983). With respect to monkey behavior, it was found that the
hand moved first toward the first target for a period of time and then
changed direction to move toward the second target. The duration of the
movement toward the first target was a linear function of the time for which
the first target remained visible. This result indicated that the arm motor
system was strongly coupled to the visual system, and faithfully followed
the changes in the location of the target. Similar results were also obtained
in human subjects (Soechting and Lacquaniti, 1983). With respect to the
neural mechanisms involved, it was found that cell activity in the motor
cortex (Georgopoulos et al., 1983) and parietal cortex (Kalaska et al., 1981)
changed promptly after the target changed location, from a pattern appropriate for a movement toward the first target to a pattern appropriate for
a movement toward the second. Indeed, the duration of the first cell response was a linear function of the duration of the first target. Thus a strong
and orderly influence of the visual condition was exerted on the neuronal

activity in the motor and parietal cortex, and that influence was later reflected on the hand movement. The delay from shifting the target to the change of neuronal discharge patterns (from the first to the second pattern) was about 130 ms (see figure 10 in Georgopoulos et al., 1983). This value can be regarded as an estimate of the delay involved in the flow of information "on-line" from the visual to the arm motor system under behavioral conditions favoring a strong dependence of the latter on the former.

In the monkey studies discussed above, the visual target was stationary and the monkeys were trained to move toward it. Under these conditions, the target shift served as a dynamic probe of visuomotor coordination. When the hand catches a moving target, however, we have a very different case of visuomotor coordination. Obviously, the drastic difference lies in the motion of the stimulus. In addition, a richer set of task instructions is possible as well; for example, to catch the target as fast as possible or to catch it at a certain location (given a predetermined stimulus trajectory). Finally, a richer set of strategies by which the task can be accomplished becomes available; for example, when the target moves slowly and the task is to catch it at a certain location, the subject can wait and make a single catching movement, or can move incrementally toward the catching point by making a number of smaller movements. Experiments in both humans (Port et al., 1997; Lee at al., 1997) and monkeys (Port et al., 2001) showed that such different strategies can indeed be adopted. Results from single-cell recordings in behaving monkeys have been published (Port et al., 2001; Lee et al., 2001).

12.2   Methods

Animals

Two male rhesus monkeys (*Macaca mulatta*, 8–11 kg body weight; referred to as "monkeys 1 and 2") were used. Monkeys 1 and 2 used their right and left hands in performing the tasks, respectively, and recordings were made from the hemisphere contralateral to the performing arm. The motor cortex of monkey 1 was recorded from in two separate sessions. In the first session (1a), the monkey was allowed to make free eye movements, whereas, in the second (1b), it was required to fixate a stationary target during task performance. For monkey 2, there were no restrictions on eye movements. Care and treatment of the animals during all stages of the experiments conformed to the principles outlined in *Principles of Laboratory*

Animal Care (NIH publication no. 86–23, revised 1995) and were approved by the relevant institutional review boards.

Apparatus

All visual stimuli were displayed on a 14-inch color computer monitor (Gateway 1020NI) located 57 cm away from the monkey at approximately eye level. The monitor was adjusted for a screen resolution of 640 horizontal and 480 vertical pixels, with a refresh rate of 60 Hz. Seated in a primate chair, the animals controlled the feedback cursor displayed on the monitor by moving a two-dimensional articulated arm on a horizontal planar working surface. The apparatus has been described previously (Georgopoulos et al., 1981). The monkeys grasped the distal end of the arm with their hand pronated while the other hand was comfortably restrained in a large acrylic tube. The position of the arm in *x-y* coordinates was digitally sampled at a rate of 100 Hz, and with a spatial resolution of 0.125 mm. The gain was set to one so that movement of the feedback cursor had a one-to-one correspondence with that of the arm. A personal computer was used for experimental control, visual presentation, and data collection.

Behavioral Task

In the interception task (figure 12.1), the stimulus (1) traveled in a straight line at 45° to the vertical from either lower corner of the computer monitor toward the interception point at 12 o'clock (two target motion directions),

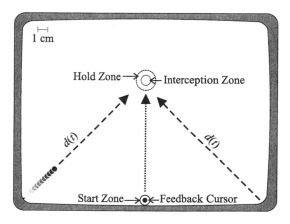

Figure 12.1
Spatial layout of the interception task.

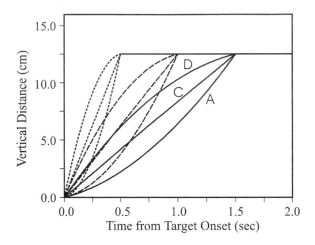

Figure 12.2
Temporal profile of stimuli used. (*Top*) Target displacement is plotted against time for all target motion times—0.5 s (dotted lines), 1.0 s (dashed lines), and 1.5 s (solid lines)—and target acceleration types (constant acceleration, constant deceleration, and constant velocity). A, C, D indicate accelerating, constant velocity, and decelerating targets, respectively.

(2) moved with constant velocity, constant acceleration, or constant deceleration (three target acceleration types), and (3) moved for a duration of 0.5 s, 1.0 s, and 1.5 s (three target motion times, or TMTs; figure 12.2). Eighteen classes of trials were generated by the combination of these three target parameters, and each combination was presented 2–3 times in a pseudo-random sequence. Accelerating targets had a starting velocity of 3.0 cm/s and underwent an appropriate constant acceleration to achieve the desired motion time. Decelerating targets had velocity profiles that were mirror images of those of the accelerating targets and underwent constant deceleration to end with a velocity of 3.0 cm/s. Constant-velocity targets traveled at the appropriate constant velocity to achieve the required motion time.

A trial in the task began when the monkey moved the feedback cursor (0.3 cm radius circle) into a start zone (1 cm radius circle for monkey 1; 0.5 cm radius circle for monkey 2) centered at the bottom of the screen along the vertical meridian (figure 12.1). After the monkey had maintained this position for a random period of 1–3 s (the start-hold period), a target (0.6 cm radius circle) appeared in the lower right or left corner of the screen. The target then traveled along a 45° path until it reached the vertical meridian of the screen, where it stopped at a location 12.5 cm directly above the center of the start zone. The monkey was required to move the feedback cursor to intercept the target just as it reached its final position at the center of the interception zone. This zone was an invisible positional window, namely, a 1.2 cm radius circle for monkey 1 and a 1.0 cm radius circle for monkey 2, centered on the final target location. The following conditions were required for a trial to be considered successful. First, the monkey had to maintain the cursor within the start zone until 130 ms after target onset. This condition was imposed to prevent anticipatory movements to the target. Second, the monkey had to move the arm so that the feedback cursor would enter the interception zone within 130 ms of the target's arrival at the interception point. And third, after the cursor entered the interception zone, the monkey had to maintain the cursor within an invisible, 2.0 cm radius, circular positional window (target-hold zone) for 0.5 s. Trials were aborted when any of the above listed conditions was violated. Monkeys were notified of unsuccessful trials with a tone, and rewarded for successful trials with a drop of juice. There were no other constraints on the animal's movements or their initiation.

Experimental Design

Eighteen combinations of two directions, three acceleration types, and three target motion times were presented in a randomized block design. In session 1a, two stimulus directions were nested within each combination of acceleration type and target motion times, and were presented in sub-blocks of 2–3 trials; in session 1b, two stimulus directions were completely randomized within a combination block. To obtain an equal number of successful trials for all target conditions, unsuccessful trials were rerandomized and repeated until correct performance was achieved.

Data Collection

Neural Recordings   After an animal was trained to perform with greater than 85% accuracy in the task, recordings of cortical neurons during task performance were initiated using a seven-electrode recording system (Thomas RECORDING, Giessen, Germany; see Mountcastle et al., 1991; Lee et al., 1998). The electrophysiological techniques used to record the extracellular electrical signals of single-cell activity, the surgical procedures and the animal care have been described previously (Georgopoulos et al.,

1982; Lurito et al., 1991). All surgical procedures were performed under general anesthesia and aseptic conditions. A lightweight metal halo (Nakasawa Works Co., Tokyo, Japan) was used to stabilize the head during recording sessions. Neural impulses were discriminated on-line using dual-time-amplitude-window discriminators (BAK Electronics, Maryland) and computer-controlled spike template matching (Alpha Omega Engineering, Nazareth, Israel).

Eye Position Recordings   For monkey 1, eye position was monitored by the sclera search coil method (CNC Engineering, Seattle); the coil was surgically implanted using the method of Judge and colleagues (1980). For monkey 2, eye position was monitored by an infrared oculometer (DR. BOUIS, Karlsruhe, Germany). Horizontal and vertical eye positions were sampled at 200 Hz. Once again, in recording from monkey 1 in session 1a and from monkey 2, there were no restrictions on eye movements; eye position data were collected throughout the trials. However, in recording from monkey 1 in session 1b, the animal was required to fixate within 2° of visual angle from the center of the start zone throughout the trials. A trial was aborted if visual fixation was broken at any time.

Histology   After the experiments were completed, the area of recording was demarcated on the cortical surface with metal pins inserted at known recording locations using a microdrive placement system. The animal was then euthanatized with a lethal overdose of sodium pentobarbital, perfused transcardially with buffered formalin, fixed, and the brain removed for histological processing.

Data Analysis

General   Standard statistical analyses (Snedecor and Cochran, 1989; Draper and Smith, 1981) were used, including multiple regression analysis. Ad hoc computer programs and commercially available statistical packages (SPSS, version 7, SPSS Inc., Chicago, 1996; BMDP/Dynamic, BMDP Statistical Software Inc., Los Angeles, 1993) were used for statistical analyses.

Analysis of Behavioral Data   The hand position was smoothed and differentiated using the finite impulse response method (pass band 0–0.5 Hz; stop band 13–50 Hz).

Spike Density Function   The spike train was converted to a spike density function for some analyses (MacPherson and Aldridge, 1979), calculated using the fixed kernel method (Richmond et al., 1987), with a Gaussian pulse width of 30 ms. Spike density functions were synchronized with target onset. Spike density functions of individual neurons were averaged to generate a population spike density function (figure 12.3A).

Multiple Linear Regression   The nature of the interception task requires a tight temporal coupling between the motion of the stimulus and the movement of the hand. A multiple linear regression model was used to relate the population spike density function to the evolving position, velocity, and acceleration of the target and hand movement. The spike density at time t was expressed as a function of the position, velocity, and acceleration of the hand at time $t + \tau_H$, and the target at time $t + \tau_S$, where τ_H and τ_S were independent time shifts in relation to the spike density function (from -130 ms to $+150$ ms). A negative shift means that the movement of the hand or the movement of the target preceded the neural activity, and a positive shift means that the target or hand movement came after the neural activity. The following model was used:

$$PSDF_t = b_0 + b_1 d^S_{t+\tau_S} + b_2 \dot{d}^S_{t+\tau_S} + b_3 \ddot{d}^S_{t+\tau_S}$$
$$+ b_4 d^H_{t+\tau_H} + b_5 \dot{d}^H_{t+\tau_H} + b_6 \ddot{d}^H_{t+\tau_H} + \varepsilon_t$$

$$t + \tau \leq T,$$

where *PSDF* is the population spike density function, d is displacement of the stimulus (S) or the hand (H) every 10 ms, $b_0, \ldots, b_6$ are regression coefficients, ε is an error term, τ_S, τ_H are time shifts for the stimulus and the hand, respectively (from -130 ms to $+150$ ms, in 10 ms intervals, see below), and T is the period of time from the onset of the target until the delivery of reward. The inequality above means that the neural data included within the shifted spike train were always contained within the behaviorally meaningful time period T. The shifting operation is illustrated in figure 12.3. To independently assess time shifts of the hand and of the target, two time shifts were used. For every time shift, the standardized regression coefficients (obtained from the raw regression coefficients by expressing them in standard deviation units, thus dimensionless) were also calculated. These coefficients allow researchers to compare the effects among the independent variables and provide information about

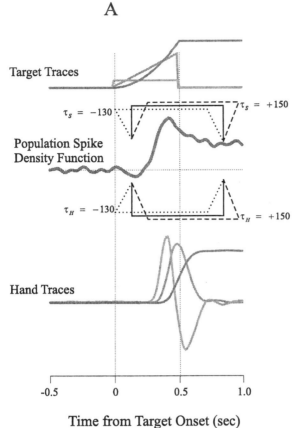

A

Target Traces

$\tau_s = -130$ $\tau_s = +150$

Population Spike
Density Function

$\tau_H = -130$ $\tau_H = +150$

Hand Traces

-0.5   0   0.5   1.0

Time from Target Onset (sec)

Figure 12.3
(*A*) Diagram of the multiple linear regression model (data from recording session
1a; accelerating target condition; target motion time 0.5 s). (*B*, *C*) Contour plots
of the R^2 for all possible shifts (τ_S, τ_H) of the multiple linear regression model for
recording sessions 1a and 1b, respectively.

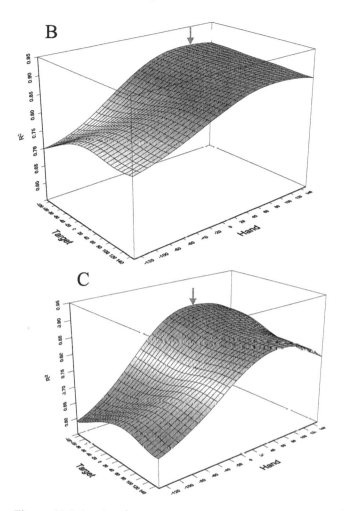

Figure 12.3 (*continued*)

the importance of a given variable in the regression equation. The coefficient of determination, R^2 (proportion of variance explained), was measured at all combinations of shifts, and the shift for which the highest R^2 was obtained, noted. The t statistic and its probability level were calculated for each coefficient. Because six simultaneous comparisons were performed, the nominal probability level was adjusted according to the Bonferroni inequality (Snedecor and Cochran, 1989) to $\alpha' = 0.05/6 \approx 0.008$; therefore, $P < .008$ was considered statistically significant. Finally, all regression analyses were run using default tolerance limits for collinearities among the independent variables; in none of the analyses were these default limits exceeded.

12.3   Results

A population spike density function from 407, 197, and 467 neurons was computed from recording sessions 1a, 1b, and 2, respectively. For some target conditions there was an early rise in the population spike density function even though the movement did not occur until several hundred milliseconds later (Port et al., 2001). At the best time shift, all coefficients in the model were significant with the exception of target acceleration in recording session 1b. The R^2 was calculated for each 10 ms shift. The results obtained are shown in table 12.1, which shows the R^2, best time shifts, and the standardized coefficients at the best time shift for each recording session. The relative importance of a particular variable on the population spike density function can be assessed by ranking the standardized coefficients. The rank-ordered standardized coefficients are listed in table 12.2. As is evident in these two tables, hand speed was generally the strongest explanatory variable for the population spike density function, followed closely by hand position and target position. Target velocity was generally fourth in the list, while hand and target acceleration had the weakest relation to the population spike density function. It is worth noting that the shifts of the target (-130 ms), t_2, are at their earliest. Shifts could not be made beyond these values due to the early onset of neural activity (130 ms for all recording sessions). The percent of variance explained (R^2) differed for different combinations of target and hand shifts. Two examples are illustrated in figure 12.3B–C, which give the R^2 values for all these combinations in recording sessions 1a and 1b, respectively. The highest R^2 (0.89, 0.86, and 0.75, for recordings 1a, 1b, and 2, respectively) were obtained

Table 12.1
R^2 and standardized coefficients of the regression model at best time shift

Recording session	Hand t_1	Target t_2	R^2	Hand			Target		
				Position	Velocity	Acceleration	Position	Velocity	Acceleration
1a	100	−130	.89	0.27	0.61	0.06	0.34	0.18	−0.08
1b	70	−130	.86	0.25	0.71	0.09	0.16	0.25	0.01★
2	50	−80	.75	−1.4	0.57	0.07	1.33	−0.08	0.07

★ Coefficient was not significant.

Table 12.2
Rank order of the standardized coefficients

Order	Session 1a	Session 1b	Session 2
1	Hand velocity	Hand velocity	Hand position
2	Target position	Target velocity	Target position
3	Hand position	Hand position	Hand velocity
4	Target velocity	Target position	Target velocity
5	Target acceleration	Hand acceleration	Target acceleration
6	Hand acceleration	—*	Hand acceleration

* Coefficient was not significant.

at time shifts $(\tau_S, \tau_H) = (-130, +100), (-130, +70),$ and $(-80, +50)$ (see table 12.1). The time shift results indicated, for all recordings, (1) that the time varying population spike density function dynamically predicted the time varying aspects of hand movement, and (2) that there was a feed-forward dynamic effect of target velocity and position on the spike density function.

As can be seen in figure 12.3B–C, the effect of the target shift was relatively flat in comparison to the shift of the hand. To test whether there was a significant effect of the target shift, a linear regression by groups (BMDP/Dynamic program 1R; see "Data Analysis" in section 12.2) was performed (this directly tests whether the regression equations for different groups differ significantly). For the optimal shift of the hand, tests were performed to identify at what point away from the best target shift the equations differed significantly. There was no difference in the regression equation for the following target shifts: -130 ms to -90 ms in recording session 1a, -130 ms to -80 ms in session 1b, and -80 ms to -20 ms in recording session 2. For target shifts greater than these, there was a statistical difference in the regression equation. Because all of the ranges listed above are negative, it may be inferred that target motion exerted a consistent feedforward effect on neural activity.

12.4   Discussion

Our results document for the first time the dynamic forward flow of information, from moving target to motor cortex to hand movement. The lags found, based on optimal time shifts in the regression analysis, were well within the range of estimates of such effects from previous neurophysiologi-cal studies. For example, the delay of visual effects on motor cortical cell activity was estimated at about 130 ms in a target shift task (Georgopoulos et al., 1983). On the other hand, an optimal time lag of about −90 ms has been found in single-cell studies during reaching movements to stationary targets; at this value, the regression model between cell activity and move-ment parameters attained the highest R^2 (Ashe and Georgopoulos, 1994). Although neither the exact pathways nor the sequence of events for this information flow are known, it is obvious that they involve a number of areas intercalated between the visual inflow and motor cortical outflow, where both anatomical and physiological studies (Caminiti et al., 1996; Schwartz, 1994b) have implicated parietofrontal pathways, and between the motor cortex and motoneuronal activation, and where corticocortical interactions as well as subcortical loops are apparently involved. Thus large circuits participate in this visuomotor coordination; our results provide an experimental estimate of the overall delays. Finally, it should be noted that these estimates may depend on the paradigm used in this study: Other esti-mates may well be obtained using different paradigms. For example, Schwartz (1994a) found the lag between the population vector and arm movement decreased as the movement curvature decreased in a tracing task. Moreover, predictive smooth tracking is usually done at minimal or zero lags between the stimulus and the movement. It is interesting that the optimal target population lag was smaller in session 2 (range: −80 ms to −20 ms) than in session 1a (−130 ms to −90 ms) or 1b (−130 ms to −80 ms), a finding that probably reflects monkey 2's using a strategy that resembled tracking (see Port et al., 2001), where one would expect a close temporal, on-line coupling between the moving stimulus and movement-related neural activity. It is also noteworthy that the optimal target popula-tion lags were very similar for sessions 1a and 1b, which differed with respect to the presence (session 1b) or absence (session 1a) of fixation requirement. This finding is in accord with monkey 1's adopting the same strategy, namely, making mostly a single precise interception movement in both conditions (Port et al., 2001). The longer lags observed in this case are close to those found following a shift of stationary targets (Georgopoulos et al., 1983).

Finally, with respect to the parameters influencing motor cortical pop-ulation activity, we found that, first, hand movement effects ranked consistently higher than those of stimulus motion; and second, that the effect of acceleration of either hand or stimulus ranked lowest. These results are in keeping with those of previous studies regarding hand movement effects (e.g., Ashe and Georgopoulos, 1994) and underscore the importance of hand velocity and position as the key parameters for the information flow in the primary motor cortex.

Acknowledgments

The work reported in this chapter was funded by U. S. Public Health Service grant PSMH48185, the U.S. Department of Veterans Affairs, and the American Legion Brain Sciences Chair.

References

Ashe, J., and Georgopoulos, A. P. (1994). Movement parameters and neural activity in motor cortex and area 5. *Cereb. Cortex* 4: 590–600.

Caminiti, R., Ferraina, S., and Johnson, P. B. (1996). The sources of visual information to the primate frontal lobe: A novel role for the superior parietal lobule. *Cereb. Cortex* 6: 319–328.

Draper, N. R., and Smith, H. (1981). *Applied Regression Analysis.* New York: Wiley.

Georgopoulos, A. P. (1990). Eye-hand coordination and visual control of reaching: Studies in behaving animals. In *Comparative Perception.* Vol. 1, *Basic Mechanisms*, M. A. Berkley and W. C. Stebbins (eds.). New York: Wiley, pp. 375–403.

Georgopoulos, A. P., Kalaska, J. F., and Massey, J. T. (1981). Spatial trajectories and reaction times of aimed movements: Effects of practice, uncertainty and change in target location. *J. Neurophysiol.* 46: 725–743.

Georgopoulos, A. P., Kalaska, J. F., Caminiti, R., and Massey, J. T. (1982). On the relations between the direction of two-dimensional arm movements and cell discharge in primate motor cortex. *J. Neurosci.* 2: 1527–1537.

Georgopoulos, A. P., Kalaska, J. F., Caminiti, R., and Massey, J. T. (1983). Interruption of motor cortical discharge subserving aimed arm movements. *Exp. Brain Res.* 49: 327–340.

Judge, S. J., Richmond, B. J., and Chu, F. C. (1980). Implantation of magnetic search coils for measurement of eye position: An improved method. *Vision Res.* 20: 535–538.

Kalaska, J. F., and Crammond, D. J. (1992). Cerebral cortical mechanisms of reaching movements. *Science* 255: 1517–1523.

Kalaska, J. F., Caminiti, R., and Georgopoulos, A. P. (1981). Cortical mechanisms of two-dimensional aimed arm movements: 3. Relations of parietal (areas 5 and 2) neuronal activity to direction of movement and change in target location. *Soc. Neurosci. Abstr.* 7: 563.

Lee, D., Port, N. L., and Georgopoulos, A. P. (1997). Manual interception of moving targets: 2. On-line control of overlapping submovements. *Exp. Brain Res.* 116: 421–433.

Lee, D., Port, N. L., Kruse, W., and Georgopoulos, A. P. (1998). Neuronal population coding: Multielectrode recordings in primate cerebral cortex. In *Neuronal Ensembles: Strategies for Recording and Decoding*, H. Eichenbaum and J. Davis (eds.). New York: Wiley, pp. 117–136.

Lee, D., Port, N. L., Kruse, W., and Georgopoulos, A. P. (2001). Neuronal clusters in the primate motor cortex during interception of moving targets. *J. Cogn. Neurosci.* 13: 319–331.

Lurito, J. T., Georgakopoulos, T., and Georgopoulos, A. P. (1991). Cognitive spatial-motor processes: 7. The making of movements at an angle from a stimulus direction: Studies of motor cortical activity at the single-cell and population levels. *Exp. Brain Res.* 87: 562–580.

MacPherson, J. M., and Aldridge, J. W. (1979). A quantitative method of computer analysis of spike train data collected from behaving animals. *Brain Res.* 175: 183–187.

Mountcastle, V. B., Reitboeck, H. J., Poggio, G. F., and Steinmetz, M. A. (1991). Adaptation of the Reitboeck method of multiple microelectrode recording to the neocortex of the waking monkey *J. Neurosci. Methods* 36: 77–84.

Port, N. L., Lee, D., Dassonville, P., and Georgopoulos, A. P. (1997). Manual interception of moving targets: 1. Performance and movement initiation. *Exp. Brain Res.* 116: 406–420.

Port, N. L., Kruse, W., Lee, D., and Georgopoulos, A. P. (2001). Motor cortical activity during interception of moving targets. *J. Cogn. Neurosci.* 13: 306–318.

Richmond, B. J., Optican, L. M., Podell, M., and Spitzer, H. (1987). Temporal encoding of two-dimensional patterns by single units in primate inferior temporal cortex: 1. Response characteristics. *J. Neurophysiol.* 57: 132–146.

Schwartz, A. B. (1994a). Direct cortical representation of drawing. *Science* 265: 540–542.

Schwartz, A. B. (1994b). Distributed motor processing in cerebral cortex. *Curr. Opin. Neurobiol.* 4: 840–846.

Snedecor, G. W., and Cochran, W. G. (1989). *Statistical Methods*. Ames: Iowa State University Press.

Soechting, J. F., and Lacquaniti, F. (1983). Modification of trajectory of a pointing movement in response to a change in target location. *J. Neurophysiol.* 49: 548–564.

Movement and Functional Magnetic Resonance Imaging: Applications in the Clinical and Scientific Environment

M. Rotte

13.1 Background

To achieve a simple movement in space is a complex task. Take, for example, a robot arm with three engines for the three axes to perform a motion from point A to B. The control program has to have a three-dimensional representation of the surrounding space. The coordinates of the start and endpoints have to be defined and a path connecting them calculated. To follow this path with the arm, three engines have to work together with great precision, integrating feedback about the position and speed of the arm. Altogether, a daunting task for the robot engineer.

To perform complex tasks like playing tennis, which involves getting to the ball (running) and hitting it with a racket (fine coordination of the tool) at the same time, is a breathtaking ability of the human body. And, even though our motor system is working at a peak level, we still have the resources to wonder how our opponent managed to return our excellent shot. We perform complex motor tasks every day without thinking; when, by reason of disability, we cannot, the resulting restrictions become obvious. Parkinson's disease is one such common neurological disability, where due to the decrease of a single transmitter in the brain, the patient experiences shaking of the limbs (tremor), a general slowing (akinesis), and a constant resistance of the skeletal muscles (rigidity).

To investigate how and where in the brain movements are controlled, researchers observed regular and disturbed motor behavior and formed hypotheses about the underlying structures. Lesions of the brain or changes detected in pathological examinations pointed toward different areas at the surface of the cortex and deeper structures. When these areas were disturbed in any way, the patient experienced a degree of malfunction in the motor system.

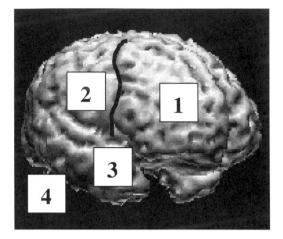

Figure 13.1
Right hemisphere of brain, with the separation of critical areas labeled by numbered squares. 1, frontal lobe; 2, parietal lobe; 3, temporal lobe; 4, occipital lobe. The central fissure is outlined by black line.

Viewed from above, the two hemispheres of the cortex are symmetrical along a central line. Each side can be divided into five large areas (see figure 13.1): the precentral area, the postcentral area, the temporal lobe, and the cerebellum.

As early as the eighteenth century, experiments were performed to reveal the kind of control for which the precentral area was responsible. Applying low-frequency faradic stimulation to the cerebral cortex of macaques, Ferrier (1875, 1876) found that locations along the precentral gyrus resulted in movements of different parts of the body. Researchers also noted that body parts were responding to stimulation of areas located on the other side of the brain (contralateral).

The neurosurgeon Penfield (see Penfield and Boldrey, 1937) investigated the distribution of primary motor areas using direct electrical stimulation on the surface of the human cortex: He observed a repeatable pattern in the distribution of body parts excited by the stimulation along the gyrus and noted that some of these representation areas covered a larger area. The hand and fingers could be easily activated over a large area in the upper third of the gyrus, whereas the arm responded only to a small area somewhat closer to the midline. Although these areas appeared to follow the same general distribution over patients, he also noted a variation of representation between patients within that distribution. Characterizing this distribution as "somatotopic," Penfield summarized his results in the picture of the motor homunculus.

Modern functional imaging methods allow us to investigate the control of body parts in a much less complicated way—at least for the patient. One of these methods, magnetic resonance imaging (MRI), uses induced magnetic changes in the brain for the reconstruction of pictures of the brain. If we want to go beyond the simple structure, to examine brain response during a specific task, these pictures have to be acquired at great speed to monitor the neuronal activation associated with the task; we therefore use functional magnetic resonance imaging (fMRI). What we actually measure are the changes in the oxygen content of blood in brain tissue due to the higher energy consumption that goes along with neuronal activation. Referred to as "blood oxygen level–dependent [BOLD] response," these are statistically calculated changes in blood oxygenation between resting and activated groups of neurons during a gradient echo imaging sequence sensitive to the paramagnetic state of deoxygenated hemoglobin. Although fMRI has no lasting biological effect on the human body (for currently used field strength of the magnet up to 3 T), application of the technique is limited by its sensitivity to head motion (a change in head position during scanning will change the relative coordinates of the brain structures within the field) and by the need to exclude subjects with implanted devices having magnetic parts (pacemakers, artificial joints, etc.). Moreover, because the differences are extremely small for a single movement—indeed, statistically not significant—the movement has to be repeated quite often to result in detectable differences between rest and exercise. Which brings up the next limitation: We can hardly suppose that most subjects will be comfortable lying on a stretcher inside the scanner with their head fixed for several hours.

Owing to the robust increase of the BOLD response to the movement of limbs, hands, or fingers and to the simplicity of instructing and training subjects to make such movements, the use of motor-related brain activation has been routine since the introduction of functional magnetic resonance imaging. Naturally, most research groups have used hand or finger movement because these are least likely to induce head motion.

Through the use of fMRI, several areas of the brain were identified as being involved in the execution of simple finger movement. Besides the expected area within the precentral gyrus contralateral to the hand, researchers found that deeper structures such as the basal ganglia and the thalamus within the same hemisphere were activated, as was the cerebellum in the ipsilateral hemisphere. The level of activation depended on the complexity, applied strength, and temporal extent of the task, with a rise in any of these factors tending to produce a rise in neuronal activation.

Not long after these initial investigations, the question arose whether movements by other parts of the body could be used to elicit detectable changes in the brain. Besides the problem of avoiding head motion, there was the problem of moving single, isolated parts of the body close to the trunk, such as an arm or leg. The goal was to create suitable tasks that would allow researchers to investigate other motor areas. Foot (Rao et al., 1995; Lehericy et al., 1998) and tongue (Yetkin et al., 1997; Corfield et al., 1999) tasks proved satisfactory, and the distribution of brain sites associated with movement of these body parts within the precentral gyrus followed the outline of Penfield's results. The foot representation area was located on the tip of the cortex, the tongue area down toward the temporal lobe, and the finger area somewhat between these two, all within the precentral gyrus. Due to the time constraints for subjects immobilized in the scanner having to remain attentive to the task, these studies were restricted to a particular part of the brain (the primary motor area and basal ganglia or the prefrontal lobe) at one time. Even so, the complete scanning procedure took several hours.

Because currently available fMRI scanners can acquire more data in less time, we can now characterize several brain structures involved in motor control and execution for a wide variety of tasks within an hour of scanning time. The next natural step would be to broaden tasks and data acquisition to cover the whole brain volume. The critical problems to solve are how to train subjects to move body parts in isolation from other body parts and how to optimize the tasks so that each takes the shortest time to elicit a significant increase of the BOLD response in the brain areas associated with the task. After investigating several tasks and scanning procedures to achieve this goal, my research group conducted a study with eight different motor tasks in healthy subjects.

13.2   Primary Motor Area: The Motor Homunculus According to Blood Oxygen Level–Dependent Response

My colleagues and I designed a protocol for a wide range of motor tasks involving the upper and lower extremities, the trunk and the face to compare the distribution of the BOLD response over the precentral gyrus with previous imaging studies and with results from direct cortical stimulation (e.g., Penfield and Boldrey, 1937). Furthermore, we intended to identify primary and secondary motor areas within the whole brain using the shortest possible scan time for each motor task, testing normal subjects for reproducibility and reliability of the activated brain areas. The study was to answer the following questions:

1. Can changes in BOLD response be detected for each of the applied motor tasks?
2. Are the detected areas for individual tasks distinguishable in location within the precentral gyrus?
3. Are secondary motor areas activated over different subjects and tasks in the same manner?

Nine healthy right-handed subjects (5 female, 4 male; mean age 24 years) participated in the study. All subjects had normal vision; neurological examination of their motor system revealed no pathology. The functional imaging was performed on a 1.5 T MR scanner with a standard GE head coil. Subjects were instructed before the session how to perform the different motor tasks and trained until inspection assured the isolated movement of the targeted body part. Finger and toe movements were performed only on the right side in a nonsequential pattern. Tongue and eye movements alternated right and left, extending to an angle of about 50°; lip movements alternated between resting and pursing. Knee movements alternated between resting and adducting with a rigid foam block between the legs; diaphragm-pelvis movements, between tensing and relaxing. All tasks had to be performed with a frequency of about 1 Hz. These tasks were selected because they reflect different functional areas of the precentral gyrus along the motor homunculus, were easy to explain and to train and involved both tasks already documented in the literature and new tasks not yet investigated.

Subjects lay on a flat scanner bed; their heads were tightly fitted into the head coil using pillows and wedge-shaped foam pieces; a strip around the forehead was used to minimize the possibility of head motion. For each subject, conventional structural images as well as echo planar functional images were acquired over a total period of about one hour. The initial structural scanning consisted of high-resolution T1-weighted images in sagittal orientation and conventional flow-weighted anatomic images with identical orientation to the functional echo planar images (16 oblique slices; 7 mm thickness). These images were used as an intermediate for off-line transformation of the functional images into the coordinate system of Talairach and Tournoux (1988), which allows the direct comparison between subjects by adjusting images of an individual brain to those of an international reference brain so that any given imaged structure will end up in roughly the same area. After transformation of each subject, the significance of each individual comparison can be combined for all subjects and compared to other studies in the field.

Functional images were acquired within separate runs for each motor task. Using single-shot gradient echo planar imaging, each run consisted of 128 time points. During each time point, whole-head volumes including the cerebellum (16 slices oriented to the plane connecting the anterior and posterior commissure; 7 mm thickness; plane resolution 3.125 mm) were recorded. The first four time points were excluded from analysis in order to eliminate magnetic saturation effects.

During each run, subjects performed four alternating, one-minute periods of rest and motor activation following acoustical start/stop instructions via intercom. The generic software allowed on-line monitoring of statistical tests contrasting rest and activation, therefore head movement–related activity could be identified and the particular run was repeated later.

Structural and functional data for each individual subject were transformed into stereotaxic space of the Talairach and Tournoux atlas, resulting in 39 axial slices of isotropic 3.125 mm voxels. Functional data were drift-corrected for the duration of single runs, and the mean of each slice adjusted to a mean value of 1,000. Activation maps for each individual and for all subjects collapsed (grand average) were calculated using nonparametric Kolmogorov-Smirnov statistics to compare movement versus rest periods in each run (for details, see Stern et al., 1996; Rotte et al., 1998), with the time course shifted 4 s to account for hemodynamic response delay.

To examine the hypothesis of task conditions, peak activation for each area with increased BOLD response was automatically detected based on the procedure described in Buckner et al., 1996, using an algorithm identifying all continuous voxels within 12 mm of the peak that reached a significance level of $p < .000001$. Multivariate analysis of variance (MANOVA) design methods were used to the hypothesis of distinctiveness of the primary motor activation for different motor tasks by taking the grand average data and standardizing the peak coordinates in the x, y, and z planes and calculating the overlap for task-related peak values within the three-dimensional distribution.

Collapsed Results across Subjects

The grand average of nine subjects showed significant increase in BOLD response in all areas involved in motor control and execution for the separate motor tasks. Activation areas were detected at different levels of significance in the precentral gyrus (M1), the postcentral gyrus, the supplementary motor area (SMA), the secondary sensorimotor areas (SM2), the basal ganglia and thalamus as well as the cerebellum.

For toe, knee, and diaphragm-pelvis movements, no primary motor cortex lateralization was detectable, whereas, for finger, eye, lip, and tongue movements, bilateral activation could be distinguished. As expected, the right-handed performance of finger movements resulted in a stronger left than right increase in BOLD response ($-\log p$ = 50,85 versus 34,15), whereas the remaining tasks showed equal levels of activation in complementary primary motor cortex. The significance levels were about the same for all tasks, with somewhat lower values for toe and eye movements ($-\log p$ values of about 45 and 30, respectively). The images shown in figure 13.2 and plate 9 summarize the distribution of peak activities detected in the precentral gyrus. The only task with activation in the postcentral gyrus was finger movement with a peak at $-33, -32, 64$ (x, y, z; $-\log p$ = 50,79). The activation during eye saccades was located somewhat deeper in the cortex compared with all other tasks resulting in significant increases of the BOLD response close to the cortical surface.

In the supplementary motor area, robust activation was detected during all tasks. The peaks were located anterior and medial in Brodmann area (BA) 6 for each separate motor activity. The secondary sensorimotor area was bilaterally activated during right-sided finger and toe movements and during bilateral movements at a similar level of significance. The peaks lay in the inferior left and right parietal lobule (BA 40).

Multiple areas showed increased BOLD response within the basal ganglia, including putamen, globus pallidus medialis and lateralis, nucleus caudatus, and different parts of the thalamus. Of the two tasks involving just one side, only the finger movement resulted in a lateralization in terms of a higher increase of the BOLD response to the contralateral side. As a result of the averaging procedure and the applied cluster analysis, a more distinct differentiation was not possible for the grand average data.

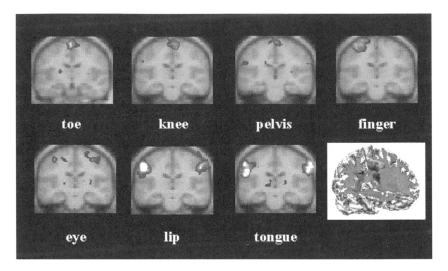

Figure 13.2
Coronal view of activated areas along the precentral gyrus. Color-coded p-values of increased blood oxygen level–dependent (BOLD) response for the different motor tasks (labeled by body part) projected on an anatomical background generated from averaged talairach. Results for the grand average of nine subjects. Inset image in the lower right corner summarizes the individual task activations from a three-dimensional perspective. See plate 9 for color version.

Within the cerebellum, both hemispheres showed increased activation in comparison to the resting state. Lateralization could be detected only for the finger movements, with a higher level of significance of the ipsilateral side to the motor task in comparison to the contralateral side ($-\log p = 52,68$ versus $38,92$).

Additional areas were activated during tongue, knee, and eye movements. Increased values at a low significance level were notable around the anterior edge of the forehead during tongue and knee movements. This pattern is related to movement artifacts during performance and reflects the difficulty of isolated motion of the targeted body part. Because these activations were spatially distinct from the areas of interest and because overall displacement of the head during these tasks did not exceed 4 mm, it is reasonable to exclude major influence on the reported areas of interest. During eye saccades, there was significant bilateral activation in the frontal eye fields ($-21, -15, 53$; $-\log p = 19,49$; $11, -9, 60$; $-\log p = 23,19$), the superior parietal lobule ($-25, -65, 59$; $-\log p = 22,09$; $29, -65, 56$; $-\log p = 25,63$), and the occipital lobe including primary and secondary visual areas.

Single-Subject Comparisons

The distribution of activated areas in single subjects was comparable to the results of the average. To compare the reliability of the areas identified in the grand average for each individual subject and task, cluster analysis was performed to identify activation within the following regions: M1, SMA, SM2, cerebellum, and basal ganglia with thalamus.

A robust and reliable activation in the precentral gyrus was detected in each subject for each motor task. For unilateral tasks (right finger and toe movement), activation of the contralateral M1, and for the other tasks, bilateral activation of M1 resulted in a significant increase of BOLD response. To correlate each motor task to a distinct area in the precentral gyrus, MANOVA analysis for different areas covering the main activation sites in the grand average for each task was applied. The factor of peak coordinate and task over subjects in single-group comparisons yielded significant effects for all except the following locations: movement of toe versus pelvis, toe versus knee, and pelvis versus knee (all others $p < .02$). To characterize the amount of overlap for the different tasks, each subject contributed one peak value within the precentral gyrus to form three-dimensional clusters for each movement. After normalization, the percentage overlap between the clusters was calculated (see table 13.1).

For the supplementary motor area, all tasks in each subject revealed significant activation. The analysis of task × peak coordinates over subjects using ANOVA design showed no significant effect ($F < 1$) for peaks related to the different body parts moved.

Table 13.1

Percentage overlap of detected peak activation within precentral gyrus between separate motor tasks

	Hand	Toe	Eye	Lips	Pelvis	Knee	Tongue
Hand	100	0	0	0	0	0	0
Toe		100	0	0	70	67	0
Eye			100	36	0	0	7
Lips				100	0	0	39
Pelvis					100	53	0
Knee						100	0
Tongue							100

Note: Each subject contributed one coordinate for each task; the distribution of these separate three-dimensional point clusters is expressed in percentage of overlap (100 equals identical cluster).

Table 13.2
Activation lateralization within basal ganglia and thalamus by motor task and subject

Motor task	Subject								
	1	2	3	4	5	6	7	8	9
Eye	R + L	R > L	—	R + L	—	—	L	L	R + L
Tongue	R + L	R + L	R < L	L	R > L	—	R > L	R > L	R > L
Lips	—	R > L	L	—	R > L	L	R + L	—	R > L
Pelvis	R + L	R < L	R > L	R + L	R + L	R > L	R + L	—	L
Knee	R + L	R < L	R + L	R < L	R > L	R > L	R < L	—	R + L
Finger	—	—	R < L	R > L	R < L	R + L	—	—	R + L
Toe	R > L	—	R < L	R + L	—	R > L	L	—	R + L

Note: Detected peaks of activation are designated by side (R, right; L, left; ">" or "<" signifies that activation of one side was stronger or weaker than other by more than 20%.

Bilateral activation in the cerebellum was detectable for all tasks in each subject with the following exceptions: Two subjects did not show significant increase in BOLD response during lip movements in either hemisphere; one subject activated only the right hemisphere during knee adduction; and another subject activated only the left hemisphere during pelvis contraction. As expected, the unilateral tasks led to a more pronounced (about 30%) increase of activation in the right hemisphere during right-sided motor activation, whereas the level of activation for the other tasks was equally distributed over the hemispheres. The analysis of task × peak coordinates over subjects did not reach significant values ($F < 1$).

Left-sided secondary sensorimotor (SM2) activation was detected in all subjects during unilateral movement tasks, while right-sided SM2 activation occurred in only two subjects during finger movement and four subjects during toe movement. Right or left SM2 activation was notable in bilateral tasks with no particular pattern over all subjects. Within the area of the basal ganglia including the thalamus, the significant level of peak activation was considerably lower than for all other areas reported. Over tasks and subjects, the distribution followed no relation to unilateral or bilateral movements or to body part (see table 13.2).

Summary

Our study confirmed the possibility of detecting changes in BOLD response in primary motor areas associated with movements of different body parts. For each subject and for the grand average, the coordinates for the applied finger, foot, and tongue movements were in line with results of previous studies. Together with the new tasks, it was possible to produce a map of the BOLD responses within the precentral gyrus. The areas were located where the direct stimulation had predicted them to be based on the motor homunculus (figure 13.2). Moreover, our study provided evidence of how and to what extent the BOLD response can be used to map the motor homunculus. It showed that changes in activation of the primary motor system can be investigated even in the case of disturbed or missing ability to exercise. For example, in the case of a paresis of the hand due to a tumor situated close to the precentral gyrus, functional brain areas can be separated by using motor tasks that elicit an activation close to the tumor side. It showed further that a variety of tasks revealing significant differences in the secondary areas involved in motor execution can be investigated within a very short scan time (5 min for one body part; table 13.3). The time subjects

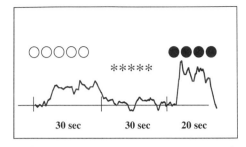

Figure 13.3
Blood oxygen level–dependent (BOLD) response over time for an example of blocked presentation of stimuli. Three different conditions (open and filled circles for different task loads; asterisks for control task). The resulting BOLD response demonstrates the temporal delay.

can be kept in the scanner is often the limiting factor, especially for elders or challenged patients who find it extremely difficult to keep their head absolutely still while performing tasks.

Our results have practical implications for brain surgery involving tumors. Before and during operations, neurosurgeons are faced with the problem of orientation within brain structures and separation of affected regions from normal (functional) areas. Cortical plasticity and variability give rise to significant individual differences in the location of language and motor areas; thus there is a pressing need for individual mapping methods. As the planning of the procedure affects its outcome, recent research has tried to develop methods to assist neurosurgeons. Today stereotaxic surgery, using frameless navigation devices, MRI, and postprocessing software, is able to visualize the tumor in a three-dimensional environment and to allow exact guidance of surgical equipment to the target location (Lumenta et al., 1997). As our study has shown, functional analysis of language (Kanowski et al., 2001) or motor areas can combine with such technical methods to facilitate neurosurgical interventions by providing additional information about affected tissue in these areas (Schulder et al., 1997).

Our results raise other questions, however. We know the level of activation in the different parts of the motor system, but nothing about the temporal dynamics and how these areas interact for a successful execution of motion, although there is converging evidence that areas separate into different functional regions whose distinctive contributions change depending on the task and the design applied.

13.3   A New Way to Look at the Blood Oxygen Level–Dependent Response: Event-Related Functional Magnetic Resonance Imaging

The study paradigm applied in the previous section is called "blocked design." Two conditions (such as motion and rest) change in an on-off kind of pattern, each lasting for about half a minute. One possible application of the paradigm with concurrent BOLD response is depicted in figure 13.3.

If we were to statistically compare the mean of each condition (open circle, filled circle, and asterisk), we would conclude that, for the area chosen, the level of activation for the filled circle condition was higher than for the open circle condition, which in turn was higher than for the resting state (asterisk condition). The disadvantage of the blocked design paradigm is that it does not let us isolate the response to a single stimulus; a serious limitation for the possible study design and subsequent data analysis.

Another paradigm, "event-related design," has been successfully applied with other imaging methods. If, say, we want to compare two conditions (A and B) in terms of the changes detected in electroencephalography (EEG), we would present them to subjects in a random pattern, such as ABAABABBAABABABABA . . . , with the subjects not able to foresee the next stimulus. The randomized presentation has several advantages. First, subjects have to pay greater attention because they cannot assume the next condition from the context. Subjects having to perform the same task over and over again for a period of time —as in the blocked design presentation—can readily fail to pay attention and drift into automatic response behavior. Second, the sum of the reaction within the block is summarized in the mean without possible differentiation of the contribution of every single event (for example, slow and fast reaction times or correct and incorrect responses). Third, for most situations in everyday life, events happen in random order (naturally, we might not expect to meet only good friends when we walk along the downtown area). Therefore, the random, event-related presentation seems to better reflect everyday demands on the system in question. And finally, the random, event-related presentation can be used even when behavior cannot be predicted. For some investigations, we need to sort single events and calculate the corresponding BOLD response. To define the level of activity for words during encoding, for example, Wagner and colleagues (1998) presented subjects words one at a time while whole-head volumes were scanned (encoding). Then, outside the

Table 13.3
Summary of peak activations for different motor tasks

Task	Toe	Knee	Pelvis	Finger	Eye	Lips	Tongue
M1 left	-3 -24 65 32,73	0 -29 61 45,51	3 -12 65 43,81	-35 -18 59 50,85	-42 -11 46 26,76	-53 -15 43 56,42	-54 -10 26 50,79
M1 right	—	—	—	37 -27 62 34,15	43 -12 53 27,2	53 -12 40 54,53	61 -12 30 48,94
SMA	2 -7 58 34,2	-3 -18 60 42,09	-3 -9 53 27,26	-5 -12 57 38,92	-2 -9 60 25,8	3 -4 63 18,19	-6 1 53 23,27
BG/T left	-18 -8 13 25,37 -6 -18 6 18,52 -25 -21 9 14,29	-3 -19 13 29,88 -15 -7 1 25,5 -25 -21 6 24,27	-16 -3 14 28,37 -25 -15 9 24,1 -3 -9 9 20,71	-9 -21 12 28,41 -18 -7 7 26,81 -18 9 9 12,16	-20 0 7 28,6 -15 -12 2 19,41 -11 -28 2 14,92	-21 -1 4 18,26 -6 -21 9 17,25 -25 -26 4 14,06	-20 -8 5 40,3
BG/T right	27 -12 10 21,62 18 -4 18 15,15 12 -27 -3 14,29	21 -15 3 28,05 15 -5 8 23,11 18 -27 9 16,24	30 -1 12 31,2 27 -15 12 31,15 13 -19 10 19,53	18 -8 14 19,53	19 -17 8 21,7 28 -3 6 20,67 25 -30 6 18,26	26 -12 12 26,85 28 -3 3 24,39 18 -9 0 16,93	24 -12 5 34,05
SM2 right	56 -30 28 27,25	40 -30 28 28,23	58 -29 28 35,81	31 -46 37 32,73	—	59 -30 28 23,31	43 -27 31 21,78
SM2 left	-53 -27 28 29,65	-43 -40 28 37,29	-59 -37 28 24,39	-46 -27 28 49	-44 -41 26 17,36	-45 -42 29 26,85	-45 -41 34 21,93

	Toe	Knee	Pelvis	Finger	Eye	Lips	Tongue
CER left	-28 -58 -15 45,4 -31 -65 -40 19,79 -34 -77 -15 14,32	-31 -55 -43 34,1 -28 -37 -25 32,44 -28 -55 -18 31,29 -8 -38 -26 25,59	-30 -67 -13 40,25 -21 -55 -21 40,09 -21 -38 -19 28,46 -31 -57 -37 28,14	-24 -56 -20 38,92 -27 -57 -41 24,19 -32 -43 -38 17,22 -40 -47 -28 16,34	-21 -58 -15 43,87 -37 -58 -15 27,2 -30 -58 -39 19,72	-15 -60 -13 45,4 -25 -56 -16 45,34 -31 -62 -40 24,02	-15 -65 -15 28,37 -35 -78 -31 13,11
CER right	31 -55 -18 45,4 19 -77 -15 28,19 15 -43 -18 23,23	31 -40 -25 40,3 25 -58 -43 32,25 28 -56 -13 24,44	27 -56 -17 47,01 6 -71 -11 38,81 15 -71 -43 31,15	21 -52 -18 52,68 25 -58 -43 43,65 9 -62 -12 40,57	18 -65 -12 45,57 2 -68 -17 40,41 25 -43 -37 18,15	21 -62 -18 43,59 6 -80 -12 27,03 31 -64 -38 25,33	25 -58 -15 24,48 43 -77 -15 24,39 43 -71 -40 20,75
Task	Toe	Knee	Pelvis	Finger	Eye	Lips	Tongue

Note: Talairach coordinates and significance level (-log(p)) of peak activations in different areas (specified in rows) for each motor task (columns) based on the average of nine subjects. Only peaks with a level of $p < .00001$ (11,5) or higher are listed.

scanner, subjects were presented with a list consisting of new words and words from the former presentation and asked to mark the old words (recognition). The idea was to define the difference between remembered old words, correctly marked as "old," and subsequently forgotten old words, which had been not marked. Wagner and colleagues sorted out the words during encoding for later remembered or forgotten words and compared the levels of activation in the brain to each other. It turned out that high levels of the BOLD response in the left medial temporal and left prefrontal region were significant for later remembered words. Because it was not possible to predict the behavior, the event-related design paradigm had to be used.

Another advantage of the event-related design paradigm is that it allows researchers to reconstruct the BOLD response of different tasks and for different regions and to compare the results in terms of amplitude as well as temporal behavior. This feature allows them to further segregate areas activated during blocked design motor tasks for distinctive functions in the applied task. Event-related studies of the supplementary motor area (SMA) and the basal ganglia (BG) are outlined below.

Single-cell recording studies of the SMA in monkeys (Matsuzaka et al., 1992; Matsuzaka and Tanji, 1996) have revealed two distinct areas in the medial frontal gyrus, with a more anterior area demonstrating a predominately stimulus-related pattern of activity and the classical SMA proper involved in motor execution. Functional imaging studies such as our previous example have failed to separate the SMA in such a manner. The SMA is involved in several aspects of motor control for sequence timing and in complex tasks of motor execution on a high level, as well as in the initiation of movements. To further investigate the exact involvement, the applied blocked design, where the task is held constant for a period as described at the beginning of this section, could not elicit the desired differences.

Humberstone and colleagues (1997) used event-related fMRI to reconstruct the BOLD response for different areas within the medial frontal gyrus. The task consisted of a random presentation of two probes displayed every 18 s on a screen in front of the subjects. If the number "5" was displayed, subject had to respond by pressing a button with the thumb (go), if the number "2" was displayed, no response was required (no-go). The reconstruction of the BOLD responses in two supplementary motor areas (SMA proper and pre-SMA, which is located more rostral and anterior to the first region) demonstrated a functional segregation. Whereas the go stimulus elicited a significant increase of activity in the SMA proper, the no-go stimulus did not. The picture was different for the pre-SMA region, where both stimuli resulted in an increase of activity independent of the motor execution. Furthermore, the hemispheric laterality was different with a higher level of activity for the SMA proper contralateral and the pre-SMA ipsilateral to the hand used for pressing the button. The authors concluded that a functional hierarchy existed in the SMA, with pre-SMA involved in decision making and SMA proper in motor execution.

From studies of several diseases having distinct movement-related symptoms, we know that the basal ganglia are more defined in terms of their anatomical separation. Looking at the literature of functional imaging thus far, however, the picture is confusing. Although animal brain lesion studies have well documented the laterality and somatotopy of the basal ganglia (BG), few human BG studies have been undertaken. Scholz and colleagues (2000), using a blocked design to elicit activation in the basal ganglia during simple and complex movements, described a somatotopically organized pattern in the caudate nucleus and the putamen. They noted— as had many other research groups before—a significant (two-thirds lower) increase in BOLD response in basal ganglia than in primary motor areas. Using the event-related design paradigm might tell us whether the low increase in activation is related to habituation during the prolonged performance or whether the basal ganglia exhibit an altogether different response behavior. In either case, applying the same function for statistical comparison as for the primary motor system would result in a lower degree of significance.

Why, if event-related techniques have fundamentally broadened the application of fMRI, did it take so long to apply them to BOLD response studies? The reason lies in the 4–6 s needed for the BOLD response to peak after stimulus presentation, and in the roughly 16 s needed for it to return to baseline. To prevent overlap with the preceding stimulus, the interstimulus interval (ISI) has to be at least 16 s. The resulting design would have to reduce the number of stimuli in a given time. The long ISI would leave subjects with nothing to do for the period, leading to poor control of what would happen while they were waiting. When we apply faster presentation rates (typically in the range of 2–3 s ISI), the overlap of stimuli is substantial. Five years ago, several research groups came up with mathematical solutions to the problem that would permit fast stimulus presentation (Dale and Buckner, 1997; Zarahn et al., 1997; for a review, see Rosen et al., 1998).

Now that the tools are available for taking a closer look at the motor-related brain activity, several questions can be addressed. Most notably, does the BOLD response correlate with the neuronal activity in a uniform pattern over the brain? A study by Schachter and colleagues (1997) detected an area in the inferior prefrontal cortex that responded to a short stimulus presentation with a delayed peak latency and a prolonged course of BOLD response, whereas all other areas measured exhibited a uniform response. Although the authors suggested these findings were due to a different cognitive load for the structure involved, they might as easily be due to regional differences arising from vascular properties or metabolic coupling. If that were the case, a direct comparison of these areas using a blocked design paradigm might be misleading: The difference in the mean over time might be caused by factors other than induced variations in the study variables.

Event-related design with spaced presentation has been used successfully to further segment regions related to their functional contribution during motor execution, especially by delayed-response task settings. With a cue for hand preparation and a go signal for the execution of a finger-tapping task, Lee and colleagues (1999) showed that the supplementary motor area can be functionally divided into an anterior and posterior part, with the first more activated during the preparation phase and both activated together during the execution phase. Cui and colleagues (2000) have applied the same design to study the role of the cerebellum during a delayed-response task. They described a similar amplitude in BOLD response in both hemispheres when a right-handed, four-step tapping task was performed. Additionally, a delay of about 1.5 s in the peak latency was observed for the cerebellar BOLD response in comparison to the primary motor area during motor execution. Toni and colleagues (1999) applied a spaced, event-related design for a simple button press task with a new method to enhance temporal resolution. Whereas the repetition time for whole-head volumes is 6.4 s, by varying the delay between visual cue and acoustic go signal, they were able to arrive at an effective time resolution of 1.28 s for reconstructed BOLD response values. These studies underscored the usefulness of event-related design in further understanding the network of areas involved in motor planning and execution. Because they were partial volume investigations, however, the studies focused only on parts of the motor system.

13.4   Investigating the Blood Oxygen Level–Dependent Response during Short Sequential Finger Movements

In this study, my colleagues and I first used rapid event-related fMRI for a sequential finger opposition task. Every 1.5 s an image of the whole brain was acquired while subjects performed the motor task (two different four-step finger/thumb sequences) with either the right or left hand every 3 s. The presentation of each condition was randomized so that the subjects could not anticipate the hand or sequence. A more complex task was used because the degree of activation in secondary motor areas is correlated to the demands of the task to perform: A single-finger exercise will not elicit significant increase in areas such as the basal ganglia, thalamus, and premotor areas. Our design permitted us to monitor areas involved in the motor execution when repetitive, short movements were performed in a natural way: Everyday motor behavior demands the fast and reliable switching of different previously learned movements. Our study addressed the following four questions:

1. Does the motor execution of short sequential finger movements elicit significant activation in all areas known to contribute to movements?
2. Are the resulting BOLD response patterns in these areas uniform over the whole brain or do they differ in shape?
3. Can notable differences in amplitude and latency be detected between the primary and secondary motor system?
4. Do hemispherical differences exist in right-handed subjects for performance with the right or left hand?

   Scanning procedure followed that of our previous study described in section 13.2; functional data acquisition consisted of 8 individual runs (23 slices per volume; TR 1.5 s; TE 40 ms; 255 volumes per run). Each run was composed of 25 presentations for each of four task conditions and a control (fixation) condition, where only a crosshair was visible for 3 s. The five different conditions—right-hand sequences 1 and 2 (R1 and R2), left-hand sequences 1 and 2 (L1 and L2), and control condition (fix)—occurred with the same frequency over the experiment, resulting in a total of 200 presentations in each condition. After selective averaging of each condition, the critical contrasts were calculated using procedures described in Herrmann et al., 2001, for each subject. To demonstrate group results, the data of each subject were averaged in Talairach space and the same contrasts calculated for the group. Because there were no significant detectable differences between the two sequences, results are presented for right hand collapsed across sequences, (R1 + R2) − (fix), and for left hand collapsed across sequences, (L1 + L2) − (fix). To reconstruct the critical areas for which the BOLD response had to be calculated, we used an automated procedure that first detected the peak coordinates for separate activated areas, and then reconstructed each area around the peak, with the restriction of significance level and distance to the peak for voxels to be included. For the resulting region of interest, the changes in BOLD response were calculated for each stimulus type over 15 s (corresponding to 10 volume images after the stimulus onset).

Results for General Activation during the Motor Task

Areas showing a significant increase in BOLD response for finger exercise versus rest were the primary motor area, premotor areas, superior parietal area, the secondary sensorimotor area, the basal ganglia and thalamus, the supplementary motor cortex, and the cerebellum. Figure 13.4 (see also plate

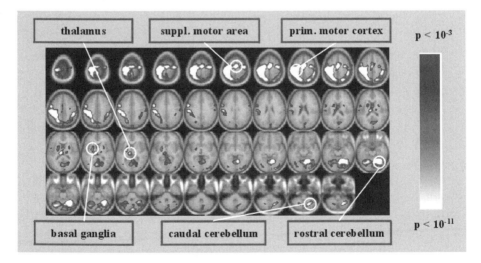

Figure 13.4
Grand average results for the selective averaging of the right-hand sequential finger exercise. Increased blood oxygen level–dependent (BOLD) response in axial view shown by color-coded *p*-values (scale on the right) projected on the anatomical background. Areas of interest are labeled for orientation within a representative slice; right is right to the viewer. See plate 10 for color version.

10) depicts the distribution of activated areas for the right-hand task (combined for R1 and R2) in an axial view; the results for the left hand are
mirror-imaged with regard to the side.

The laterality of the individual areas follows the expected pattern, as
described in the literature, with all of the most prominent areas activated
contralateral to the limb exercised, except for the cerebellum, where the
side ispilateral to the limb exercised showed the more significant increase
in BOLD response. These results verify the design in terms of distinguishable event related activation for different stimulus types, presented randomized with short intervals.

The Reconstruction of Areas and the Blood Oxygen Level–
Dependent Response

Was the BOLD response the same in all different motor areas involved
in the execution of finger exercise? Let us first consider the primary
motor area. We reconstructed the primary motor region based on the main
peak for the right-hand task (x, y, $x = -27$, -20, 54). Because the area
covered several slices along the z-axis, we moved the region of interest
toward a higher and a lower z-value (59 and 50, respectively) for comparison. Shown in figure 13.5 and plate 11 is the percentage signal change
plotted against time in seconds for the comparison sequence R1 or R2
versus rest.

At different z-values, the amplitude changes but not the general shape,
with a peak latency at 4.5 s after stimulus onset. Because the demand to
perform the movements is the same, the two different motor tasks (R1 and
R2) elicit identical responses over time. The detected peak and consequent
region of interest thus represent the most active part within the primary
motor area, despite an extended distribution along the z-axis.

In view of these results, the question arises whether the BOLD response patterns for the secondary motor system will be comparable to those
for the primary motor area. Figure 13.6 depicts the results of different regions of interest for the right-hand task (combined for R1 and R2) with
the Talairach coordinates of the detected peak and the anatomical name
specified at the upper right corner and the reconstructed area at the upper
left corner. Furthermore, the BOLD response patterns for the left-hand
task are included based on the same region of interest; thus they describe
the amount of activation in the hemisphere involved in movements of the
limb on the same side.

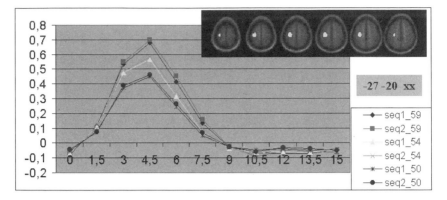

Figure 13.5
Reconstruction of the blood oxygen level–dependent (BOLD) response values for
the primary motor cortex, with three different talairach coordinates for the z-value
(rostral to caudal values 59, 54, and 50). Example for $z = 54$ is shown in the upper
left corner. The individual BOLD response values are labeled in the lower right
corner, with "seq1" and "seq2" representing sequential finger movements of the
right-hand version 1 and version 2, respectively. The y-axis is scaled in percentage
signal changes; the x-axis, in seconds after stimulus presentation. Because the different sequences showed identical responses, it was reasonable to collapse the results
of the study. The different z-values did not affect the general shape even though
the amplitude varied. See plate 11 for color version.

Figure 13.6 ▶
Reconstruction of the blood oxygen level–dependent (BOLD) response values for
eight different areas of interest. Grand average results for right-hand exercise and
the BOLD response values during left-hand exercise in the same areas are shown.
In the upper left corner are the reconstructed areas of interest in axial view; in the
right upper corner, the talairach coordinates and the functional area name. M1,
primary motor cortex; SM2, secondary sensorimotor area; PMr, premotor area
rostral; PMc, premotor area caudal; THAL, thalamus; BG, basal ganglia; and CEB1,
CEB2, two areas within the cerebellum. The BOLD response values are expressed
as percentage signal change values over the time period following the stimulus
presentation (in seconds). Although no major differences are notable for the general shape, SM2, BG, CEB1, and CEB2 demonstrate a significant delay of about
1.5 s. See plate 12 for color version.

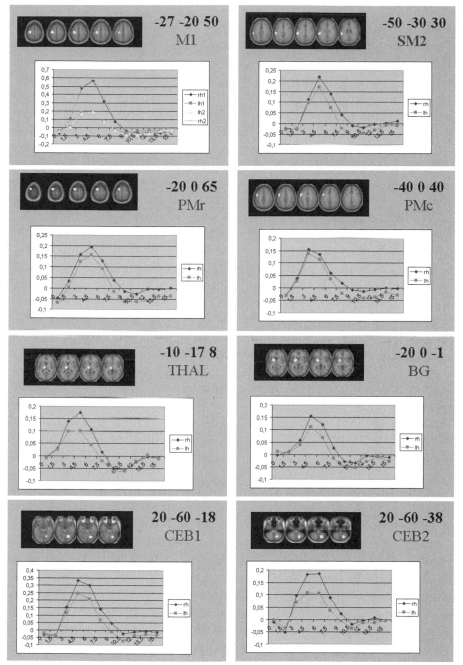

In general, the shape and latency of the BOLD response patterns in the secondary motor system were about the same with a peak delay of about 4.5 s after stimulus onset. Only the two regions within the cerebellum showed a somewhat longer peak, ranging from 4.5 to 6 s after onset. The BOLD response for the secondary sensorimotor areas and the basal ganglia demonstrated a delay in onset of about 1.5 s, whereas all other areas in the hemisphere started to rise immediately after the stimulus onset. Again, the cerebellum demonstrated a different behavior, with an initial decrease in the BOLD response before a steep rise. The pattern was identical—also mirrored along the interhemispheric gap—in all aspects for the left-hand task.

To compare the distribution of the activation within the left hemisphere for the right hand (contralateral to the movement) and for the left hand (ipsilateral to the movement), my colleagues and I first calculated the area under the curve for each response after the baseline had been corrected to zero. We then calculated the percentage of activation for the ispilateral movement with respect to the contralateral movement.

We can see at a glance in figure 13.6 and plate 12 that the primary motor system (M1) displayed only about one third (32%) of the activation in the hemisphere ispilateral to the movement, whereas the other regions displayed about one half of the activation. The values for each secondary region were thalamus: 45%; basal ganglia: 61%; premotor rostral: 84%; premotor caudal: 70%; secondary sensorimotor: 63%; rostral cerebellum (CEB1): 59%; and caudal cerebellum (CEB2): 45%. This distribution points toward the functional connectivity of the motor areas, as a high specialization of the primary motor area for short sequential finger movements in the contralateral hemisphere contrasted with the bilateral hemispheric distribution for the secondary motor system. The same results were calculated for the right hemisphere, where the left-hand movements gave rise to higher activity in all areas and where a considerable amount of ispilateral activity was noted as well.

The total amount of activation followed the previous description with a considerable, more significant increase in BOLD response within the primary motor area (up to 0.6% signal change) than within the secondary motor system (up to 0.2% signal change) for the left hemisphere and for the right hemisphere (0.5% and 0.3% signal change, respectively).

These observations support the hypothesis of the study, that short, sequential finger exercises—performed at fast pace with randomized changes of the hand and the sequence—elicit similar BOLD response values in primary and secondary motor brain areas. Differences can be detected—within the given temporal resolution of 1.5 s—in latency and rise time as well as in hemispheric distribution (bilateral activation of secondary areas in contrast to primarily contralateral activation for the primary motor area). Characterizing how the brain in healthy young subjects manage the short motor task helps us better investigate how the brain in subjects with diseases that disturb the function of the motor system (e.g., Parkinson's disease, multiple sclerosis, and amyotropic lateral sclerosis) fails to manage that task. Furthermore, the effect of treatment can be monitored directly at the level of individual areas, given the opportunity to follow the changes during therapy and along the course of the disease. First steps into this direction have been taken by Haslinger and colleagues (2001) using spaced event-related design to investigate the effect of levodopa in Parkinson's disease.

Although the results discussed above allow us to hypothesize about how the brain copes with the performance of short movements, they can tell us nothing about how the different locations interact for voluntary movements. The question then arises, are there other, more productive ways to look into timing and connectivity issues beside the classical statistical evaluation of differences between rest and motion over the brain?

13.5 Functional and Effective Connectivity: A New Perspective on the Motor System at Work

If we look at the temporal pattern for the BOLD response in blocked design studies (see figure 13.3), simply calculating the mean for the two conditions and comparing these leaves out the behavior of the region over time. How, then, can we use the temporal course of the BOLD response for information of interaction between regions?

One successful approach, which emerged from a study using multi-unit microelectrode recordings in monkeys (Gerstein et al., 1989), is strikingly easy. If two groups of neurons demonstrate the same pattern of stimulus-induced oscillation, it can be assumed that these groups are linked functionally in the process of information processing and execution. The comparison cannot tell us whether the link is direct or indirect, through a common third group that provides input to both groups simultaneously (see figure 13.7).

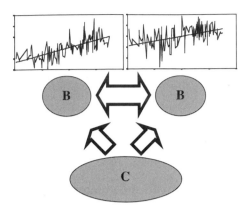

Figure 13.7
Applying the functional connectivity method to two areas (A and B). (*Top*) Correlation of the blood oxygen level–dependent (BOLD) response. (*Bottom*) Consequential implications for the possible interaction of areas A and B.

In the following subsection, I will present the concept of using the temporal behavior of different brain areas during blocked paradigm to archive information about the functional connectivity of these areas.

Functional Connectivity and Functional Magnetic Resonance Imaging

Using the temporal quantities of the BOLD response instead of a single property (mean value) provides us with a more distinct tool to investigate activation of brain areas. The approach to functional connectivity in blocked data presentation is easy. We simply apply regression analysis methods to the different activated areas for a given task. Taking our example for blocked design and motor tasks, we might compare primary and supplementary motor areas when finger tapping was performed. Because the nature of the connection cannot be inferred, however, the approach is limited in terms of interpretation.

How can we use the information functional connectivity provides? One application is in patient studies. For Parkinson's patients, the decrease of dopamine production in the substantia nigra leads to a change of balance within the motor system resulting in tremor, rigor, and akinesis. At the onset of the disease, oral dopamine supplements (levodopa) can reverse the symptoms. Functional MRI studies have shown that, in response to simple hand exercise, the pattern of activation in Parkinson's patients differs from that in healthy, age-controlled subjects (Sabatini et al., 2000). The dopamine deficit in the putamen disorganizes the motor system in such a way that the supplementary motor area becomes less activated and the primary motor and premotor areas more activated in patients than in control subjects.

It is still unknown whether medication can bring the motor systems of Parkinson's patients back to normal balance or at least make them able to simulate normal proportions even though major detectable differences remain between their motor systems and those of healthy persons. Haslinger et al., 2001, supports the hypothesis that levodopa reverses the disturbances in the motor system observed by fMRI. Using a spaced, event-related design for joystick-guided movements, Haslinger and colleagues compared Parkinson's patients with healthy control subjects, and Parkinson's patients on with those off levodopa therapy. Activation in the investigated regions (partial volume scan covering the primary and supplementary motor areas) was observed to be at a higher level in patients than in normal subjects, but became normalized after initiation of levodopa therapy. By comparing the level of activation and the underlying functional connectivity in normal subjects and in early-stage Parkinson's patients on and off medication, we should be able to infer changes in the motor system related to dopamine deficiency.

My colleagues and I are currently investigating the effects of levodopa; I can provide our first results (Rotte et al., 2002) for the correlation of the primary and supplementary motor areas. In a blocked design presentation, Parkinson's patients performed simple hand movements (clenched their fist) over 30 s, with rest periods in between. The task was performed in separate runs for the left and right hand in de novo Parkinson's patients before and after initiation of levodopa therapy. Data were then analyzed following the procedures described in the first part of this chapter. Regions of interest were automatically defined for peaks of activation within the whole head. For normal subjects, the connectivity values were high between primary and supplementary motor areas ($r > 90$), whereas for untreated Parkinson's patients the correlation was lower ($r \sim 80$). When we recalculated the correlation between the same areas after patients were treated with oral dopamine until their symptoms were reduced to near normal, it increased to near normal levels ($r \sim 86$).

The use of functional connectivity extends our ability to investigate BOLD response patterns during motor tasks. Despite initial imaging studies that used or discussed the functional connectivity approach in the early 1990s (Grafton et al., 1994; Friston, 1994), since then, few studies have made use of this approach (Friston et al., 1996; Buchel and Friston, 1997; Buchel et al., 1999). In the coming years, it is expected to receive greater attention, especially among those investigating changes over time in degenerative diseases.

Effective Connectivity

In the social sciences, the effects of interaction between different groups have been investigated using structural equation modeling. The idea is to first build a hypothesis about a system including each contributing part and the connections between them and then to apply the resulting model to the measurements taken from a sample. Translated into functional imaging, two different models have to be combined to form the hypothesis of how one or more areas are influenced by other areas within the model: a mathematical model defining the nature of connections to be investigated and a neuroanatomical model specifying the areas known to contribute in the course of the experimental situation. Several studies of effective connectivity have been undertaken for brain areas where our knowledge about the underlying cortical tracts and physiology is greatest, namely, the primary visual system, the motor system, and the hippocampus area (Maguire et al., 2000, 2001; Friston and Buchel, 2000).

References

Buchel, C., and Friston, K. J. (1997). Modulation of connectivity in visual pathways by attention: Cortical interactions evaluated with structural equation modelling and fMRI. *Cereb. Cortex* 7: 768–778.

Buchel, C., Coull, J. T., and Friston, K. J. (1999). The predictive value of changes in effective connectivity for human learning. *Science* 283: 1538–1541.

Buckner, R. L., Raichle, M. E., Miezen, F. M., and Petersen, S. E. (1996). Functional anatomic studies of memory retrieval for auditory words and visual pictures. *J. Neurosci.* 16: 6219–6235.

Corfield, D. R., Murphy, K., Josephs, O., Fink, G. R., Frackowiak, R. S., Guz, A., Adams, L., and Turner, R. (1999). Cortical and subcortical control of tongue movement in humans: A functional neuroimaging study using fMRI. *J. Appl. Physiol.* 86: 1468–1477.

Cui, S. Z., Li, E. Z., Zang, Y. F., Weng, X. C., Ivry, R., and Wang, J. J. (2000). Both sides of human cerebellum involved in preparation and execution of sequential movements. *NeuroReport* 11: 3849–3853.

Dale, A. M., and Buckner, R. L. (1997). Selective averaging of rapidly presented individual trials using fMRI. *Hum. Brain Map.* 5: 329–340.

Ferrier, D. (1875). Experiments on the brain of monkeys. *Proc. R. Soc. Lond. B Biol. Sci.* 23: 409–430.

Ferrier, D. (1876). *The Functions of the Brain.* New York: Putnam.

Friston, K. J. (1994). Functional and effective connectivity in neuroimaging: A synthesis. *Hum. Brain Mapp.* 2: 56–78.

Friston, K. J., Frith, C. D., Fletcher, P., Liddle, P. F., and Frackowiak, R. S. (1996). Functional topography: Multidimensional scaling and functional connectivity in the brain. *Cereb. Cortex* 6: 156–164.

Friston, K. J., and Buchel, C. (2000). Attentional modulation of effective connectivity from V2 to V5/MT in humans. *Proc. Natl. Acad. Sci. U. S. A.* 97: 7591–7596.

Gerstein, G. L., Bedenbaugh, P., and Aertsen, M. H. (1989). Neuronal assemblies. *IEEE Trans. Biomed. Eng.* 36: 4–14.

Grafton, S. T., Sutton, J., Couldwell, W., Lew, M., and Waters, C. (1994). Network analysis of motor system connectivity in Parkinson's disease: Modulation of thalamocortical interactions after pallidotomy. *Hum. Brain Mapp.* 2: 45–55.

Haslinger, B., Erhard, P., Kampfe, N., Boecker, H., Rummeny, E., Schwaiger, M. Conrad, B., and Ceballos-Baumann, A. O. (2001). Event-related functional magnetic resonance imaging in Parkinson's disease before and after levodopa. *Brain* 124: 558–570.

Herrmann, M., Rotte, M., Grubich, C., Ebert, A. D., Schiltz, K., Munte, T. F., and Heinze, H. J. (2001). Control of semantic interference in episodic memory retrieval is associated with an anterior cingulate-prefrontal activation pattern. *Hum. Brain Mapp.* 13: 94–103.

Humberstone, M., Sawle, G. V., Clare, S., Hykin, J., Coxon, R., Bowtell, R., Macdonald, I. A., and Morris, P. G. (1997). Functional magnetic resonance imaging of single motor events reveals human presupplementary motor area. *Ann. Neurol.* 42: 632–637.

Kanowski, M., Fernandez, G., Heinze, H.-J., and Rotte, M. (2001). Fast and robust localization of Broca and Wernicke areas by fMRI. *NeuroImage* 13: 548.

Lee, K. M., Chang, K. H., and Roh, J. K. (1999). Subregions within the supplementary motor area activated at different stages of movement preparation and execution. *NeuroImage* 9: 117–123.

Lehericy, S., van de Moortele, P. F., Lobel, E., Paradis, A. L., Vidailhet, M., Frouin, V., Neveu, P., Agid, Y., Marsault, C., and Le Bihan, D. (1998). Somatotopical organization of striatal activation during finger and toe movement: A 3 T functional magnetic resonance imaging study. *Ann. Neurol.* 44: 398–404.

Lumenta, C. B., Gumprecht, H. K., Leonardi, M. A., Gerstner, W., and Brehm, B. (1997). Three-dimensional computer-assisted stereotactic-guided microneurosurgery combined with cortical mapping of the motor area by direct electrostimulation. *Minim. Invasive Neurosurg.* 40: 50–54.

Maguire, E. A., Mummery, C. J., and Buchel, C. (2000). Patterns of hippocampal-cortical interaction dissociate temporal lobe memory subsystems. *Hippocampus* 10: 475–482.

Maguire, E. A., Vargha-Khadam, F., and Mishkin, M. (2001). The effects of bilateral hippocampal damage on fMRI regional activations and interactions during memory retrieval. *Brain* 124: 1156–1170.

Matsuzaka, Y., and Tanji, J. (1996). Changing directions of forthcoming arm movements: Neuronal activity in the presupplementary and supplementary motor area of monkey cerebral cortex. *J. Neurophysiol.* 76: 2327–2342.

Matsuzaka, Y., Aizawa, H., and Tanji, J. (1992). A motor area rostral to the supplementary motor area (presupplementary motor area) in the monkey: Neuronal activity during a learned motor task. *J. Neurophysiol.* 68: 653–662.

Penfield, W., and Boldrey, E. (1937). Somatic motor and sensory representation in the cerebral cortex of man as studies by electrical stimulation. *Brain* 60: 389–443.

Rao, S. M., Binder, J. R., Hammeke, T. A., Bandettini, P. A., Bobholz, J. A., Frost, J. A., Myklebust, B. M., Jacobson, R. D., and Hyde, J. S. (1995). Somatotopic mapping of the human primary motor cortex with functional magnetic resonance imaging. *Neurology* 45: 919–924.

Rosen, B. R., Buckner, R. L., and Dale, A. M. (1998). Event-related functional MRI: past, present, and future. *Proc. Natl. Acad. Sci. U. S. A.* 95: 773–780.

Rotte, M., Koutstaal, W., Schacter, D. L., Wagner, A. D., Rosen, B. R., Dale, A. M., and Buckner, R. L. (1998). Left prefrontal activation correlates with levels of processing during verbal encoding. *NeuroImage* 7: 813.

Rotte, M., Eckert, T., and Heinze, H.-J. (2002). L-Dopa related changes in early Parkinson disease: An fMRI study. *NeuroImage Hum. Brain Mapp.* 2002 Meeting, 849.

Sabatini, U., Boulanouar, K., Fabre, N., Martin, F., Carel, C., Colonnese, C., Bozzao, L., Berry, I., Montastruc, J. L., Chollet, F., and Rascol, O. (2000). Cortical motor reorganization in akinetic patients with Parkinson's disease: A functional MRI study. *Brain* 123: 394–403.

Schacter, D. L., Buckner, R. L., Koutstaal, W., Dale, A. M., and Rosen, B. R. (1997). Late onset of anterior prefrontal activity during true and false recognition: An event-related fMRI study. *NeuroImage* 6: 259–269.

Scholz, V. H., Flaherty, A. W., Kraft, E., Keltner, J. R., Kwong, K. K., Chen, Y. I., Rosen, B. R., and Jenkins, B. G. (2000). Laterality, somatotopy and reproducibility of the basal ganglia and motor cortex during motor tasks. *Brain Res.* 879: 204–215.

Schulder, M., Maldjian, J. A., Liu, W. C., Mun, I. K., and Carmel, P. W. (1997). Functional MRI-guided surgery of intracranial tumors. *Stereotact. Funct. Neurosurg.* 68: 98–105.

Stern, C. E., Corkin, S., Gonzalez, R. G., Guimaraes, A. R., Baker, J. R., Jennings, P. J., Carr, C. A., Sugiura, R. M., Vedantham, V., and Rosen, B. R. (1996). The hippocampal formation participates in novel picture encoding: Evidence from functional magnetic resonance imaging. *Proc. Natl. Acad. Sci. U. S. A.* 93: 8660–8665.

Talairach, J., and Tournoux, T. (1988). *Coplanar Stereotaxic Atlas of the Human Brain.* New York: Thieme Medical.

Toni, I., Schluter, N. D., Josephs, O., Friston, K., and Passingham, R. E. (1999). Signal-, set- and movement-related activity in the human brain: An event-related fMRI study. *Cereb. Cortex* 9: 35–49. (See also corrected erratum in *Cereb. Cortex* 9: 196.)

Wagner, A. D., Schacter, D. L., Rotte, M., Koutstaal, W., Maril, A., Dale, A. M., Rosen, B. R., and Buckner, R. L. (1998). Building memories: Remembering and forgetting of verbal experiences as predicted by brain activity. *Science* 281: 1188–1191.

Yetkin, F. Z., Mueller, W. M., Morris, G. L., McAuliffe, T. L., Ulmer, J. L., Cox, R. W., Daniels, D. L., and Haugton, V. M. (1997). Functional MR activation correlated with intraoperative cortical mapping. *Am. J. Neuroradiol.* 18: 1311–1315.

Zarahn, E., Aguirre, G., and D'Esposito, M. (1997). A trial-based experimental design for fMRI. *NeuroImage* 6:122–138.

Contributors

Emilio Bizzi
Department of Brain and Cognitive
Science
Massachusetts Institute of Technology
Cambridge, Massachusetts

Laurel J. Buxbaum
Moss Rehabilitation Research
Institute and Thomas Jefferson
University
Philadelphia, Pennsylvania

James A. Danckert
Department of Psychology
University of Waterloo
Waterloo, Ontario

Elena Daprati
Institut des Sciences Cognitives
Centre National de la Recherche
Scientifique
Lyon, France

Michel Desmurget
Espace et Action
INSERM Unit 534
Bron, France

Richard T. Dyde
Department of Psychology
University of Durham
Durham, England

Elizabeth A. Franz
University of Otago
Dunedin, New Zealand

A. P. Georgopoulos
Brain Sciences Center
Veteran Affairs Medical Center and
University of Minnesota
Minneapolis–Saint Paul, Minnesota

Pascal Giraux
Institut des Sciences Cognitives
Centre National de la Recherche
Scientifique
Lyon, France

Melvyn A. Goodale
CIHR Group on Action and
Perception
Department of Psychology
University of Western Ontario
London, Ontario

Scott Grafton
Center for Cognitive Neuroscience
Dartmouth College
Hanover, New Hampshire

Laura L. Helmuth
Department of Psychology
University of California
Berkeley, California

Marco Iacoboni
Ahmanson-Lovelace Brain Mapping
Center
Department of Psychiatry and
Biobehavioral Sciences
University of California
Los Angeles, California

Richard B. Ivry
Department of Psychology
University of California
Berkeley, California

Marc Jeannerod
Institut des Sciences Cognitives
Bron, France

Scott H. Johnson-Frey
Center for Cognitive Neuroscience
Dartmouth College
Hanover, New Hampshire

W. Kruse
Brain Sciences Center
Veteran Affairs Medical Center and
University of Minnesota
Minneapolis–Saint Paul, Minnesota

D. Lee
Brain Sciences Center
Veteran Affairs Medical Center and
University of Minnesota
Minneapolis–Saint Paul, Minnesota

A. David Milner
Department of Psychology
University of Durham
Durham, England

Camillo Padoa-Schioppa
Department of Brain and Cognitive
Science
Massachusetts Institute of Technology
Cambridge, Massachusetts

N. L. Port
Brain Sciences Center
Veteran Affairs Medical Center and
University of Minnesota
Minneapolis–Saint Paul, Minnesota

Pascale Pradat-Diehl
Service de Réeducation de
Neurologie
Hôpital de la Salpetriere
Paris, France

Yves Rosetti
Espace et Action
INSERM Unit 534
Bron, France

M. Rotte
Department of Neurology II
Otto-von-Guericke University
Magdeburg, Germany

Angela Sirigu
Institut des Sciences Cognitives
Centre National de la Recherche
Scientifique
Lyon, France

Index